IMMUNOHEMATOLOGY FOR MEDICAL LABORATORY TECHNICIANS

IMMUNOHEMATOLOGY FOR MEDICAL LABORATORY TECHNICIANS

Sheryl A. Whitlock, MA, MT (ASCP) BB

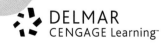

DELMAR
CENGAGE Learning™

Australia • Brazil • Japan • Korea • Mexico • Singapore • Spain • United Kingdom • United States

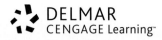

**Immunohematology for Medical
Laboratory Technicians**
Sheryl A. Whitlock

Vice President, Career and Professional
Editorial: Dave Garza

Director of Learning Solutions:
Matthew Kane

Senior Acquisitions Editor: Sherry Dickinson

Managing Editor: Marah Bellegarde

Product Manager: Natalie Pashoukos

Editorial Assistant: Anthony Souza

Vice President, Career and Professional
Marketing: Jennifer McAvey

Marketing Director: Wendy Mapstone

Senior Marketing Manager: Kristin McNary

Marketing Coordinator: Erica Ropitzky

Production Director: Carolyn Miller

Production Manager: Andrew Crouth

Senior Content Project Manager:
James Zayicek

Content Project Management:
Pre-PressPMG

Senior Art Director: David Arsenault

Compositor: Pre-PressPMG

For product information and technology assistance, contact us at
Professional & Career Group Customer Support, 1-800-648-7450

For permission to use material from this text or product,
submit all requests online at **cengage.com/permissions.**
Further permissions questions can be e-mailed to
permissionrequest@cengage.com.

Library of Congress Control Number: 2009931319

ISBN-13: 978-1-4354-4033-3

ISBN-10: 1-4354-4033-1

Delmar
5 Maxwell Drive
Clifton Park, NY 12065-2919
USA

Cengage Learning products are represented in Canada by Nelson Education, Ltd.

For your lifelong learning solutions, visit **delmar.cengage.com**

Visit our corporate website at **cengage.com.**

Notice to the Reader
Publisher does not warrant or guarantee any of the products described herein or perform any independent analysis in connection with any of the product information contained herein. Publisher does not assume, and expressly disclaims, any obligation to obtain and include information other than that provided to it by the manufacturer. The reader is expressly warned to consider and adopt all safety precautions that might be indicated by the activities described herein and to avoid all potential hazards. By following the instructions contained herein, the reader willingly assumes all risks in connection with such instructions. The publisher makes no representations or warranties of any kind, including but not limited to, the warranties of fitness for particular purpose or merchantability, nor are any such representations implied with respect to the material set forth herein, and the publisher takes no responsibility with respect to such material. The publisher shall not be liable for any special, consequential, or exemplary damages resulting, in whole or part, from the readers' use of, or reliance upon, this material.

Printed in the United States of America
1 2 3 4 5 6 7 13 12 11 10 09

Contents

UNIT 2

Blood Group Systems

UNIT 3

Patient Pre-Transfusion Testing

UNIT 4

Blood Components and Their Administration

Preface

INTRODUCTION

Immunohematology for Medical Laboratory Technicians was written with clinical laboratory technology (CLT) students as a focus audience. Historically, students in CLT programs have been an underserved population. Immunohematology textbooks have been written at a level and depth most appropriate for clinical laboratory science students. CLT students and instructors have found themselves adapting to the text, rather than using a text appropriate for their level of course instruction.

This text has been authored with CLT instructors and students as a primary focus. The text should not only serve as a resource but also provide novice teachers with a firm course structure. Individual chapters are structured to provide an organized and detailed approach to the instruction of Immunohematology.

The text may also serve as a reference for laboratory science students of all levels. The material is presented at an appropriate level to serve as a resource for certification exams review. Review questions at the end of each chapter are presented to reinforce material presented in the text. A supplemental instructor's manual will be available with additional instructional and organizational materials.

ORGANIZATION AND FEATURES

While standard textbook features are included in all chapters, the text has been organized to facilitate the learning process. *Immunohematology for Medical Laboratory Technicians* is not only a text for technical reading, but provides interactive and critical thinking activities to enhance study. Web activities are included to provide computer savvy students the opportunity to reinforce concepts with visual and interactive aids.

Sample procedures are included not only to provide conceptual understanding of test methods, but also to be readily adapted to the student laboratory as necessary. These sample procedures are featured and strategically placed within each chapter to optimize learning and conceptualization. Technical concepts are included in all chapters with visual reinforcement when appropriate.

ANCILLARY MATERIALS

The instructor's manual includes answers to all of the critical thinking activities and review questions from the text. A midterm and final exam have been included in the manual, as well as the answers to both exams. Additional completion, short answer, and matching questions and crossword puzzles are included for use as review activities.

Case studies with explanations and sample problem-solving activities are included to reinforce and enhance understanding of both technical and clinical concepts. Opportunities to focus on technical and interpretative concepts are provided in critical thinking activities throughout the text. These activities may be adaptable for either classroom or "dry" laboratory activities. Review questions are included at the end of each chapter. Answers to questions are provided in the instructor's manual.

AUTHOR

Sheryl Whitlock has a bachelor of science in medical technology from the University of Delaware. Additional education includes a master of arts in education from

Arcadia University. The author has more than 30 years of work experience as an educator for both Clinical Laboratory Science and Clinical Laboratory Technology Programs and in all areas of laboratory medicine. Currently, the author is the laboratory coordinator for Student Health Services at the University of Delaware. Additionally, she works as a CLS at Union Hospital in Elkton Maryland. Previous publications include authoring laboratory manuals in Immunohematology, Urinalysis, and Clinical Chemistry for Delmar, Cengage Learning, and chapter or section contributor for additional textbooks and exam review books.

Supplemental author Kevin E. Whitlock also has a bachelor's degree in Clinical Laboratory Science from the University of Delaware. Kevin is currently employed at A. I. DuPont Hospital for Children in Wilmington, Delaware.

ACKNOWLEDGMENTS

Special thanks to:

1. My colleagues at Student Health Services including Debra Kenaley, MT (ASCP) who diligently read and edited every chapter at least once, and Susan Locke MLT (ASCP) who was my primary contact with the Blood Bank of Delmarva.

2. Michael J. Healy, MT (ASCP) SBB at the Blood Bank of Delmarva who never failed to answer my questions and allowed me to visit the Blood Bank and benefit from his vast experience.

3. Blood Bank supervisors at the Health Care Center at Christiana and A. I. DuPont Hospital for Children who allowed me to visit their facilities and shared their expertise with me.

4. Edith Thompson MT (ASCP), laboratory manager, and Rebecca Collins MT (ASCP), Blood Bank supervisor at Union Hospital, Elkton, Maryland who shared procedures, publications, and other technical information with me as the text developed.

DEDICATION

To my husband, Stephen, who assumed additional household responsibilities, patiently cheered me on from the sidelines, and served as my IT support person on many occasions. Also to my children Adam Whitlock, BSN, Rachel Williams, DPT, and Kevin Whitlock, MT

(ASCP) who were supportive and at times served as my technical advisors during the development and production of this text.

REVIEWERS

Nancy T. Beamon, MS, MT, BB (ASCP)
Certified Allied Health Instructor (AMT)
Director MLT, HT, and PBT Programs
Darton College
Albany, Georgia

Susan L. Conforti, EdD, MT (ASCP) SBB
Assistant Professor
Medical Laboratory Technology
Farmingdale State College
Farmingdale, New York

Michelle L. Gagan, MSHS, BSMT (ASCP)
MLT Clinical Coordinator
York Technical College
Rock Hill, South Carolina

Karen Golemboski, PhD, MT (ASCP)
Assistant Professor
Bellarmine University
Louisville, Kentucky

Loretta L. Gonzales, MAEd, CLS (NCA) C, MLT (ASCP)
Medical Laboratory Technician Program Director
University of New Mexico, Gallup Campus
Gallup, New Mexico

Candy Hill, MT (ASCP) CLS (NCA) MAEd
CLT Program Coordinator
Jefferson State Community College
Birmingham, Alabama

Jessica Mantini, MT (ASCP)
Clinical Instructor
School of Allied Medical Professions, Medical Technology Division
College of Medicine, The Ohio State University
Dublin, Ohio

Judy Miller, MT (ASCP)
MLT Clinical Coordinator
Medical Laboratory Technology
Barton Community College
Great Bend, Kansas

UNIT 1

Introduction to Immunohematology

Basic Immunology

LEARNING OUTCOMES

Upon completion of this chapter, the student should be able to:

■ Diagram and list the components in each layer of a tube of anticoagulated blood.
■ Explain the components and functions of the immune system.
■ List and differentiate the cells and mediators involved in immunologic reactions.
■ Define antigens, antibodies, and complement.
■ Prepare a detailed list of characteristics of antigens.
■ Identify and explain specific details of the structure and function of antibodies.
■ Diagram the complement cascade and label all of the components.
■ Explain the role of complement in antigen-antibody reactions.
■ Interpret antigen-antibody interactions and relate these concepts to final results.
■ Diagram and explain primary and secondary immune response.
■ Define and differentiate active and passive immunization.

GLOSSARY

acquired immunity   response by lymphocytes in response to antigen exposure; response is specific for the stimulating antigen

active immunization   stimulation of antibody production by direct antigen contact

agglutination   clumping of red blood cells or particulate matter resulting from the interaction of the antibody and the corresponding antigen

allele   one or more forms of a gene that occupies a specific locus on a chromosome

anamnestic response   antibody response stimulated by secondary exposure to an antigen; the response is accentuated and a rapid rise in antibody is exhibited

antibody   proteins produced in response to stimulation by an antigen and interacts with the stimulating antigen

anticoagulant   chemical substance that prevents or delays the clotting (coagulation) of blood

antigen   biochemical substance recognized as foreign; stimulates an immune response

atypical antibodies   antibodies found either in the serum or on the cells that are unanticipated or not found under normal circumstances

autoantibodies   antibodies directed against one's own red cell antigens

cell-mediated immunity   immunity involving cellular components such as macrophages, natural killer cells, T lymphocytes, and cytokines

chemical mediators   substances secreted by cells that are then involved in an inflammatory response

complement   a series of proteins in the serum that are activated sequentially; following activation, bacterial and red cell lysis may occur

cytokines   chemical mediators that stimulate tissue response to invading pathogens

decline phase   phase of antibody production where the level of detectable antibody is decreasing due to catabolism

erythrocyte   mature red blood cell; cell that transports oxygen and carbon dioxide

flocculation   soluble antigen and soluble antibody combine to "fall out" of solution in flakes

foreign   recognized by the immune system as non-self

graft versus host disease (GVHD)   functional immune cells received from a donor that become engrafted in the recipient; these cells then recognize the recipient as "foreign" and mount an immunologic attack

hapten   a small molecule that can elicit an immune response only when attached to a large carrier such as a protein

hemagglutination   the clumping of red blood cells; used to visualize antigen-antibody reactions

hemolysis   disruption of the membrane of a red blood cell; results in release of the contents into the plasma

human leukocyte antigens (HLA)   antigens present on leukocytes and tissues. Genes that code for these antigens are part of the major histocompatibility complex (MHC) gene systems

humoral immunity   immune response resulting in the production of antibodies

immune antibody   antibody produced by direct stimulation with an antigen

immunogen   synonym for antigen; substance that prompts the generation of antibodies and can cause an immune response

immunoglobulin   gamma globulin protein found in blood or bodily fluids and used by the immune system to identify and neutralize foreign objects, such as bacteria and viruses

immunohematology   study of blood related antigens and antibodies as applied to situations in blood bank and the transfusion service

immunology   study of components and processes of the immune system

innate immunity   first line of defense for invading pathogens; cells and mechanisms that defend the host from invasion by other organisms; a non-specific defense

lag phase   first phase of an immune response; the level of antibody is not detectable by testing

leukocytes   white blood cells

log phase   second phase of an immune response; antibody levels steadily increase in a linear fashion

lymphocyte   mononuclear leukocyte that mediates cellular and humoral immunity

major histocompatibility complex (MHC)   a group of linked genes on Chromosome 6 that determine the expression of complement proteins and leukocyte antigens

mononuclear phagocytes   leukocytes involved in phagocytosis and antigen presenting; these include monocytes (circulating cells) and macrophages (fixed cells)

natural antibody   antibody produced without known exposure to the antigen

passive antibody   antibody administered to an individual

plasma   liquid portion of whole blood containing water, electrolytes, glucose, proteins, fats, and gases; refers also to the liquid portion of a blood sample collected with an anticoagulant

plateau phase   response phase where antibody production is constant and detectable at stable levels

polymorphic   system possessing multiple allelic forms at a single locus

polymorphonuclear neutrophil   a granulocytic white blood cell that phagocytizes invading microorganisms to provide protection to the host

precipitation   formation of an insoluble compound when soluble ions in separate solutions are combined. The insoluble compound settles out of solution as a solid. The solid is called a precipitate

primary response   antibody response following initial antigen exposure

proenzyme   an inactive enzyme precursor; requires a chemical change to become active

prozone phenomenon   incomplete lattice formation with a lack of agglutination; results from antibody excess in comparison to antigen

refractory   resistant to ordinary treatment

rouleaux   coin like stacking of red cells in the presence of abnormal plasma proteins

[CGLO] secondary response (anamnestic response)   antibody response that follows any antigen exposure other than initial exposure

serum   liquid portion of the blood after coagulation

solid phase adherence   testing method where one component of testing is adhered (attached) to a solid phase such as a microtiter plate; the patient's sample is added; a final assessment is made by examination of the test wells of the plate

T cytotoxic (T_C) cells   a sub-group of lymphocytes that kill other cells

T helper (T_H) cells   a sub-group of lymphocytes that play an important role in activating and directing other immune cells

thrombocytes   anucleate cell fragments called platelets; these cells play a key role in blood clotting

titer   measurement of antibody strength by testing its reactivity with decreasing amounts of the corresponding antigen; reciprocal of the highest dilution that shows agglutination represents the titer

zeta potential   difference in charge density between the inner and outer ion cloud surrounding the surface of the red blood cells in an electrolyte solution

zone of equivalence   when both reactants are present in amounts to create optimal reaction conditions

INTRODUCTION

Immunohematology as a defined term can be broken into two components: "immuno" is related to immune response and "hematology" is the study of blood. This chapter examines basic **immunology** and applies the concepts to the testing and transfusion of blood and blood components. Learning about immunologic principles and conceptual information, regarding components of whole blood, will provide a knowledge base for specific topics discussed throughout all chapters in the text. Topics to be covered include: blood group antigen systems and their associated antibodies, pretransfusion testing, blood component donors, principles of blood collection, recipients of blood products, clinical conditions requiring transfusion, and potential adverse effects of transfusion.

The immune system is one of the most diverse systems in the human body. The basic function of this system is protection of the host organism. Specific defense mechanisms begin with the external body surfaces and portals of entry, which extend inward to include tissues, organs, and cellular defenses. The immune system differentiates self from non-self and removes potentially harmful organisms. Non-self organisms range from uni- to multicellular and include bacteria, viruses, fungi, and parasites.

The immune system is not autonomous. Elements of the immune system are integrated with other systems in the body. Systems that interact with the immune system include the hematopoietic, digestive, respiratory, and nervous systems. Without the immune system, these other systems would be at risk of attack by invading organisms. These systemic interactions help explain the complexity of the immune system and emphasize its vital role in the human body.

COMPONENTS OF BLOOD

Blood is composed of cellular components suspended in a liquid portion called plasma. Plasma comprises approximately 55% of the blood volume. Plasma is composed of more than 90% water and carries suspended elements including proteins, nutrients, and electrolytes. Blood is the major transport system in the body. Suspended elements are present in the blood because they are in transport within the body.

When a blood sample is collected for analysis in the laboratory, it is necessary to distinguish the liquid portion as plasma or serum. Plasma is the fluid portion of a sample collected with an anticoagulant, while serum results from a clotted sample. Figure 1-1 represents a comparison of anticoagulated blood and clotted blood. Either serum or plasma may be used for blood bank testing. Anticoagulants and their actions are summarized in Table 1-1.

Specimens for Blood Bank Testing

Blood specimens acceptable for blood bank testing can include anticoagulated whole blood or a clotted sample. The anticoagulant used for blood bank testing is ethylenediaminetetra-acetate (EDTA). EDTA is the anticoagulant used for hematology testing as well as some chemistry analyses. The collection tube commonly used for hematology testing has a lavender or purple stopper. To provide a unique sample tube for blood bank, some manufacturers of evacuated tubes have produced a tube with a pink stopper containing EDTA. See Figure 1-2 for a comparison of these tubes.

Screening of donor blood for ABO, Rh, red-cell stimulated antibodies, and infectious diseases is performed prior to release of blood or blood components for transfusion. The summary of blood collection

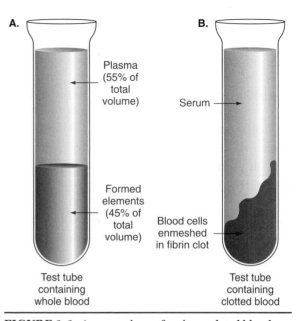

FIGURE 1-1 A comparison of anticoagulated blood and clotted blood. Test tube A contains anticoagulated whole blood. Plasma is separated from the formed elements. Test tube B contains clotted blood. The clot is cellular components enmeshed in fibrin. The liquid portion is serum.
Source: Delmar, Cengage Learning

tubes provided in Figure 1-3 include those that may be used for routine blood bank testing and screening of donor blood.

Cellular Components of Blood

The blood's cellular components, and their specific functions, are summarized in Table 1-2. The erythrocyte is the major cellular component considered in this

---

TABLE 1-1 Common Anticoagulants and Their Actions

- ethylenediaminetetra-acetate (EDTA)—binds calcium preventing anticoagulation
- sodium citrate—binds calcium preventing anticoagulation
- sodium heparin—anti-thrombin; acts to inhibit thrombin that is a component of the coagulation process

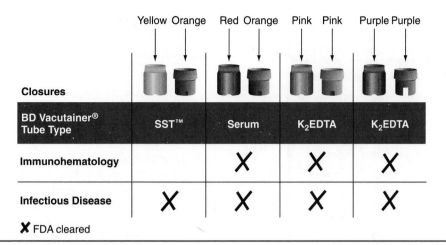

Closures								
	Yellow	Orange	Red	Orange	Pink	Pink	Purple	Purple
BD Vacutainer® Tube Type	SST™		Serum		K₂EDTA		K₂EDTA	
Immunohematology			X		X		X	
Infectious Disease	X		X		X		X	

X FDA cleared

FIGURE 1-2 Lavender or purple top tubes are designated for hematology and chemistry analyses. Pink top tubes with paper labels are designated for blood bank testing. *Reprinted with Courtesy and © Becton, Dickinson and Company.*

text. Leukocytes and thrombocytes will be considered briefly. Five types of leukocytes are found in circulation. Some are also deposited in tissues for specific phagocytic and immunological functions.

IMMUNE SYSTEM

The immune system is a collection of tissues, organs, cells, mechanical barriers, and chemical substances that interact to protect the body from invasion by foreign agents. Organs involved in immune processes include the lymph nodes, spleen, and thymus. See Figure 1-4 for a view of the primary and secondary lymphoid organs. Some tissues, such as bone marrow and lymphatic tissue, also play a role in the immune process. The two major immune system components are innate immunity and acquired immunity. These components work simultaneously to protect the human body from the adverse effects of invasion of a vast number of foreign substances.

Innate and Acquired Immunity

Innate immunity is a nonspecific immunity that provides the first line of defense from invading pathogens. Innate immunity is composed of mechanical barriers, chemical barriers, and normal bacterial flora. The mechanical barriers are skin, mucus membranes, chemical secretions, and normal bacterial flora. Chemical barriers include lysozyme, lactoferrin, and the low pH of stomach secretions. The second line of natural defense is activated after the invading substances have passed mechanical barriers.

The second line of defense is an inflammatory response. This inflammatory response utilizes chemical mediators of inflammation and phagocytic cells. The effects of the chemical mediators are cell migration and the concentration of cells in the affected area. The phagocytic cells function to remove foreign organisms and debris.

Chemical mediators, or cytokines, stimulate an immune response to the invading pathogen. Cardinal signs of the inflammatory response include redness, heat, swelling, and pain. Edema, an accumulation of fluid, is caused by an increase in permeability of the capillaries. Part of the cellular response is induced by the migration of phagocytes into the tissues. Neutrophils, monocytes, and macrophages accumulate in the tissues and phagocytize invading pathogens. This phagocytosis plays a major role in the nonspecific immune response.

Cumulatively, these nonspecific responses occur in the same manner each time the system is activated. Since the response is nonspecific, the mechanism does not incorporate memory of recognition for a specific microorganism or pathogen.

Acquired immunity or adaptive immunity is a specific immune response enlisted when the innate system is unable to stop the invading pathogen or foreign substance. The acquired immune response includes lymphocytes and highly specific antibodies.

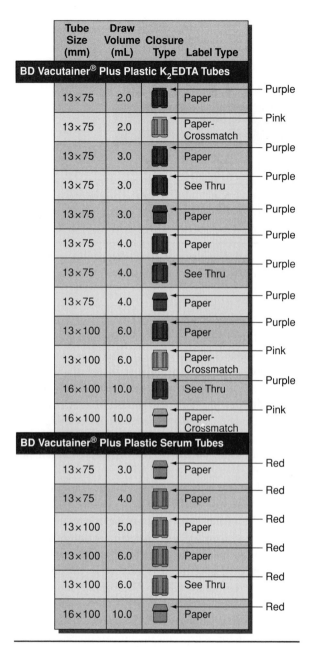

Tube Size (mm)	Draw Volume (mL)	Closure Type	Label Type	
BD Vacutainer® Plus Plastic K₂EDTA Tubes				
13×75	2.0		Paper	Purple
13×75	2.0		Paper-Crossmatch	Pink
13×75	3.0		Paper	Purple
13×75	3.0		See Thru	Purple
13×75	3.0		Paper	Purple
13×75	4.0		Paper	Purple
13×75	4.0		See Thru	Purple
13×75	4.0		Paper	Purple
13×100	6.0		Paper	Purple
13×100	6.0		Paper-Crossmatch	Pink
16×100	10.0		See Thru	Purple
16×100	10.0		Paper-Crossmatch	Pink
BD Vacutainer® Plus Plastic Serum Tubes				
13×75	3.0		Paper	Red
13×75	4.0		Paper	Red
13×100	5.0		Paper	Red
13×100	6.0		Paper	Red
13×100	6.0		See Thru	Red
16×100	10.0		Paper	Red

FIGURE 1-3 A summary of collection tubes that may be used for blood bank testing and infectious disease testing. *Reprinted with Courtesy and © Becton, Dickinson and Company.*

The acquired immune response supplements the innate mechanisms to provide a wider range of immunological protection. Acquired immunity and its components are discussed in subsequent sections.

TABLE 1-2 Cellular Components Suspended in Plasma

- Erythrocytes (red blood cells)—carry oxygen to tissues and transport waste products to the lungs for expulsion
- Leukocytes (white blood cells)
- Types of Leukocytes
- Neutrophils—most abundant type of white blood cells; phagocytize bacteria
- Lymphocytes—play an integral role in the body's cellular and humoral defenses
- Monocytes—found in small numbers in the circulation; in tissues may mature into macrophages; phagocytize bacteria; and present antigens
- Eosinophils—found in small numbers in the circulation; involved in allergic reactions
- Basophils—predominantly in the tissues; few circulate and are involved with histamine releasing reactions
- Thrombocytes (platelets)—anucleate cells that play a key role in clot formation during blood coagulation

CELLS AND MEDIATORS OF IMMUNITY

Phagocytes

Phagocytes provide a cellular defense for the host. **Mononuclear phagocytes** include monocytes in the peripheral circulation and macrophages in the tissues. Monocytes phagocytize bacteria and other foreign material and serve as precursors for macrophages. Macrophages are antigen-presenting cells. They present a foreign antigen to the circulating lymphocytes. The lymphocytes process the presented material and respond with the appropriate adaptive immune response. See Figure 1-5 for a summary of development and maturation of cells of immunity.

Polymorphonuclear neutrophils (PMN) are found in the peripheral circulation. They migrate to tissues in response to chemical mediators, and phagocytize microorganisms. The cells contain intracellular granules, which contain bactericidal substances and lytic enzymes

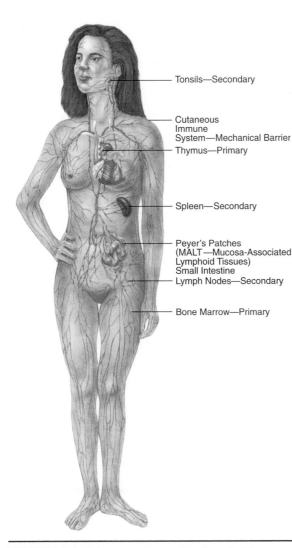

Tonsils—Secondary

Cutaneous
Immune
System—Mechanical Barrier
Thymus—Primary

Spleen—Secondary

Peyer's Patches
(MALT—Mucosa-Associated
Lymphoid Tissues)
Small Intestine
Lymph Nodes—Secondary

Bone Marrow—Primary

FIGURE 1-4 Primary and secondary lymphoid organs. These organs play a vital role in cellular immunity and antibody protection. Collectively cellular immunity and antibodies provide global protection from foreign substances and pathogens.
Source: Delmar, Cengage Learning

that kill the ingested microorganisms. When the granules are released externally, they will damage healthy tissues and host cells. The release of increased numbers of PMNs from the bone marrow occurs in response to the chemical mediators of inflammation.

Lymphocytes

Lymphocytes are white blood cells that play a major role in the body's immune system. There are two major

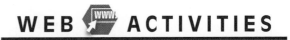

1. Go to www.cellsalive.com
2. In the left column choose "Immunology."
3. In the table of contents choose: Making Antibodies.
4. Note the "Antigen Processing" for a video view of the antigen presentation.

types of lymphocytes: T cells and B cells. These cells originate in the bone marrow from the same stem cell, but mature, in separate locations. Precursors of T lymphocytes migrate to the thymus for maturation while B lymphocyte precursor cells mature in the bone marrow. See Figure 1-5 for a summary of lymphocyte development.

Immunological roles of lymphocytes include:

1. Following contact with cells, chemical substances, proteins, and other biological substances, they differentiate "self" from "non-self."
2. B cells provide **humoral immunity** by producing a specific **antibody** in response to stimulation with a foreign substance.
3. T cells provide **cell-mediated immunity**, inactivating and removing foreign substances with cell-to-cell interactions.
4. Interaction of these two types of immunity provides protection from invasive substances.

B Cells

B lymphocytes (B cells) develop and mature in the bone marrow. Lymphocytes in the peripheral circulation are 10–20% B lymphocytes. Mature B cells are found in bone marrow, lymph nodes, spleen, and other lymphatic organs. Antibody production occurs as follows:

1. B lymphocytes have receptor sites on their surface.
2. Specific **antigens** attach to these receptors.
3. Following antigenic attachment, B lymphocytes differentiate into plasma cells or memory cells.

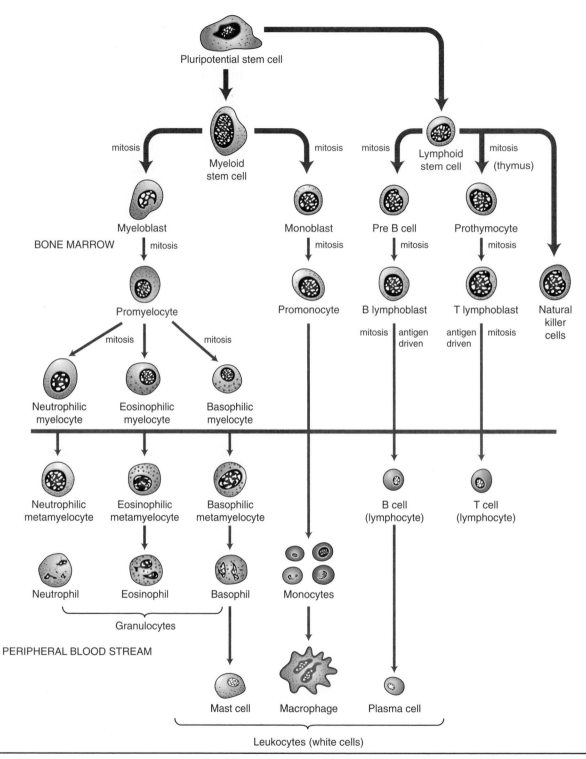

FIGURE 1-5 All immunologically active white blood cells originate from a pluripotential stem cell. The cells of the lymphoid line differentiate into B lymphocytes and T lymphocytes. The myeloid lines differentiate into neutrophils, eosinophils, and basophils. Neutrophils are a key player in removal of foreign substances.
Source: Delmar, Cengage Learning

a. Plasma cells produce antigen-specific antibodies. These antibodies react with the specific antigens. This combination neutralizes the offensive substance.

b. Memory cells provide lasting immunity for that antigenic determinant.

T Cells

T lymphocytes (T cells) mature. Some remain in the thymus gland while some circulate to perform immunological functions. T cells comprise the remainder of the circulating lymphocytes. Mature T lymphocytes are stored in bone marrow, lymph nodes, spleen, and other secondary lymphoid organs. They also circulate in the bloodstream and the lymphatic system.

There are two populations of T cells. Each population has a unique function. T helper cells (T_H) recognize and interact with antigens. The cytokines produced as a result of this interaction activate other cells that participate in the immune response. Cells that may be activated include T cytotoxic cells (T_C), B lymphocytes, and macrophages.

T lymphocytes are not activated directly by soluble antigens. Major Histocompatibility Complex (MHC) antigens on the macrophage surfaces are involved antigen processing. Macrophages process antigens and present them to T cells. This presentation of processed antigens activates the T cells initiates the stimulation of T cells and, hence, the induction of cell mediated immunity.

Cytokines

Cytokines are molecules secreted by cells that have been stimulated by potentially infectious materials. Cytokines perform a variety of functions in the immune response. These functions include regulation of the intensity and duration of the immune response, as well as, specific regulatory functions such as providing initiation signals for immune cells such as T cells and macrophages. Activated cells travel to the site of invasion where each performs a specific function. In addition, cytokines stimulate cells to produce additional cytokines. Refer to Table 1-3 for a list of specific cytokines and their functions.

TABLE 1-3 Cytokines and Their Functions

CYTOKINE	PRODUCED BY	FUNCTION
Interleukin 1 (IL-1)	Macrophages, Endothelial Cells, B cells	T Cell activation, Inflammation, Fever Acute phase protein Stimulation
Interleukin 2 (IL-2)	T cells	T cell, Chemotaxis Macrophage activation
Interleukin 3 (IL-3)	T cells	Colony stimulating factor
Interleukin 4 (IL-4)	T cells	T and B cell differentiation, B cell activation, T-cell growth
Interleukin 5 (IL-5)	T cells	Differentiation of B cells and Eosinophils
Interleukin 6 (IL-6)	Macrophages, T cells, B cells	Cell differentiation, Fever, Acute phase protein synthesis
Interleukin 8 (IL-8)	Macrophages, Endothelial Cells	Inflammation, Cell migration, Chemotaxis
Interleukin 10 (IL-10)	Macrophages, T cells	Suppression of T cells, Inhibits antigen presentation Inhibits cytokine production
Tumor Necrosis Factor (TNF)	Macrophages and Lymphocytes	Inflammation, Fever, Production of adhesion molecules, Acute phase protein synthesis
Interferon γ (INF-γ)	T cells	Immunoregulation, Antiviral, Phagocyte activation
Colony Stimulation Factors (GM-CSF, M-CSF, G-CSF)	Macrophage, Fibroblasts	Growth and activation of phagocytic cells

Complement Proteins

The complement system is a group of circulating plasma proteins that perform multiple functions in the immune response. Primary functions include lysis of cells, bacteria, and viruses. Peptide fragment split products are the result of complement activation and are involved in mediating inflammatory and immune responses. The outcomes of the mediation include: vascular permeability, smooth muscle contraction, chemotaxis, and migration.

Complement components circulate in inactive forms as **proenzymes**. As each complement component is activated, it is converted from an inactive or proenzyme form to an active form. This activated form initiates the next step. Multiple steps, each catalyzed by the product of the previous step, produce a cascade effect that may progress through one of two pathways: the classical pathway or the alternative pathway (see Figure 1-6). An antigen-antibody complex activates the classical pathway. In contrast, the alternative pathway does not require a specific antibody but rather high molecular weight molecules with repeating units. Examples include carbohydrates and lipopolysaccharides. Foreign cells including, but not limited to, viruses and bacteria or other foreign proteins may also activate it.

TABLE 1-4 Functions of Complement Proteins	
SERUM PROTEIN	**FUNCTION**
C1q	Binds to Fc area of IgM and IgG Molecules
C1r	Activates C1s
C1s	Cleaves C4 and C2
C4	Part of C3 Convertase
C2	Binds to C4 to form C3 convertase
C3	Intermediate component in all pathways
C5	Initiator of membrane attack unit
C6	Part of membrane attack unit
C7	Part of membrane attack unit
C8	Initiates pore formation on membrane
C9	Lyses cell

Complement proteins and their specific functions are summarized in Table 1-4.

The classic pathway is involved in blood bank testing outcomes. The major role of complement is red cell hemolysis. When an antigen-antibody complex involves

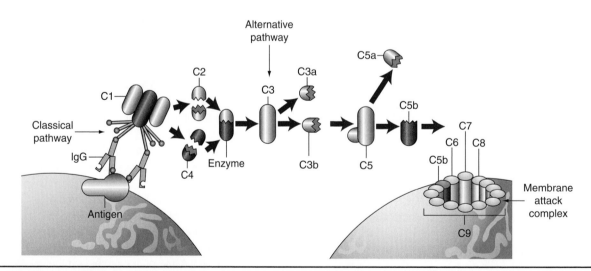

FIGURE 1-6 Complement cascade including the classical and alternative pathways. A bound antigen-antibody complex activates the complement cascade. C1 binds to this complex to begin activation. This event starts a cascade effect with each step activating the next step. Once activation occurs and reaches C3, two pathways may be followed. The alternate pathway ends with C3a, while the classical pathway proceeds to C9. C9 results in cell lysis (Redrawn from Schindler LW: *Understanding the Immune system*. NIH Pub No 92-529, Bethesda, MD 1991, U. S. Department of Health and Human Services, p. 11.)

an antigen on the red cell surface, bound complement may proceed to hemolysis of the red cells. This lysis of the membrane occurs when the pathway proceeds to completion (C9).

ANTIGENS
Antigen Characteristics

An antigen is a foreign substance that either combines with an antibody or is processed and binds to a T lymphocyte to stimulate an immune response. An antigen that stimulates an immune response is an **immunogen**. The immune response results in antibody production (B lymphocytes) or cellular reaction (T lymphocytes). Properties of molecules that contribute to immunogenicity are summarized in Table 1-5.

To stimulate antibody production, a substance must have a molecular weight of greater than 10,000. As the molecular weight increases, the immunogenicity of the substance also increases. **Haptens** are small chemical substances that must be bound to a larger molecule to provide sufficient molecular weight for stimulation of antibody production.

The chemical nature of an antigen can be protein, carbohydrate, or lipopolysaccharide. Proteins are the most immunogenic followed by complex carbohydrates. Lipopolysaccharides are the least immunogenic.

Complexity is an important characteristic for immunogenicity. The more complex the molecule, the greater the likelihood that antibody will be produced. Stability also plays an important role. A molecule that is unstable and easily degraded is less likely to stimulate an antibody response.

Foreignness is another important factor for antigenicity. Foreign antigens originate outside of the body. A substance recognized by the immune system as foreign or "non-self" is most likely to stimulate an antibody response. When antibodies are produced to antigens that are "self," these antibodies are autoantibodies. Recognition of "non-self" or foreign substances will stimulate the production of protective antibodies.

Antigen location

Antigens are found ubiquitously in nature. In human beings, microorganisms, viruses, fungi, and chemical substances such as proteins may serve as antigens. Human antigens are found on cells, organs, and tissues as well as in plasma and other body fluids. Physical location on the cell membrane varies, and it is antigen-specific. Some antigens protrude from the cell surface, while others are an integral part of the membrane. Physical location impacts antibody stimulation as well as the physical ability of the antigen to react with an antibody once it is produced. Physical accessibility of the antigen impacts its ability to stimulate antibody production and subsequently react with the formed antibody.

Red Blood Cell Antigens

Red blood cell antigens and corresponding antibodies provide the foundation for blood bank testing. Every individual's red blood cells contain a unique, genetically determined set of antigens. There are more than 20 blood group systems that contain greater than 200 red blood cell antigens. The ABO and Rh antigens are matched between donor and recipient. Additional red blood cell antigens are not considered in routine pretransfusion testing unless a red cell stimulated antibody is present in the individual's plasma.

Red blood cell antigens are protein (or proteins) in combination with lipids, glycolipid, carbohydrate, or glycoprotein. Antigen location on the red cell surface varies by blood group. For example, ABO antigens protrude from the red cell surface while Rh antigens are an integral part of the membrane. Antigens that are less physically accessible will require the use of enhancement agents to aid in visible antigen-antibody reactions.

TABLE 1-5 Properties of Molecules that Contribute to Immunogenicity	
PROPERTY	**DESCRIPTION**
Foreignness	Non-self more likely to stimulate antibody production
Size	>10,000 M.W.
Chemical Composition	Protein—best immune response
	Complex carbohydrate—second best immune response
	Lipids—weak immune response
	Nucleic acid—weak immune response
Complexity	More complex molecules produce better immune response

Specific characteristics of antigen-antibody systems are discussed in Chapters 5, 6, and 7.

Leukocyte Antigens

Human leukocyte antigens (HLA) are found predominantly on nucleated cells such as leukocytes and tissues. These antigens are antigenic and stimulate antibody response when presented to an antigen-negative recipient. The genes encoding for the HLA antigens are part of the **Major Histocompatibility Complex (MHC)** genes located on Chromosome 6 (see Figure 1-7).

The MHC region of chromosome 6 is divided into three categories or classes. Class I are A, B, and C locus. Class II loci are DR, DP, and DQ. Class III genes code for secreted proteins, such as complement components and cytokines. These proteins have immunological functions but are not exposed on cell surfaces.

Multiple alleles are possible at each of these loci. Alleles are variant forms of a gene. Since multiple alleles are possible at each loci, the MHC system may be described as **polymorphic.**

HLA antigens and antibodies have applications in transfusion medicine as well as transplantation. Applications include: organ and tissue transplant, bone marrow and stem cell transplants, paternity testing, and blood component matching in some situations. Specific applications will be discussed throughout the text, as appropriate.

An individual exposed to foreign antigens via transfusion may produce antibodies in response to one or more of the antigens. These antibodies may be incriminated in future transfusion reactions as well as in the destruction of transfused components such as platelets. Transfusion reactions and administration of blood components will be discussed in Chapters 11 and 12.

Finally, the role of HLA matching in donor and recipient is vital for an organ transplant. **Graft versus host disease (GVHD)** may occur in persons for whom an HLA match is not similar. GVHD is a condition where a transplant or transfusion recipient becomes engrafted with cells from the donor. These cells then mount an immune response *against* the recipient. GVHD will be discussed in more detail in Chapter 12.

Platelet Antigens

Proteins that may stimulate an immune response are present on the surface of platelets. These antibodies are found infrequently. The presence of a platelet antibody is suspected when the post-transfusion increase in the recipient's platelet count does not achieve the anticipated level.

ANTIBODIES
Antibody Characteristics

An antibody is a protein. It is produced in response to stimulation with an antigen. The antibody is specific for the stimulating antigen and will react with that antigen. An antibody molecule is also called an **immunoglobulin.**

Immunoglobulin Structure

An antibody molecule is four polypeptide chains joined by disulfide bonds. The number of disulfide bonds ranges from 1 to 15 with the exact number variable by class and subclass of immunoglobulin. The chains consist of two identical heavy chains and two identical light chains. The chains are joined by disulfide bridges (S-S) (see Figure 1-8). The molecule is a Y shape with a flexible hinge area. Each of the four chains has two areas (or domains). These are designated constant and variable domains (see Figure 1-8). The constant domain of the heavy chains imparts the biological function to the antibody molecule. This is the portion of the molecule that attaches the antibody to cells and serves to activate complement. The variable portions of the molecule provide the specificity for antigen binding. The variable portions of both the heavy and light chains attach to individual antigen molecules.

The hinge region consists of disulfide bonds (see Figure 1-8). These disulfide bonds provide physical flexibility. The hinge can "open up" or spread apart. This spread allows each antigen-binding site to attach to a separate antigen on *different cells*. The hinge also permits an inward folding of the antibody molecule. This inward folding provides physical flexibility allowing the

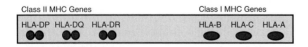

FIGURE 1-7 Location of Class HLA Class I and II genes on Chromosome 6
Source: Delmar, Cengage Learning

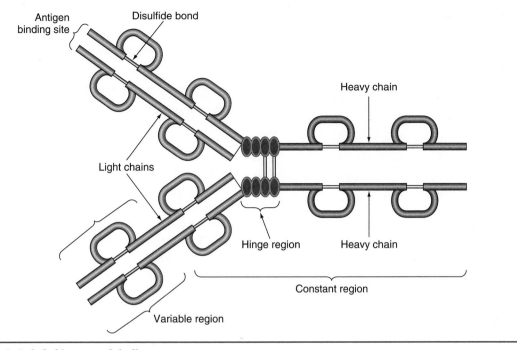

FIGURE 1-8 Labeled immunoglobulin monomer
Source: Delmar, Cengage Learning

two antigen-binding sites to attach to two different antigen sites on the *same* cell.

Monomeric units may be combined to form polymers. Polymeric units produced may be dimers (two units) or pentamers (five units). These polymeric units have a higher molecular weight and a large physical size. The polymeric units can bind more antibody molecules based on the number of antigen-binding sites.

Immunoglobulin classes

Five distinct classes of immunoglobulins have been identified and named according to the specific heavy chain of the immunoglobulin molecule. These classes are designated IgG, IgM, IgA, IgD, and IgE. The heavy chains are gamma, mu, alpha, delta, and epsilon, consecutively. The characteristics of immunoglobulin include biological and physical properties. See Table 1-6 for a summary

TABLE 1-6 Characteristics of Immunoglobulin Molecules

CHARACTERISTIC	IgM	IgG	IgA
Molecular Weight	900,000	150,000	180,000–500,000
H-chain isotype	μ	γ	α
L-chains, types	κ, λ	κ, λ	κ, λ
Sedimentation Coefficient	19S	7S	11S
Structure	pentamer	monomer	dimer
HalfLife (days)	5	23	6
% Total Immunoglobulin	5	80	15
Present in Secretions	No	No	Yes
Fixes Complement	Yes	Yes	No
Crosses Placenta	No	Yes	No

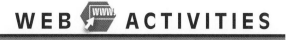

WEB ACTIVITIES

Immunoglobulin Molecules
1. Paste the link http://bio-alive.com into your browser.
2. Choose Immunology.
3. Scroll down the page and click on: *Immunoglobulins Animation* by W.H. Freeman.

of the immunoglobulin classes significant to the blood bank. Antibodies detected in the blood bank are primarily IgG and IgM. IgG is a monomer, whereas IgM is a pentamer. This structural difference makes IgM a much larger molecule (see Figure 1-9).

IMMUNOLOGICAL PRINCIPLES

As discussed previously, primary immunological components are antigens and antibodies. These two components provide the basis for blood bank testing and reactions. There is a cardinal rule for antigens and antibodies as they relate to the blood bank. Antigens are

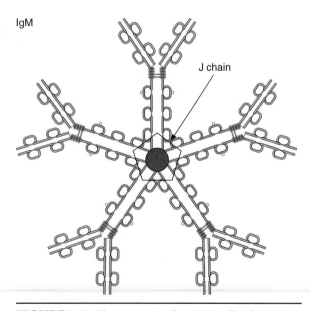

IgM

J chain

FIGURE 1-9 The structure of an IgM molecule
Source: Delmar, Cengage Learning

located on red blood cells and antibodies are found in the serum or plasma. Rare exceptions to this rule will be noted throughout the text.

Primary and Secondary Immune Response

Antibody production begins with initial antigen exposure, which stimulates the primary response. During the primary response, antibody production begins slowly with a lag phase (see Figure 1-8). During this phase, the antibody concentration is very low and no antibody is detectable. The timing of the lag phases varies, but typically lasts five to seven days.

The log phase follows the lag phase. It represents a period of time when the antibody is produced in a linear fashion (see Figure 1-10). During this phase, the titer of IgM antibody increases initially followed by a rise in the IgG titer.

The third phase of the primary response represents stable antibody production and is labeled the plateau phase, where the antibody production remains stable. This is followed by the final decline phase. During this phase, antibody is being catabolized and the detectable level of antibody is decreasing.

Following the first or initial exposure, a subsequent exposure results in a secondary or anamnestic response (see Figure 1-10). This response differs from the primary response in several ways. The primary antibody class produced in the secondary response is IgG, not IgM. During the log phase, the antibody titer rises higher and remains elevated longer than in a primary response. This increase may be as much as tenfold over the primary response. The secondary response has a shorter lag phase and longer plateau and decline phases.

ANTIGEN-ANTIBODY REACTIONS

Once an antibody is produced, it has the capability to react with its specific antigen. This specificity provides the basis for blood bank tests. Combination of antigen and antibody results in the formation of an immune complex. Factors influencing antigen-antibody reactions are summarized in Table 1-7.

The factors summarized in Table 1-7 influence antigen-antibody reactions. Visualization of antigen-antibody reactions may be agglutination,

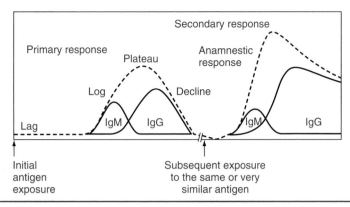

FIGURE 1-10 Primary and secondary immune response
Source: Delmar, Cengage Learning

hemagglutination, precipitation, flocculation, hemolysis, or solid phase adherence. In blood bank testing, antigen-antibody reactions are classically visualized by hemagglutination and/or hemolysis.

TABLE 1-7 Factors Influencing Antigen-Antibody Reactions

Specificity—each antibody reacts with the antigen that stimulated its production

Bonding—noncovalent bonds are involved in the attachment of antigens to antibodies

Physical fit—the fit of the antigen and antibody depend on compatible shapes that allow the antigen and antibody to physically touch. This physical contact allows for strong bonds to form. This is called a lock and key mechanism.

Concentration of antigen and antibody—antigens and antibodies must be present in optimal concentrations; excess antibodies will result in a situation known as prozone phenomenon

Temperature—optimal temperature of reactivity for a specific antibody will expedite the combination of antigen and antibody

Time—incubation time must be that which is optimal for the specific antibody. General guidelines are a range of 15–60 minutes for optimal antigen-antibody attachment

pH—a pH range of 7.2–7.4 is maintained for most antigen-antibody reactions

Surface charge—a net negative charge known as zeta potential surrounds the red cells. The reduction of this charge influences the ability of antigen and antibody to combine.

Specificity

Antigens and their specific antibodies physically combine, and the physical binding plays a role in the strength of the complex. The number of points of attachment corresponds to the strength of the complex. This is known as a "Lock and Key" mechanism (see Figure 1-11).

Optimum Concentrations of Antigens and Antibodies

As with any reaction (chemical, physical, or biological), the concentration of the reactants is vital to the final

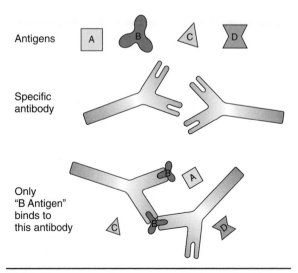

FIGURE 1-11 Lock and Key mechanism: The affinity of antibody for its corresponding antibody will be greater when the physical fit is the best (i.e. more physical contact points will lead to a more secure attachment of the antigen and antibody).
Source: Delmar, Cengage Learning

outcome. Antigen-antibody reactions in the blood bank are no exception. With few exceptions, the antigens are present on the red cells and the antibodies are found in the serum/antiserum. When the optimal concentration of both reactants occurs in combination with optimum reaction conditions, the zone of equivalence is reached. The zone of equivalence represents the formation of the maximum number of immune complexes (see Figure 1-12).

On either side of the zone of equivalence the concentration of one of the reactants, antigen or antibody, is not optimal. Fewer immune complexes are formed resulting in fewer red cell agglutinates and a reaction that may not be visible. Antibody excess is known as prozone phenomenon. Most of the accessible antigen sites on each cell are combined with an antibody molecule. Since this results in few antigen sites being available on each red blood cell, crossbridging between two cells is prevented. Agglutination cannot occur due to the lack of lattice formation. See Figure 1-13 to see lattice formation.

Antigen Location

The physical location of the antigens plays a practical role in immune complex formation. Some antigens protrude from the surface (e.g. ABO antigens), while

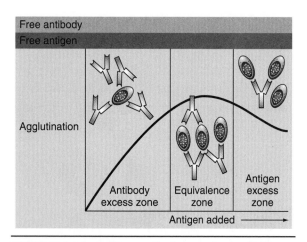

FIGURE 1-12 Antigen-antibody complexes will form agglutinates or precipitates when the concentration of both antigen and antibody are equal. In the presence of either antigen or antibody excess, the amount of precipitate formed will be decreased. *Reproduced with permission from Blaney and Howard (2000), "Basic and Applied Concepts of Immunohematology." St. Louis, Mosby.*

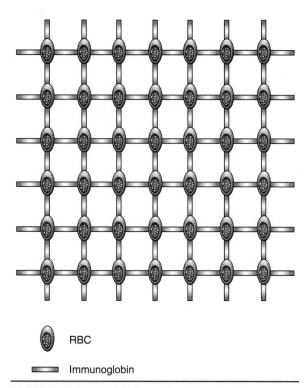

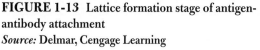

FIGURE 1-13 Lattice formation stage of antigen-antibody attachment
Source: Delmar, Cengage Learning

others are an integral part of the red blood cell membrane (e.g. Rh). Physically accessible antigens are more readily available for attachment of the antigen-binding site of the immunoglobulin molecule.

Environmental Factors
Ionic Strength

Red blood cell suspensions used for testing are prepared with isotonic saline. The saline contributes ions that attach to oppositely charged groups on the antigen and antibody molecules. After this ionic coating occurs, the formation of immune complexes will be hindered. A reduction in the ionic environment allows efficient formation of immune complexes.

pH

The physiologic pH is 7.2–7.4. This pH with small variances is optimum for formation antigen-antibody reactions. Hemagglutination, the most common method for viewing antigen-antibody reactions in the blood bank, also occurs optimally at physiologic pH.

Temperature of Reaction

Antibodies have an optimum temperature of reactivity. Clinically significant antibodies are IgG class and react at 37°C. Incubation at 37°C enhances the formation of the immune complex. Since clinically significant antibodies exhibit optimum reactivity at 37°C, incubation is imperative for detection of problematic or dangerous antibodies in a transfusion setting. Antibodies with reactive temperatures of 22°C or colder are historically IgM antibodies and are not usually clinically significant.

Incubation Time

Time of incubation also impacts the strength of antigen-antibody reactions. Elapsed time allows for equilibration of components and formation of the antigen-antibody complex. As these steps are completed, a reaction is visible. The optimum time is dependent upon the specific antigen and antibody involved, reagents used, and the test procedure employed.

AGGLUTINATION

Agglutination of red blood cells or hemagglutination and hemolysis are classic methods for visualization of antigen-antibody reactions in blood bank tests. Agglutination differs from precipitation. In a precipitation reaction, the antigen is dissolved in the reacting solution. This soluble antigen combines with the antibody and forms a complex. The complex cross-links with other

CRITICAL THINKING ACTIVITY

Create a list of at least five negative consequences of extended incubation for an antigen-antibody reaction and/or not using an optimal temperature of incubation. Explain *why* each of the negative results occurs. Consolidate these into a combined list with classmates.

complexes resulting in the formation of small particles that "precipitate" or fall out of the solution. This makes the reaction visible.

Agglutination involves a particulate antigen or an antigen that is attached to a particle (such as a red blood cell). Agglutination occurs in when:

1. An antibody molecule attaches to a single antigen on a single cell with one antigen-binding site.
2. The free arm of the immunoglobulin molecule attaches to an antigen on a second red cell. This creates a crosslink.
3. Multiple cross links create a lattice.
4. The lattice is visualized as agglutination.

Zeta Potential

The cross-linking of cells is affected most by zeta potential (see Figure 1-14). When cells are suspended

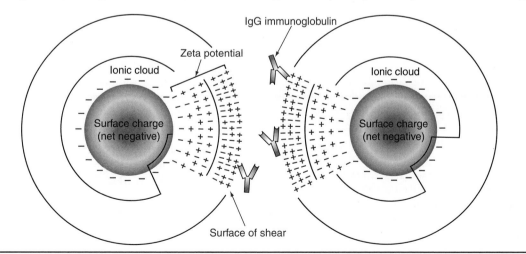

FIGURE 1-14 Zeta potential
Source: Delmar, Cengage Learning

in isotonic saline, a cloud of negative ions surrounds the red cell. The cloud of negative charge surrounding the cells causes them to repel one another. Zeta potential is the difference in negative charge between the inner and outer surfaces of the cloud. The distance between the red cells is proportional to the zeta potential. Reduction of zeta potential allows the red cells to approach one another and aids in lattice formation. Zeta potential may be reduced by suspension of the cells in isotonic saline; addition of a potentiating substance such as albumin, low ionic strength substance (LISS), or polyethylene glycol (PEG); or treatment of the cells with enzymes. Additional forces that are involved in antigen-antibody reactions are summarized in Table 1-8.

Grading Agglutination Reactions

After agglutination has occurred in a test tube or gel matrix, it is necessary to determine the strength of the reaction. The reaction mixture of cells and serum (or antisera) are centrifuged for the appropriate amount of time. A serological centrifuge is represented in Figure 1-15. When the centrifugation is complete, the cells form a compressed cell button in the bottom of the tube. Surrounding this button is the remaining serum or antisera.

Each tube is first observed for hemolysis by examining the supernatant fluid for red or pink color. If present, hemolysis is noted and considered a positive reaction.

Examination of the reactants for agglutination requires good lighting, preferably with a magnification mirror. An agglutination viewer that may be used for lighting and magnification is represented in Figure 1-16.

SAMPLE PROCEDURE 1-1

1. Centrifuge all tubes for the designated time for that specific serofuge.
2. Tilt each tube with a gentle motion that allows the liquid to flow approximately 2/3 of the distance to the top of the tube.
3. While tilting, observe the reflection of the tube in the reflecting mirror.
4. As the cell button becomes dislodged and the tube is tilted, focus on the reflection of the fluid as it flows up the side of the tube. Be sure to look into the mirror and not examine the tube itself.
5. The fluid is examined for agglutinates or clumps of red cells.
6. During the tilting process, the cell button is also observed.
7. As the button is dislodged, note whether clumps of cells break off *or* the cells swirl off of the bottom of the tube with no apparent clumping.
8. The final assessment of agglutination strength is made when the entire cell button has been dislodged from the bottom of the tube.

A sample procedure for examination of blood bank tubes is summarized in Sample Procedure 1-1.

The final step is to grade the agglutination. This grading method uses a standard system with results ranging from a negative reaction graded as a 0 (zero) to a complete agglutination reaction, graded as 4+ (four plus) (see Figure 1-17). The grading scheme and criteria for making a final determination are outlined in Table 1-9. When recording the results, a negative reaction must be recorded as a 0 (zero), never as a negative mark (−). Negative marks may be readily transformed to positive marks. Worksheets, whether paper or electronic, are legal documents that may be used as evidence in court cases. For this reason, the use of the negative sign is unacceptable. The positive reactions are recorded using either a number followed by a plus (+) sign or hash marks (see Table 1-9).

Gel testing systems have been developed to perform antigen-antibody testing. The premise behind

TABLE 1-8   Forces Involved in Antigen-Antibody Reaction

Ionic Bonding (Electrostatic Forces)—opposite charges on two molecules attracting each other

Hydrogen Bonding—attraction of two electronegative atoms to a positively charged hydrogen atom

Hydrophobic Bonding—bond between antigen and antibody that excludes a water molecule; usually a weak bond

Van der Waals Forces—attractive or repulsive forces between molecules or parts of molecules; excludes covalent bonds or electrostatic forces

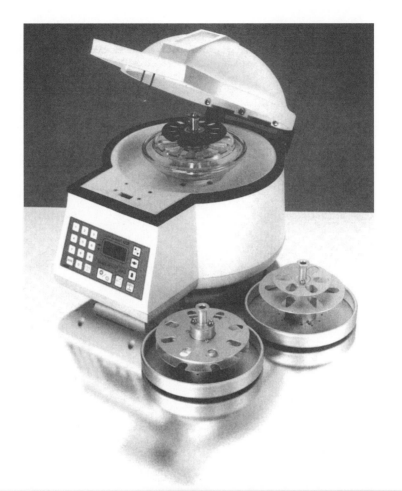

FIGURE 1-15 Serological centrifuge *(Courtesy of Becton Dickinson Primary Care Diagnostics; Clay Adams and Serofuge are trademarks of Becton Dickinson and Company)*

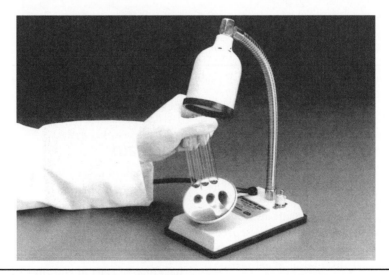

FIGURE 1-16 Agglutination viewer with magnifying mirror *(Courtesy of Becton Dickinson Primary Care Diagnostics; Clay Adams and Serofuge are trademarks of Becton Dickinson and Company)*

Reaction Grading

The degree of red cell agglutination observed in any blood bank test procedure is significant and should be recorded. A system of grading is illustrated

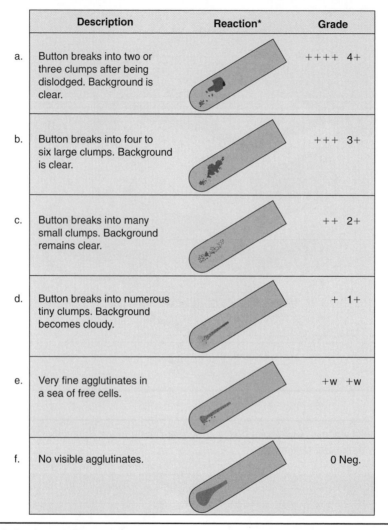

	Description	Reaction*	Grade
a.	Button breaks into two or three clumps after being dislodged. Background is clear.		++++ 4+
b.	Button breaks into four to six large clumps. Background is clear.		+++ 3+
c.	Button breaks into many small clumps. Background remains clear.		++ 2+
d.	Button breaks into numerous tiny clumps. Background becomes cloudy.		+ 1+
e.	Very fine agglutinates in a sea of free cells.		+w +w
f.	No visible agglutinates.		0 Neg.

FIGURE 1-17 Agglutination grading: a. 4; b. 3+; c. 2+; d 1+; e + weak; f. negative
Source: Delmar, Cengage Learning

these testing methods is a card with gel-filled wells that resemble test tubes. Each well on the card contains gel mixed with a specific testing reagent. The patient's serum or cells is added to the wells. Incubation takes place and, if necessary, additional reagents are added. The final interpretation is made. Results are scored on the same scale as tube methods (see Figure 1-18). Chapter 2 contains further discussion of gel testing methods.

Rouleaux

Agglutination is seen macroscopically as clumping in the tube, in a gel matrix, or on a slide. When visible microscopically, agglutination appears as clumps of cells arranged in random patterns. A cellular interaction that macroscopically may mimic agglutination is **rouleaux** (see Figure 1-19). Microscopically, rouleaux is the appearance of cells in coin-like stacks. The presence of

TABLE 1-9 Grading of Agglutination

GRADE	DESCRIPTION
Negative	No clumps of aggregates
Weak (+)	Very fine agglutinates in a sea of free cells
1+	A few small aggregates visible macroscopically; background supernatant cloudy
2+	Medium size aggregates; clear background
3+	Several large aggregates; clear background
4+	One solid aggregate; clear supernatant

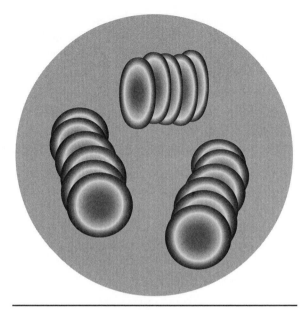

FIGURE 1-19 Rouleaux: Red cells resemble stacks of coins
Source: Delmar, Cengage Learning

rouleaux does not represent agglutination or an antigen-antibody reaction. Rouleaux, when present, is not considered a positive reaction.

ACTIVE IMMUNIZATION VERSUS PASSIVE IMMUNIZATION

When antibodies are stimulated by direct contact with the antigen, it is called active immunization. With regard to the blood bank testing, active immunization or sensitization with foreign antigens may occur either via transfusion or during pregnancy. Initial antigen exposure stimulates lymphocyte processing of the antigen and subsequent production of antibodies. These antibodies

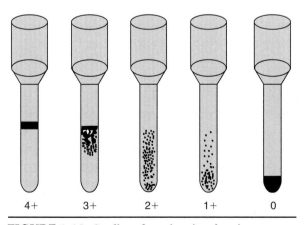

FIGURE 1-18 Grading of reactions in gel testing systems
Source: Delmar, Cengage Learning

are immune antibodies. Immune antibodies will be discussed and referred to as atypical antibodies or red cell stimulated antibodies. Atypical antibodies, when produced, will appear in the patient's serum and can prove problematic in testing. Clinical conditions or circumstances resulting from active immunization include hemolytic disease of the fetus and newborn (HDFN) and hemolytic transfusion reaction (HTR).

An example of active immunization without direct application to blood bank is antibody stimulation by natural exposure. Exposure to the *Varicella* virus during active chicken pox infection is a specific example of this process. An immune antibody is produced and offers immunologic protection for subsequent exposures.

In contrast, antibody formation may occur without apparent antigen exposure. An antigen or antigen-like substance is responsible for stimulation of antibody production. The exact nature of the antigen stimulant is often not known. These antibodies are natural (or non-red cell stimulated) antibodies. Antibodies to ABO blood group system antigens provide an example of non-red cell stimulated antibodies. These antibodies will be discussed in Chapter 5.

Antibodies may be obtained from an external source and serve a temporary protective role. Passive antibodies are either administered via injection *or* cross the maternal-placental barrier. Examples of injected passive antibodies include Rh immune globulin, used to prevent hemolytic disease of the fetus and newborn, and Hepatitis B immune globulin used to counteract exposure to the hepatitis B virus. In addition, numerous antibodies cross the placental barrier. These serve a protective role for neonates until their own immune system matures.

SUMMARY

- The components of blood consist of the liquid or plasma with suspended cellular components: red cells, white cells, and platelets.

- There are two types of lymphocytes involved in the immune process. B lymphocytes produce antibodies and T lymphocytes are involved in cellular responses.

- Chemicals or cytokines serve as mediators in immunological reactions. The roles of cytokines are varied and at times, nonspecific.

- Complement is a group of plasma proteins that circulate in the body as proenzymes. An antigen, a complex molecule or a cellular stimulus activates the proenzyme. The active form of each proenzymes serves to activate the next complement component. The series of reactions continues in a cascade. Some antibodies will bind complement only to the C3 component.

- Following activation of complement, the reactions may proceed by one of two pathways: Classic or alternate. Some antibodies will activate complement only to C3 while others will activate complement through C9, resulting in red cell hemolysis.

- Innate immunity consists of barrier immunity and inflammatory response.

- Antigens are substances that stimulate antibody production and react with the antibody that is formed.

- Antibody production occurs as primary and secondary immune responses. The timing of response and amount of antibody produced varies. Primary response starts more slowly and wanes more quickly. Secondary or anamnestic response rapidly produces a high level of antibody and the titer or level of antibody remains high for a longer period of time.

- There are five classes of immunoglobulins. These classes all have the same basic monomeric structure, but some classes exist as polymers. Polymers are larger molecules. The size of the molecule may be beneficial in the initiation of agglutination, but may also hinder functions such as placental passage.

- Immunoglobulin monomers are composed of four chains: two heavy and two light chains. Each monomer has two sites where antigens bind. These sites incorporate both the heavy and light chains. The heavy chains are involved in functions such as complement binding and placental passage.

- Characteristics of antigens that impact on an antigen-antibody reaction include: Size, chemical composition, and location on cell surface.

- Factors influencing antigen-antibody reactions include: specificity, bonds, physical fit, concentration of antigen and antibody, temperature, time, pH, and surface charge.

- Antigen-antibody reactions are visualized by agglutination, hemagglutination, hemolysis, flocculation, or precipitation.

- Blood bank testing classically uses hemagglutination and hemolysis for test resulting. These reactions are graded using a system where the results can be compared with one another using a scale of negative to 4+.

- Acquired immunity is composed of two components: Active and passive immunity. Active immunity is antibody production stimulated by exposure to an antigen or an antigen-like substance while passive immunity is acquiring immunity by administration from an external source or passage from the mother to fetus. Passive immunity is a less permanent immunity.

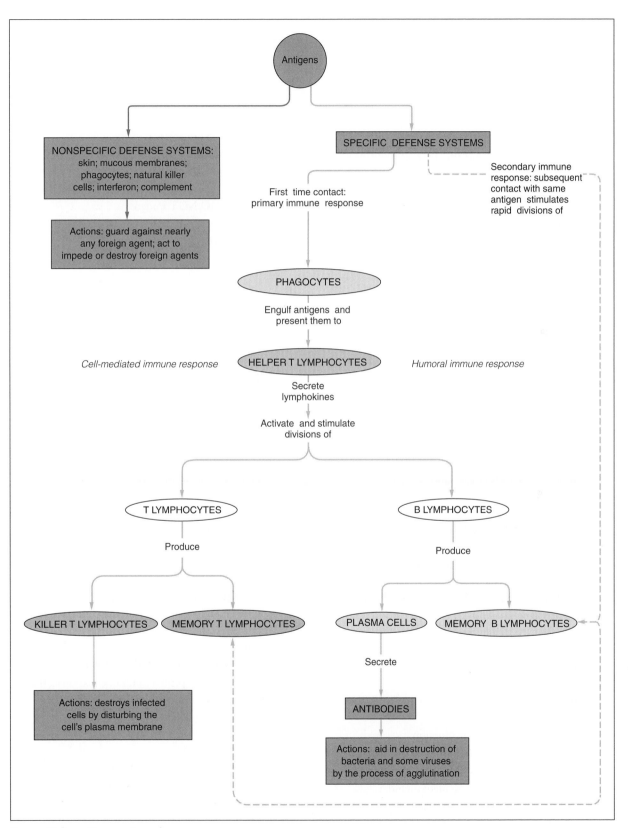

Antigens

NONSPECIFIC DEFENSE SYSTEMS: skin; mucous membranes; phagocytes; natural killer cells; interferon; complement

Actions: guard against nearly any foreign agent; act to impede or destroy foreign agents

SPECIFIC DEFENSE SYSTEMS

Secondary immune response: subsequent contact with same antigen stimulates rapid divisions of

First time contact: primary immune response

PHAGOCYTES

Engulf antigens and present them to

Cell-mediated immune response   **HELPER T LYMPHOCYTES**   *Humoral immune response*

Secrete lymphokines

Activate and stimulate divisions of

T LYMPHOCYTES

Produce

B LYMPHOCYTES

Produce

KILLER T LYMPHOCYTES   **MEMORY T LYMPHOCYTES**

PLASMA CELLS   **MEMORY B LYMPHOCYTES**

Actions: destroys infected cells by disturbing the cell's plasma membrane

Secrete

ANTIBODIES

Actions: aid in destruction of bacteria and some viruses by the process of agglutination

Source: Delmar, Cengage Learning

Lake Superior College Library

REVIEW QUESTIONS

1. Plasma cells perform which of the following functions?
   a. phagocytize bacteria
   b. produce complement components
   c. produce antibody
   d. transform into B lymphocytes

2. The antigen binding portion of the antibody molecule is the:
   a. constant region of the light chains
   b. constant regions of the heavy and light chains
   c. variable regions of the heavy and light chains
   d. variable region of the light chains

3. The cells that perform the antigen presenting function are:
   a. B cells
   b. T cells
   c. polymorphonuclear phagocytes
   d. macrophages

4. Complement proteins circulating are in the form of:
   a. cytokines
   b. lysozymes
   c. proenzymes
   d. epitopes

5. Lattice formation occurs when:
   a. excess antibody is present in the serum-cell mixture and the cells are antibody coated
   b. most antibody molecules span two cells with multiple antibodies attached to each cell
   c. antigen-antibody reactions occurring in a tube are dislodged to three large clumps
   d. the cells lyse and hemolysis is seen in the supernatant

6. Complement activation that results in red blood cell lysis ends at component _____.
   a. 3
   b. 4
   c. 5
   d. 9

7. Active immunization occurs following:
   a. transfusion of red cells
   b. injection of Rh immune globulin
   c. antibody transfer across the placental barrier
   d. hepatitis B immune globulin administration

8. Primary functions of complement include:
   1. cell lysis
   2. inflammation

3. phagocytosis
   4. degranulation of white cells mediating immune responses
   a. 1, 2, and 5 are correct
   b. 1, 3, and 4 are correct
   c. 2, 3, and 4 are correct
   d. 2, 4, and 5 are correct

9. Cytokines have multiple immunologic functions. Cytokines DO NOT initiate:
   a. chemotaxis
   b. cell migration
   c. antibody secretion
   d. fever

10. A substance is most antigenic when its biochemical composition is:
    a. carbohydrate
    b. lipoprotein
    c. polysaccharide
    d. protein

11. Choose the correct statement regarding primary vs secondary immune response.
    a. Primary immune response contains more IgG antibody than the secondary response.
    b. Antibody produced in a primary immune response remains increased for a longer period of time than the secondary immune response.
    c. IgM and IgG antibodies are produced in the same amounts in primary and secondary responses.
    d. IgG antibodies rise higher and stay higher longer in the secondary immune response.

12. Prozone phenomenon occurs when:
    a. antigen and antibody are equal concentrations
    b. antigen is in excess
    c. antibody is in excess
    d. either antigen or antibody is missing

13. Compared to the primary immune response, the secondary response is characterized by:
    a. a longer lag phase
    b. production of less IgG antibody
    c. a longer plateau
    d. less total antibody production

14. 2+ agglutination may be described as:
    a. one large clump with a clear background
    b. many small clumps with a clear background

c. numerous tiny clumps with a cloudy background
d. very fine agglutinates in a sea of free cells

15. Zeta potential serves to:
    a. assist in agglutination of red blood cells
    b. cause rouleaux or coin-like stacking of red cells
    c. prevent red cell agglutination
    d. decrease the isoelectric constant of saline solutions

16. A technologist has centrifuged a tube and wishes to observe the button for agglutination. This observation should be done by:
    a. agitating and looking for hemolysis
    b. tilting the tube and watching the button
    c. inverting the tube and watching for swirling cells
    d. tapping the tubes on the magnifying mirror

17. The correct statement related to Major Histocompatibility Complex is:
    a. class I genes are coded for at a single loci
    b. class II genes are found in the C region
    c. class III genes code for complement components
    d. class I, II, and III genes code for substances found on the red cell surface

18. Skin, mucus membranes, and normal bacterial flora are part of:
    a. innate immunity
    b. passive immunity
    c. acquired immunity
    d. active immunity

19. The classical pathway of the complement system is initiated by:
    a. complexing of antigen and its specific antibody
    b. contact with the polysaccharide coating of a microorganism
    c. release of cytotoxic granule contents from polymorphonuclear neutrophils
    d. major histocompatibility
    e. complex antigens

20. Lattice formation is the establishment of cross links between:
    a. antigens and antibodies
    b. antibodies and complement
    c. B lymphocytes and antibodies
    d. white blood cells and MHC antigens

Match the following factors in antigen-antibody reactions with their descriptors:
_____ 21. exactness of fit   a. Van Der Wahls
_____ 22. bonds   b. Lock and Key
_____ 23. surface charge   c. Zone of Equivalence
_____ 24. optimum concentration of antigens and antibodies   d. Temperature
_____ 25. environmental condition   e. Zeta potential

REFERENCES

Brecher, Mark, editor. *American Association of Blood Banks Technical Manual* 15th edition. AABB, 2005.

Blaney, Kathy and Howard, Paula. *Basic and Applied Concepts of Immunohematology*. Mosby, Philadelphia, 2000.

Henry, John Bernard, *Clinical Diagnosis and Management by Laboratory Methods*. W. B. Saunders Co. 2001.

Harmening, Denise. *Modern Blood Banking and Transfusion Practices*. F. A. Davis, Philadelphia, 2005.

Issitt PD, Anstee DJ (1998). *Applied Blood Group Serology*. 4th edition, Durham, NC, USA: Montgomery Scientific Publications.

McCullough, Jeffrey. *Transfusion Medicine* 2nd edition. Elsevier. 2005.

Reid, Marion E. and Lomas-Francis, Christine. *The Blood Group Antigen: Facts Book*. Elsevier, 2004.

Schenkel-Brunner, Helmut. *Human Blood Groups: Chemical and Biochemical Basis of Antigen Specificity*. Springer Wien, 2000.

Sheehan, Catherine. *Clinical Immunology, Principles and Laboratory Diagnosis*. Lippincott, Philadelphia, 1997.

Stevens, Christine. *Clinical Immunology and Serology, a Laboratory Perspective*. F. A. Davis, Philadelphia. 2003.

Turgeon, Mary Louise. *Fundamentals of Immunohematology*. Williams and Wilkins, Media, PA, 1995.

Reagents and Methods Used for Immunohematology Testing

Contributions by: Kevin E. Whitlock, MT (ASCP)

LEARNING OUTCOMES

At the completion of this chapter, the student should be able to:

- List and describe antisera used in blood bank testing.
- List and describe reagent red cells used in blood bank testing.
- Compare and contrast enhancement media used in blood bank testing.
- Describe the principles behind gel testing methodology.
- List applications for gel testing methodologies.
- Describe microplate and solid phase technologies used in blood bank testing.
- Describe the principles behind the indirect and direct antiglobulin tests.
- Apply the principles of indirect antiglobulin tests to specific test methods.
- Outline the production and use of anti-human globulin reagents.
- List instrumentation used for blood bank testing in the past and present.
- Describe molecular diagnostic techniques applicable to blood bank testing.
- Explain the different types of molecular methods used in the blood bank.
- List the components and steps involved in polymerase chain reaction (PCR), Real-Time PCR, and microarray methods.
- Identify the clinical uses of molecular biology in the blood bank.

GLOSSARY

antibody identification panel   test performed using a panel of cells with known antigen content; when reacted with serum, eluate, or other body fluid the panel of cells creates a pattern of reactivity that can be used to identify the specific antibody or combination of antibodies in the fluid being tested

antibody screen   test performed by mixing patient or donor plasma with cells of known antigen content to detect the presence of atypical antibodies

antigram   chart describing the antigen content of the cells used for antibody screen and antibody identification tests

anti-human globulin (AHG) sera   reagent sera produced in a species other than human (usually a rabbit) that contains antibodies directed against human globulins; used to aid in the detection of antibody coated cells in test procedures

29

anti-human globulin test test method that uses antibodies directed against human globulins to aid in detection of antibody-coated cells; used in specific tests in the blood bank

atypical antibodies antibodies found either in the plasma or on cells that are unanticipated or not found under normal circumstances

autoantibodies antibodies directed against antigens on an individual's own cells

compatibility testing (crossmatch) the mixing of donor red cells and recipient plasma to determine if *in vitro* reactions that may indicate potential for an *in vivo* reaction between the donor's cells and the recipient's plasma

Coombs control cells (check cells) cells coated with an antibody used to confirm negative results obtained in indirect or direct antiglobulin tests

direct antiglobulin test (DAT) test that detects the presence of antibody on the surface of red cells

gene chip glass or a silicon chip to which the probes are attached

in vitro outside of the body; in glass

in vivo in the body

microarray A DNA detection method in which a probe is attached to solid surface and binds to the target sequence of DNA, allowing for detection, usually through fluorescence

monospecific AHG anti-human globulin sera containing only a single component

murine related to a mouse

polymerase chain reaction (PCR) a molecular technique for the amplification of a specific target sequence of DNA

polyspecific AHG anti-human globulin with multiple components; usually anti-IgG, anti-IgM, IgA, and anti-complement

primer pieces of single-stranded DNA that are complementary to the end sequences of the target, and mark the sequence of DNA to be amplified

probe single-stranded piece of labeled DNA that is complementary to the target sequence, and binds to a targeted DNA site to allow for the detection of a specific DNA

single nucleotide polymorphism (SNP) a genetic variation in which only one base pair differs between two strands of DNA

INTRODUCTION

The major focus of blood bank testing is constructed around detecting antigens and antibodies. Historically, this testing has been visualized by observation of agglutination or hemolysis in test tubes or in microplates. The introduction of gel testing, solid phase adherence, molecular techniques, and automation have changed the work practices of some laboratories while the original test methods continue to be widely used. Regardless of the techniques, with the exception of molecular methods, the test methods share common premises. Antigen and antibody detection and identification are an integral part of blood bank testing. Understanding the testing processes and outcomes requires an understanding of the test reagents. General categories of reagents, their production and applications will be outlined in the following sections. Some test methods employ the **anti-human globulin (AHG) test**. Understanding the principles and applications of this methodology is vital to performing and interpreting blood bank testing.

Molecular diagnostic techniques have become a valuable tool in the blood bank. These techniques provide an in-depth and accurate look at antigen specificity and structure and will be discussed later in this chapter. This area of the blood bank testing is rapidly developing as applications, instrumentation, and methodologies become available and affordable.

SUMMARY OF ROUTINE BLOOD BANK TESTING METHODS

Blood bank testing includes evaluation of potential transfusion recipients, donors, maternal and cord specimens, and patients exhibiting transfusion reaction symptoms. The blood bank also performs testing on donor units and components. This testing includes determination of antigens and antibodies and screening of each unit for infectious diseases. Specific test methods detect the presence of antigens on cells and antibodies in plasma or coating the red blood cells. In each blood bank test methodology, there are two factors: one is unknown and the other is known. The known factor is contained in the test reagent being used. The recipient or donor contributes the unknown factor. This concept is summarized in Figure 2-1.

Routine Testing in the Blood Bank Laboratory

Standard blood bank test menus include universal test procedures. These tests are performed to screen patients for pre-transfusion, maternal prenatal and postnatal samples, and donors. Testing for antigens on the red cell surface uses commercially prepared antisera containing a known antibody. Conversely, the test method for antibodies in the plasma uses known antigens on the surface of the commercially prepared red cells. The combination of antigen and antibody will result in a reaction if the unknown component is present. This reaction is visualized by hemagglutination, hemolysis, or solid phase adherence. A summary of the basic procedures is:

1. **Typing for ABO and Rh Antigens:** Commercial antisera is combined with red cells from the recipient or donor.

2. **Typing for Antigens of Other Blood Group Systems:** Commercial antisera is combined with red cells from the recipient or donor.

3. **Antibody Screen:** Recipient or donor plasma combined with commercial red blood cells with known antigen content.

4. **Antibody Identification:** Recipient or donor plasma combined with commercial red blood cells with known antigen content; an expansion of the antibody screen.

5. **Compatibility Test (crossmatch):** Donor red cells and recipient plasma are combined; usually identical ABO and Rh types, but additional antigens on donor red cells and antibody status of recipient plasma is unknown. The potential for other incompatibilities exists between donor cells and atypical antibodies in the recipient's plasma.

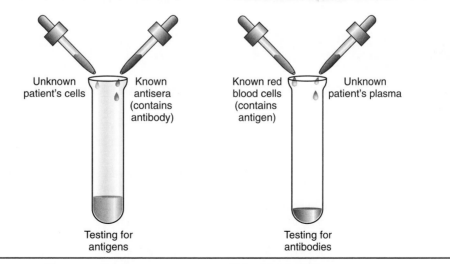

Unknown patient's cells   Known antisera (contains antibody)

Testing for antigens

Known red blood cells (contains antigen)   Unknown patient's plasma

Testing for antibodies

FIGURE 2-1 **Summary of known and unknown components of blood bank testing.**
Antigen testing includes unknown red cells from the patient combined with known antibody from the antisera.
Antibody testing includes unknown plasma from the patient combined with known antigens from reagent red blood cells.
Source: Delmar, Cengage Learning

6. Direct Antiglobulin Test: Recipient or donor is tested for the presence of *in vivo* sensitization of red cells; recipient or donor is tested for the presence of antibodies coating the red cells; antibody detected is a specific antibody, but this screening method cannot identify the specific etiology.

A summary of routine blood bank testing and the sources of antigens and antibodies is provided in Table 2-1.

Antisera

Antisera is defined as an antibody titered to an optimal concentration for the detection of the corresponding antigen. Most antisera used in blood bank testing are monoclonal in origin. Monoclonal antibodies originate from a single clone of cells versus polyclonal that originate from multiple cell clones. See Figure 2-2 for a summary of monoclonal versus polyclonal antibodies. The specific origin of most blood bank antisera is **murine**. Mice are used to produce antibodies that are harvested and titered to appropriate levels to allow for optimum antigen detection. Some are lectins or seed extracts that have antibody specificity for one of the red cell antigens. Regardless of origin of the antisera, the Food and Drug Administration (FDA) governs the manufacturing processes.

Historically, antisera were human in nature. Human antisera have been made obsolete by the implementation of monoclonal antisera. Monoclonal antisera have greater specificity and are free of some of the biohazardous issues associated with human blood products.

Monoclonal antisera are used for all antigen testing methods. This includes tube, slide, microplate, gel, and automated methods. Specific reagents may not be interchangeable, but are similar in titer and constitution. The package insert should always be consulted before beginning any testing regimen. Daily quality control is required for antisera. This will be discussed further in Chapter 3. See Table 2-2 for a summary of monoclonal antisera.

ABO Antisera

ABO typing sera are historically the mainstay of blood bank testing. Landsteiner discovered the human version of these antisera when he did his "typing" of employees by mixing cells and serum of various individuals. ABO antisera are standardized by colors. See Table 2-3 for a summary of the colors of these antisera. This standardization aids in the interpretation of agglutination patterns of the three antisera used for this testing.

Rh Antisera

The RhD antigen is the primary Rh antigen. The D antigen is historically important in all donors, recipients, prenatal patients, and newborns of RhD negative mothers. The AABB's *Standards for Blood Banks and Transfusion Services, 25th Edition,* requires that all donors and recipients be typed for this highly immunogenic antigen.

TABLE 2-1 Source of Known and Unknown Components in Routine Blood Bank Tests

TEST PROCEDURE	DETECTION	ORIGIN OF ANTIGEN	ORIGIN OF ANTIBODY
ABO forward group	A and B antigens	Patient or donor red blood cells (unknown)	Commercial anti-A, anti-B, anti-A, B (known)
ABO reverse group	Anti-A and anti-B antibodies	Commercial red blood cells (known)	Patient or donor serum (unknown)
Rh Type	Rh(D) antigens	Patient or donor red blood cells (unknown)	Commercial anti-A, anti-B, anti-A,B (known)
Antibody screen	Atypical antibodies to antigens on red cells	Commercial antibody screen cells (known)	Patient or donor serum (unknown)
Antibody identification	Identification of atypical antibodies to antigens on red cells	Commercial antibody screen cells (known)	Patient or donor serum (unknown)
Crossmatch	Compatibility between donor and recipient	Donor red blood cell (unknown)	Recipient's serum (unknown)

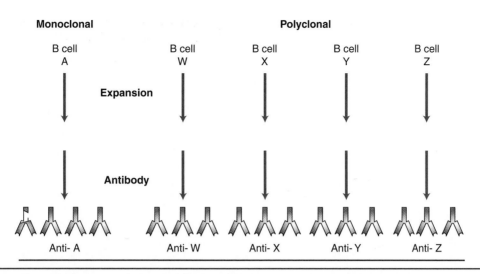

FIGURE 2-2 Monoclonal versus polyclonal antibody production—a single clone of cells used to produce monoclonal cells. Multiple clones produce an antibody "blend" of antibody molecules.
Source: Delmar, Cengage Learning

Rh antisera is monoclonal and usually does not require the use of a parallel control. Comparison of the testing results in the RhD test to the ABO forward grouping is sufficient to determine validity of the test. When the ABO forward group is positive in all three tubes, (group AB) and the Rh test is positive, it is impossible to determine if the test results are valid. In this case, 6 to 8% bovine albumin may be used as a parallel control. In this circumstance, lack of agglutination in the parallel control indicates a valid RhD test. In addition when the patient has a positive direct antiglobulin test (DAT), the same parallel control should be included in the RhD testing. Daily quality control is required for all Rh antisera. These methods will be discussed in Chapter 3. Figure 2-3 represents anti-D antisera.

Historically, Rh (anti-D) antisera were protein suspended and required a parallel control to determine the accuracy of the typing of the red cells. When this high protein solution is used to suspend the antisera, there are incidences of false positive tests due to the high protein diluent. If the parallel control is positive, the test is considered invalid. See Table 2-4 for a summary of these reactions.

False positive reactions occur most frequently when antibodies are coating the patient's red cells. These antibodies are called **autoantibodies**. The antibodies on the red cell surface are protein. When combined with the high protein antisera, the cells agglutinate. This constitutes an invalid test. When an invalid test occurs, it is not possible to determine if the positive results are true positives or false reactions.

In addition to the high protein antisera, there are other categories of reagents available for RhD typing. These include saline antisera (IgM) and chemically modified (IgG) reagents. Before pursuing any Rh testing, it is imperative to refer to the package insert to determine the type of antisera and the test method for the specific antisera. These antisera are summarized in Table 2-5. With the expansion of testing methods, the antisera currently in use are adaptable to multiple test methods, e.g. slide method, tube method, automated method, and so forth.

Antisera for Other Blood Groups

Commercial antisera exist for most antigens encountered in the blood bank. These antisera are almost exclusively monoclonal. Their temperature and media of reactivity vary by manufacturer and cell line. Most are IgM and do not require 37°C incubation or indirect antiglobulin technique to produce accurate results. The package insert should be consulted for proper test methods. Positive and negative controls are required each day of use. These procedures will be discussed further in Chapter 3.

Reagent Red Blood Cells

Reagent red blood cells are human cells processed for specific use in blood bank testing. All reagent red cells are manufactured by washing the cells to remove

TABLE 2-2 Clones Used in the Manufacturer of Reagents

	GAMMA		IMMUCOR		ORTHO		
Antisera	**Clone**	**Ig Class**	**Ig Class**	**Clone**	**Clone**	**Ig Class**	**Gel Card Clone**
Anti-A	BIRMA 1	IgM	IgM IgM	BIRMA 1A26A2	M1104 3D3	IgM IgM	BIRMA 1
Anti-B	GAMA110	IgM	IgM	ES4	NB10 5A5 NG10.3B1 NB1.19	IgM IgM IgM	LB-2
Anti-A,B	BIRMA 1 ES4 ES15	IgM IgM IgM	IgM IgM IgM IgM IgM	B95.3 LB-2 BIRMA 1 ES4 ES15	MH04 3D3 NB10.3B1 NB1.19	IgM IgM IgM IgM	ES4 ES15
Anti-D	GAMA401 GAMA401 P8D8	IgM IgM IgG	IgM IgM IgG IgM IgG	Series 5 TH28 MS26 Series 4 MS201 MS26	MAD2 HUMAN	IgM IgG	MS201
Anti-C	MS24	IgM	IgM	MS24	MS24	IgM	MS24
Anti-E	GAMA402	IgM	IgM	MS12	C2	IgM	MS258 MS260
Anti-CDE			IgM IgM IgM	MS201 MS258 MS24			
Anti-c	951	IgM	IgM	MS33	MS42	IgM	MS33
Anti-e	MS16 MS21 MS63	IgM IgM IgM	IgM	MS16	MS16	IgM	MS16 MS21 MS63
Anti-Le[a]	GAMA701	IgM	IgM	LM112/161	LM112/161	IgM	
Anti-Le[b]	GAMA704	IgM	IgM	LM129/181	LM129/181	IgM	
Anti-Jk[a]					MS15	IgM	
Anti-Jk[b]					MS8	IgM	
AntiK1	MS56	IgM	IgM	MS56			
Anti-M	M2A1	IgM	IgM	F23			
Anti-N	12E.A1	IgG1					
Anti-P1	OSK17	IgM					
Anti-IgG	16HB	IgM					
Anti-C3b	055A.305GA MA003	IgM			F7G3	IgG1	
Anti-C3d	053A.714GA MA004	IgG1			C4C7	IgG1	

Reprinted with permission from Immunohematology.

TABLE 2-3 ABO Antisera Color Standardization

ANTISERA	COLOR
Anti-A	Blue
Anti-B	Yellow
Anti-A,B	Colorless

TABLE 2-4 Summary of RhD Typing Results Using High Protein Antisera

RHD TYPE	EXPECTED RESULTS WITH ANTI-D	EXPECTED RESULTS WITH RH CONTROL
Rh positive	+	negative
Rh negative	negative	negative
Invalid	+/ negative	positive

residual plasma antibodies. The cells are resuspended to a concentration of 2 to 5% in saline and a preservative solution. The cells are typed for the specific antigens of choice and are selectively negative for antigens with a high incidence of interference. Package inserts for each product should be referenced for specific directions for use.

A and B Reverse Grouping Cells

Testing for naturally occurring ABO antibodies in the plasma of donors and recipients requires the use of reagent red blood cells. These cells are prepared from specific blood groups and are processed as described in the previous section. The cells are packaged in different combinations, but the combination of A_1 and B cells is the most common combination. Figure 2-4 represents a set of three reverse grouping cells. Each cell is the specific

ABO group and Rh negative. The cells are usually D, C, and E antigen negative. Remaining antigens are random and not considered significant to testing regimens. Daily quality control is performed as required in the AABB's *Standards for Blood Banks and Transfusion Services, 25th Edition.* Therefore, a parallel control is not required for these tests. Chapter 4 will outline ABO reverse grouping and expected findings for specific blood groups.

Antibody Screen Cells

Patient and donor plasma is screened for **atypical antibodies** using commercially prepared cells. These antibodies are formed in response to antigens *not* present on the individual's red cells. Antibody stimulation occurs by

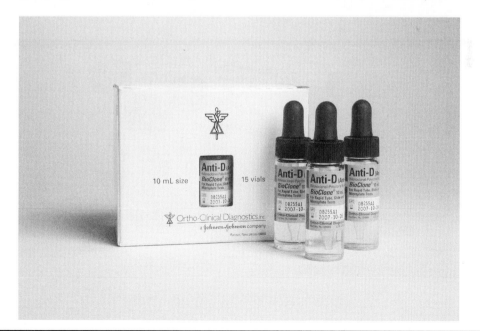

FIGURE 2-3 Anti-D is a monoclonal antisera that is used for the detection of RhD antigen on the surface of red blood cells. *Reproduced with permission of Ortho Clinical Diagnostics, Raritan, NJ.*

TABLE 2-5 Anti-RhD Antisera

TYPE OF ANTISERA	DESCRIPTION	USE OF PARALLEL DILUENT CONTROL
Monoclonal-Polyclonal Blend	Source: Human and Murine Human IgG Polyclonal mixed with Human-Murine IgM monoclonal	No
High Protein (Polyclonal)	Source: Human IgG in a high protein diluent	Yes
Monoclonal	Source: Human/Murine heterohybridoma IgM blend	No
Chemically Modified	Source: Human Hinge of IgG molecule	No

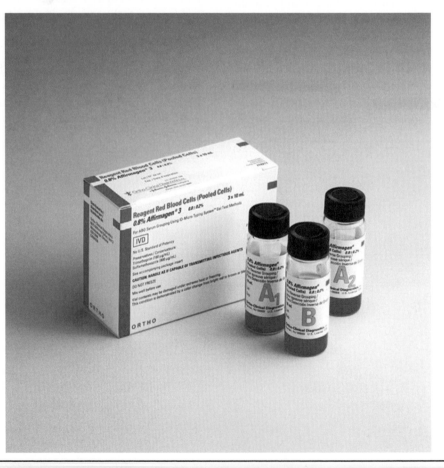

FIGURE 2-4 A set of three reverse grouping cells, A_1, A_2, and B cells, used to detect ABO antibodies in the plasma. *Reprinted with permission of Ortho Clinical Diagnostics, Raritan, NJ.*

exposure to a foreign antigen either through transfusion or pregnancy. The resulting antibodies are innocuous unless the individual is exposed to red cells with the antigen that stimulated the production of the antibodies. If this subsequent exposure occurs, the potential for a life-threatening transfusion reaction exists. Pre-transfusion screening of an individual's plasma aids in prevention of these reactions.

Antibody screen cells are human products. They are group O cells tested for the presence of the most commonly encountered antigens. This provides a product with a known antigen content. The cells are packaged by the manufacturer in sets of either two or three vials. See Figure 2-5 for a set of antibody screen cells. Each vial contains cells from a single, unique donor. The vials are supplied with a description of the antigen content of each of the cells. This description is provided in a chart known as an **antigram**. See Figure 2-6 for a sample antigram.

The antibody screen test is performed by testing the cells in each vial with the plasma of the patient or

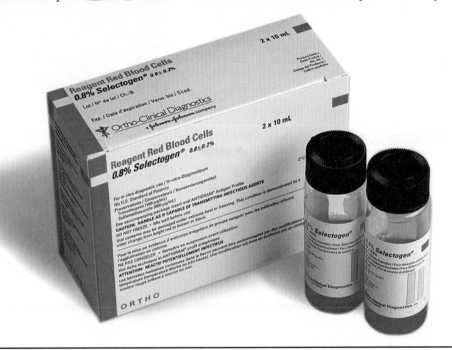

FIGURE 2-5 A set of two-antibody screen cells for determination of atypical antibodies in the plasma. *Reprinted with permission of Ortho Clinical Diagnostics, Raritan, NJ.*

Cell #	Rh-hr	Donor Number	D	C	E	c	e	f*	Cw	V	K	k	Kpa	Kpb	Jsa	Jsb	Fya	Fyb	Jka	Jkb	Xga	Lea	Leb	S	s	M	N	P1	Lua	Lub	Special Antigen Typing	Cell #	Test Results
					Rh-hr								KELL				DUFFY		KIDD		Sex Linked	LEWIS		MNS				P	LUTHERAN				
1	R1R1	303777	+	+	0	0	+	0	0	0	0	+	0	+	0	+	0	+	+	+	+	0	+	0	+	+	+	+s	0	+		1	
2	R2R2	300515	+	0	+	+	0	0	0	0	0	+	0	+	0	+	+	0	+	0	+	0	+	+	0	+	+	0	+	0	+		2	
3	rr	303377	0	0	0	+	+	+	0	0	0	+	0	+	0	+	+	0	+	0	0	0	+	+	+	+	0	0	0	0	+		3	
	Patient Cells																																	

Shaded columns indicate those antigens which are destroyed or depressed by enzyme treatment.

*f antigen status may have been determined presumptively based on Rh-hr phenotype

Lot No. 3SS816
Exp. Date 2008-06-17
CCYY-MM-DD

Antigram® Antigen Profile

Ortho-Clinical Diagnostics, Inc. a *Johnson-Johnson* company
Reagent Red Blood Cells Surgiscreen®
© OCD 1989   Raritan, NJ 08869
635200303

FIGURE 2-6 A sample antigram that is included with a set of antibody screen cells. The antigram represents the antigen composition of each of the cells. *Reprinted with permission of Ortho Clinical Diagnostics, Raritan, NJ.*

donor. Temperature and media of reactivity are varied during the testing procedure. The media of reactivity includes saline immediate spin, incubation at 37°C with a potentiating substance such as LISS, and the indirect antiglobulin (IAT) phase. Variations in the reaction media used are made at the discretion of the institution.

Results are recorded at the end of each phase of testing. Since this is a screening test, the results indicate the presence of an antibody, but do not identify the specific antibody. By using the antigrams and knowing the temperature and media of reactivity of the potential antibodies, the possibilities may be narrowed. A more definitive identification is provided by the use of the **antibody identification panel.**

Antibody Identification Cells

Antibody identification cells are also human products. As with the antibody screen cells, these are group O cells that have been tested for the presence of the most commonly encountered antigens. The cells are provided from the manufacturer in sets of 8 to 16 vials. Each vial

contains cells from a single donor. See Figure 2-7 for an an antibody identification panel. The vials are provided with an antigram. See Figure 2-8 for a sample antigram.

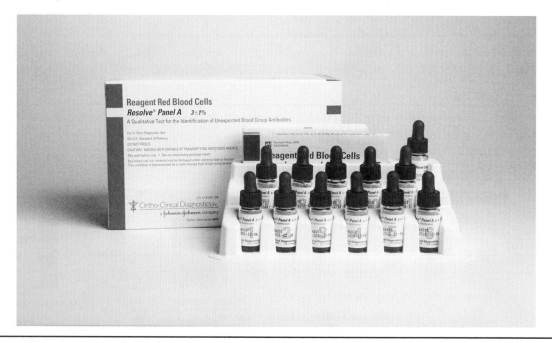

FIGURE 2-7 A sample antibody identification panel used for the identification of atypical antibodies in the plasma. Antibody identification panels have 8 to 16 unique cells. *Reprinted with permission of Ortho Clinical Diagnostics, Raritan, NJ.*

Ortho-Clinical Diagnostics, Inc.
a *Johnson&Johnson* company
© OCD 1989   Raritan, NJ 08869

Cell 2 of this lot is designated with an A. Cell 5 of this lot is designated with an A.

PATIENT NAME: _____
PATIENT ID: _____
DATE: _____ TECH: _____
CONCLUSION: _____

Lot No. _RA639_   Exp. Date _2008-07-15_
CCYY-MM-DD

Panel A

Reagent Red Blood Cells
Resolve® Panel A
Antigram® Antigen Profile

635200323

Cell #	Rh-hr	Donor Number	D	C	E	c	e	f*	Cw	V	K	k	Kpa	Kpb	Jsa	Jsb	Fya	Fyb	Jka	Jkb	Xga	Lea	Leb	S	s	M	N	P1	Lua	Lub	Special Antigen Typing	Cell #	Test Results
						Rh-hr					KELL						DUFFY		KIDD		Sex Linked	LEWIS		MNS				P	LUTHERAN				
1	R1wR1	106004	+	+	0	0	+	0	+	0	0	+	0	+	0	+	0	+	+	+	0	0	+	0	+	0	+	0	0	+		1	
2	R1R1	300688	+	+	0	0	+	0	0	0	+	+	0	+	0	+	+	+	+	0	0	0	0	0	+	0	+	+s	0	+		2	
3	R2R2	303941	+	0	+	+	0	0	0	0	0	+	0	+	0	+	0	+	+	0	+	0	+	+	0	+	0	+	0	+		3	
4	Ror	116382	+	0	0	+	+	+	0	0	0	+	0	+	0	+	+	+	+	+	0	0	+	+	0	0	+	+	0	+		4	
5	r'r	111143	0	+	0	+	+	+	0	0	0	+	0	+	0	+	0	+	+	0	0	+	0	+	+	+	+	+	0	+	@	5	
6	r"r	303924	0	0	+	+	+	0	0	0	0	+	0	+	0	+	+	0	0	+	+	0	+	0	+	0	+	+s	0	+	@	6	
7	rr	113318	0	0	0	+	+	+	0	0	+	+	0	+	0	+	0	+	0	+	0	0	0	+	+	0	+	+	0	+	@	7	
8	rr	117830	0	0	0	+	+	+	0	0	0	+	0	+	0	+	+	0	0	+	+	+	0	+	+	+	0	+s	0	+		8	
9	rr	113027	0	0	0	+	+	+	0	0	0	+	0	+	0	+	0	+	0	+	+	0	+	+	0	+	0	+	0	+		9	
10	rr	118280	0	0	0	+	+	+	0	0	0	+	0	+	0	+	+	0	+	+	+	0	+	0	+	0	+	0	0	+		10	
11	R1R1	23759	+	+	0	0	+	0	0	0	+	+	0	+	0	+	0	+	0	+	+	0	+	0	+	+	0	+s	0	+		11	
	Patient Cells																																
Mode of Reactivity		37°C/Antiglobulin									Antiglobulin						Variable					Cold				Var.							

*f antigen status may have been determined presumptively based on Rh-hr phenotype.

Shaded columns indicate those antigens which are destroyed or depressed by enzyme treatment.

Additional Cells Cell #	Rh-hr	Donor Number	D	C	E	c	e	f*	Cw	V	K	k	Kpa	Kpb	Jsa	Jsb	Fya	Fyb	Jka	Jkb	Xga	Lea	Leb	S	s	M	N	P1	Lua	Lub	Special Antigen Typing	Cell #	Test Results
						Rh-hr					KELL						DUFFY		KIDD		Sex Linked	LEWIS		MNS				P	LUTHERAN				

FIGURE 2-8 A sample antigram that is included with a set of antibody identification cells. The antigram represents the antigen composition of each of the cells. *Reprinted with permission of Ortho Clinical Diagnostics, Raritan, NJ.*

In the same manner as the antibody screen test, the previously screened plasma is tested with the cells in each vial. The test is performed with variation in the temperature and media of reactivity. The reactive media includes saline immediate spin, incubation at 37°C with a potentiating reagent such as LISS, polyethylene glycol (PEG), or albumin, and the IAT phase. Choice of appropriate reaction media is made at the discretion of the institution. Results are recorded and evaluated at the end of each phase of testing. Evaluation of the test results involves the use of the antigrams and comparison of the temperature and media of reactivity of the potential antibodies. Possible antibodies may be narrowed, although further testing may be required. This process will be described in detail in Chapter 8.

CRITICAL THINKING ACTIVITY

In small groups, students will evaluate a sample antigram in Figure 2-8. For each of the following antibodies, answer questions 1 and 2.

Anti-C
Anti-K
Anti-Lea

1. With which screening cell(s) does the antibody react?
2. List three additional antibodies that would react with the same cell(s).

Coombs Control Cells

The antiglobulin test will be described later in this chapter. A cellular reagent, Coombs control cells or check cells are used as a confirmatory step in the anti-human globulin test. These are group O cells that are coated with human globulin. Specifically, the cells are Rh (D) positive cells coated with anti-D. These cells are, then, used to test the viability of anti-human globulin serum in negative tests. This process will be described later in this chapter.

Anti-human Globulin Sera (AHG)

AHG sera are reagents used for the detection of human globulin that has coated the surface of red blood cells. The sera were originally produced in rabbits or other animals immunized with human sera. As with typing sera, the most commonly used anti-human globulin is now monoclonal. It is generated from a single clone of cells. The anti-human sera is collected, processed, and packaged for distribution.

Anti-human globulin sera can be divided into two broad categories: polyspecific AHG and monospecific AHG. Polyspecific AHG is a combination of multiple types of anti-human globulin. Most often polyspecific AHG is composed of anti-IgG and anti-C3 (complement component three) while monospecific AHG is a single component, anti-IgG, or anti-C3. Less commonly used monospecific AHG include anti-IgM and anti-IgA.

Enhancement Media

Enhancement media assists in the attachment of an antibody to the specific antigen on the red cell. Multiple enhancing reagents are available. The choice of reagents is made at the discretion of the individual blood bank. These reagents include LISS, PEG, bovine serum albumin (BSA) and proteolytic enzymes (ficin and papain). See Box 2-1 for examples of test procedures that include the use of enhancement media.

Box 2-1

Antibody Screen
Antibody Identification
Compatibility Testing (Crossmatch)

TABLE 2-6 Summary of Enhancement Agents

ENHANCEMENT MEDIA	ACTION
Bovine Serum Albumin	Affects the second stage of agglutination
Low-Ionic Strength Solution	Increases rate of antibody uptake; first stage of agglutination
Polyethylene Glycol	Concentrates the antibody in a low-ionic strength solution
Enzymes (Ficin and Papain)	Reduces negative charges from surface of red cell; first stage of agglutination

Specific actions of enhancement agents can be divided into two broad categories: enhancement of the first stage of agglutination, also known as antibody uptake, or enhancement of the second stage of agglutination by promoting direct agglutination. A summary of these potentiators and their actions is provided in Table 2-6.

Low Ionic Strength Solution (LISS)

LISS is a mixture of sodium chloride, glycine, and salt-poor albumin. These constituents provide a low-ionic environment that will enhance antibody uptake. This enhanced uptake improves the rate of antibody detection in the anti-human globulin phase of testing.

LISS influences the first stage of agglutination. It increases the rate of antibody binding to the specific antigen on the red cell surface. The attachment of an antibody to antigens on the surface of the red cells is impacted by negative charges surrounding the red cells. These negative charges create an environment for the red cells to repel each other. By adding LISS, negative charges are reduced and the cells are able to approach each other. This allows the antibody molecules to bridge multiple red cells. LISS may be used in one of the following ways:

- Suspending the test red cells with LISS.
- Using LISS as an additive to the testing method.

Polyethylene Glycol (PEG)

PEG is an additive solution that removes water from the test environment. The removal of water concentrates the antibody and increases the likelihood of molecule collision. As the number of collisions increases, the amount of antibody uptake by the red cells also increases. In addition, PEG creates a low-ionic strength environment that enhances the antigen-antibody complex formation. Since PEG directly affects the aggregation of the red blood cells, it is used exclusively in the indirect antiglobulin test. Nonspecific agglutination has been documented when PEG is used in combination with polyspecific AHG reagents. Therefore, only IgG anti-human globulin should be used with PEG.

Bovine Serum Albumin (BSA)

BSA is commercially available in either 22% or 30% concentration. Historically, this reagent has been used as an enhancement media. It affects the second phase of agglutination. Theory suggests that albumin increases the dielectric constant of the medium. This change in dielectric constant disperses some of the positively charged ions that gather around each of the negatively charged red cells. Antibody-coated red cells may then approach each other and agglutination is enhanced.

Proteolytic Enzymes

Proteolytic enzymes, such as ficin and papain, are used to enhance or eliminate the activity of atypical antibodies in plasma. Enzymes act by removing negatively charged molecules from the surface of the red cell. The removal of negative charges reduces zeta potential. This enhances the agglutination of IgG immunoglobulin molecules. Because of the discriminating nature of enzymes, this is a method that may be used in the identification of antibodies. The specifics of antibody identification will be discussed in Chapter 8. A summary of clinically significant antibodies destroyed and enhanced by enzymes is found in Box 2-2.

Box 2-2

Red Cell Antibodies Enhanced and Destroyed by Enzymes

Enhanced	Destroyed
Rh	Duffy
Lewis	M,N,S
Kidd	

ANTI-HUMAN GLOBULIN (AHG) TEST

The AHG test is a method that employs AHG sera to aid in visualization of antigen-antibody reactions. Some antibodies are capable of making a single attachment to an antigen present on the surface of the cell, but are not able to bridge the distance between two red cells. Hence, lattice formation and agglutination cannot occur. See Chapter 1 for a review of agglutination and characteristics of antibodies.

When antibody molecules are unable to bridge cells to produce agglutination, it is necessary to provide assistance in the agglutination process. AHG sera creates this bridging effect. Once the bridging is in place, the antigen-antibody interactions may be observed. The anti-human globulin test may be divided into two broad categories: indirect and direct tests.

Indirect Antiglobulin Testing

Indirect method of anti-human globulin testing usually combines a known antigen or antibody with either plasma or cells that have an unknown component. This test is indirect because the cells are coated with antibody *in vitro*. This is compared to the direct antiglobulin test that detects cells coated with antibody *in vivo*. The indirect test is used to determine the presence of either antibodies or antigens. See Figure 2-9 for a visual explanation of the indirect antiglobulin technique.

After combining the reactants, the steps of testing are continued as outlined in Sample Procedure 2-1. Following the incubation step, the tubes are washed three times. The saline is decanted between each wash and completely decanted following the final wash. This washing phase removes and dilutes antibodies not bound to the antigens on the red cells. The washing steps are vital to obtaining correct test results. Automated cell washers are typically employed for this purpose. However, manual washing parallels the automated process. Sample Procedure 2-2 summarizes the wash procedure.

At the completion of the wash phase, AHG serum is added to each tube. Each tube is mixed and centrifuged. The cell button is resuspended and observed for agglutination and hemolysis. If no agglutination and/or hemolysis are seen, the interpretation of the results is negative. A five-minute incubation and re-examination for observation of agglutination or hemolysis is performed. Negative results in the incubated tubes require

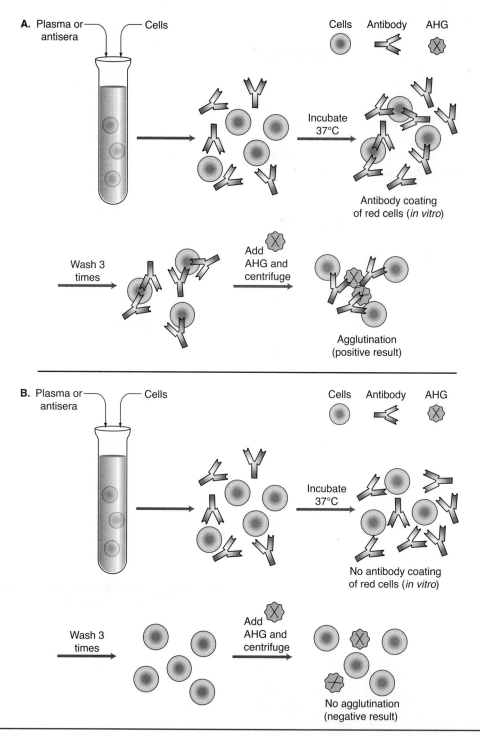

FIGURE 2-9 Indirect antiglobulin test.
a. Positive result = Antibodies present in the plasma attach to specific antigens on the red cells. The antihuman globulin serum attaches to the antibodies on the red blood cells and produces a bridging effect. Agglutination is the positive result.
b. Negative result = Antibodies in plasma are not specific for antigens on red cells. No antibodies attach to cells. The antihuman globulin serum has no antibodies to bridge.
Source: Delmar, Cengage Learning

SAMPLE PROCEDURE 2-1

Method for Using the Indirect Antiglobulin Test

1. Combine sera (or antisera) and cells. Either the sera or the cells comprises the known factor in the test scheme.
2. Centrifuge tubes.
3. Examine, interpret, and record the results.
4. Add enhancement media, if indicated.
5. Incubate for the appropriate time designated by the enhancement media. Do not incubate beyond the upper limit for the enhancement media, as the antigen-antibody complexes may begin to dissociate.
6. Centrifuge tubes.
7. Examine, interpret, and record results.
8. Wash tubes three times.
9. Add AHG sera.
10. Centrifuge tubes.
11. Examine, interpret, and record results. If results are negative, incubate for five minutes and re-examine.
12. Add check cells to all negative tubes.
13. Centrifuge tubes.
14. Examine, interpret, and record results.

SAMPLE PROCEDURE 2-2

Manual Wash Technique for the Anti-Human Globulin Test

1. Using a wash bottle filled with 0.85% saline, add saline to the tubes until approximately 2/3 full. Forcefully add the saline to ensure mixing. Be certain not to contaminate the dropper of the wash bottle.
2. Place the tubes in the serofuge. The serofuge must be balanced.
3. Spin the tubes for one minute or the amount of time designated for a wash spin.
4. Remove the tubes when the serofuge comes to a complete stop.
5. Completely decant the tubes by quickly turning them upside down over a beaker of disinfectant. DO NOT IMMEDIATELY TURN THE TUBES BACK TO AN UPRIGHT POSITION. While still inverted, shake the tubes several times to remove the saline.
6. Return tubes to an upright position. Mix.
7. Repeat steps 3 to 6 two additional times. On the third wash, remove the excess saline by blotting the opening of the tubes with a piece of gauze or absorbent material.

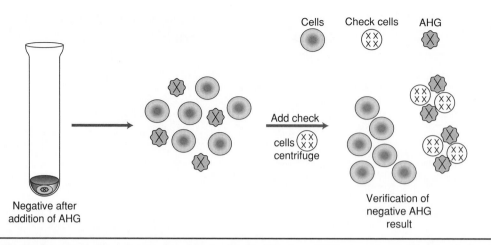

FIGURE 2-10 Confirmation of negative results with check cells. The free AHG serum is combined with the check cells (antibody coated) to create a positive reaction. This reaction confirms that the AHG is viable and that the negative reaction is legitimate.

Source: Delmar, Cengage Learning

that check cells be added as a form of quality control. After adding a drop of coated cells to each negative tube, the tubes are centrifuged and examined. Agglutination should be seen. Figure 2-10 summarizes this procedure.

This step confirms that test procedures were performed in a manner that left the unused anti-human globulin sera viable. It also proves that the AHG was not neutralized by human globulins not washed away in the wash phase. Table 2-7 summarizes errors that may cause check cells not to agglutinate.

Applications of the Indirect AHG Test

The AHG test has many test applications. Applications of the indirect method include the antibody screen test, antibody identification panel, compatibility test (also known as the crossmatch), and antigen typing with some AHG reactive antisera. These applications will be discussed in future chapters.

TABLE 2-7 Sources of Error Resulting in Negative Check Cell Results
Inadequate washing of cells
Omission of AHG sera from test
Omission of check cells from test
Contaminated AHG
Contaminated saline

Direct Antiglobulin Test

A second test performed for the detection of antibodies is the direct antiglobulin test or DAT. Historically, this test was the direct Coombs test (DCT). It is a test that detects antibodies coating the surface of the red blood cells *in vivo*. Coating substances may be globulins, complement or both. The attached antibody may be identified after it is removed from the surface of the red cell. These procedures will be discussed in Chapter 8.

ALTERNATE TEST METHODS FOR ANTIGEN-ANTIBODY REACTION TESTING

Automation

Automation of blood bank tests has been in the developmental stage for more than thirty years. Historically, tests have been automated with limited success. Several instruments were developed and used but are no longer in use due to expense of operation and lack of suitability for antibody detection and crossmatching. Automation has, however, become affordable and more user friendly. This has resulted in an extended use of automated systems. Immucor has developed an instrument, Galileo, which mimics manual testing (see Figure 2-11). This instrument is a "microprocessor-controlled instrument designed to fully automate Immunohematology in vitro diagnostic

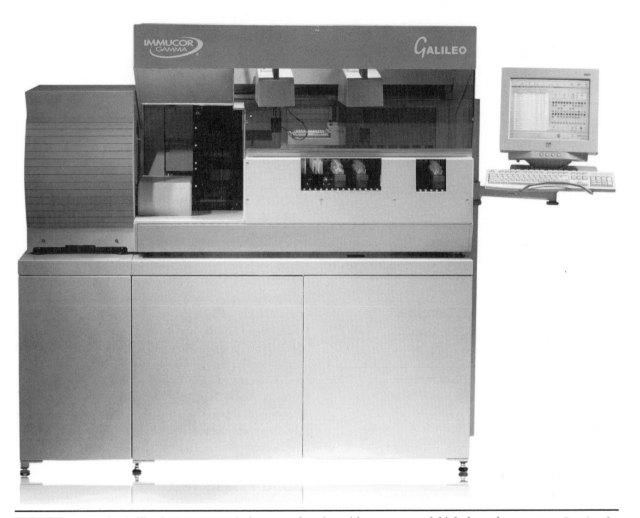

FIGURE 2-11 The Galileo by Immucor mimics manual testing with an automated, high throughput system. *Reprinted with permission by Immucor, Inc. Atlanta, GA.*

testing of human blood." (Gallileo Echo Revised 510(k) Summary.) The functions are fully automated and include "ABO grouping and RhD typing, detection/identification of IgG red blood cell antibodies, compatibility testing and red blood cell phenotyping." (Gallileo Echo Revised 510(k) Summary.) The advantages of automation include volume testing, reduced hands-on technologist time, process controls, and error detection mechanisms.

Gel Technology

Gel technology was developed as an alternative to tube testing. Use of gel testing has increased due to increased

accuracy and ease of use compared to tube testing, smaller sample size, as well as decreased exposure to biohazardous blood samples and breakable glassware.

The test method parallels tube testing. The technology utilizes dextran acrylamide gel particles. The gel particles are spherical beads. The beads function both as a reaction media, parallel to saline in the tube test, and a filter. Gel is packaged in pre-filled cards. There are specific gel cards for each type of test performed. See Figure 2-12 for an example of a gel card. The appropriate patient sample is added to the reagent tubes in each card. Directions for test performance are provided in each package insert. Table 2-8 summarizes the applications of gel testing.

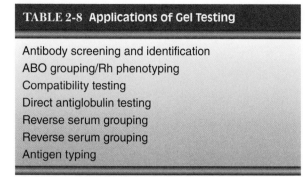

TABLE 2-8 Applications of Gel Testing

Antibody screening and identification
ABO grouping/Rh phenotyping
Compatibility testing
Direct antiglobulin testing
Reverse serum grouping
Reverse serum grouping
Antigen typing

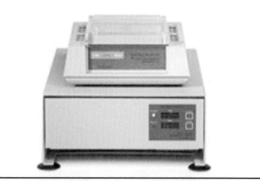

FIGURE 2-13 MTS Pro-Vue workstation. *Reproduced with permission from Ortho Clinical Diagnostics, Raritan, NJ.*

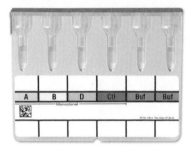

FIGURE 2-12 Ortho gel card for ABO forward grouping. *Published with permission from Ortho Clinical Diagnostics, Raritan, NJ.*

Endpoints of gel testing are recorded by observation of red cell agglutination or lack of reaction. The red cell agglutinates are trapped and visualized to interpret the endpoint. Large agglutinates are seen at the top layer of the gel tube. Smaller agglutinates are trapped in lower sections of the gel tubes. Unagglutinated cells travel through the gel and form a button in the bottom of the tube. This is identical to a negative reaction in the test tube.

Gel testing may be performed manually or by an automated system. The automated system consists of several parts. These parts include: centrifuge, incubator, worktable, reagent dispensers, and pipettor. Automation permits walk-away testing as well as analysis of large test volumes. See Figure 2-13 for a photo of the Ortho Pro-Vue™.

Microplate Testing

The use of microplates for blood bank testing became popular in the 1990s. These plates have 96 wells and allow multiple patients or donors to be tested concurrently. Methods may be adapted for red cell or plasma testing. Plasma and cells are added to the individual wells of the microplates. Plates are mixed and centrifuged and results are interpreted by examining the button on the bottom of each well. A solid-formed button indicates positive reactions. Negative reactions are indicated by cell dispersion throughout the well. Results are read manually or on a microplate reader. This method permits a higher volume testing and has also been adapted for automated testing. See Figure 2-14 for an example of microplate interpretation.

Solid Phase Testing

Solid phase testing has been in use in the blood bank since the 1980s. This testing employs a microplate wells coated with reagent red blood cells. The patient/donor samples are added to the plates. The antibodies

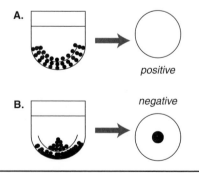

FIGURE 2-14 Interpretation of Microplate Testing.
a. Positive result—cells dispersed throughout the well
b. Negative result—cell button in the bottom or the well
Source: Delmar, Cengage Learning

from the patient/donor samples are captured by the red cells. As with tube testing, a wash phase removes and dilutes excess immunoglobulins. Indicator cells, are added and the mixture centrifuged. In this centrifugation step, the indicator cells come into contact with the attached immunoglobulins.

Interpretation of solid phase testing is the reverse of standard blood bank tube tests. Since the antibody complexes are attached to the side of the wells, positive reactions are indicated by the adherence of the indicator cells to the attached complexes on the sides of the wells. Hence, no cell button is formed in the bottom of the well. If a button is formed in the bottom of the well, this is the indicator cells that have *not* adhered to the immunoglobulins bound to the sides of the well. Therefore, the unattached indicator cells will fall to the bottom of the tube. See Figure 2-15 for a pictorial explanation of positive and negative reactions in solid phase adherence testing.

MOLECULAR BIOLOGY

Since the discovery of ABO antigens, traditional blood bank testing has been based on simple hemagglutination methods. These methods rely on the antibodies contained in the plasma or the antigens present on the surface of the cells being known to the tester. A positive reaction indicates that an antigen or antibody is present, while a negative reaction confirms an absence of the antibody or antigen. With the emergence of molecular technology, the gold-standard of hemagglutination testing may become a method of the past.

Molecular diagnostics has the potential to completely transform pretransfusion testing. As molecular methods have evolved, it has become evident that great

potential exists for resolving discrepancies previously out of the scope of available test methods. Applications of molecular testing methods in blood bank are summarized in Box 2-3. The use of low to high throughput methods, such as **polymerase chain reaction (PCR)** and **microarray**, is gradually transforming blood bank methods from the traditional hemagglutination assays to specific DNA tests.

BOX 2-3

Applications of Molecular Testing in Blood Bank

Donor center
Genotype RBC products
Product for special patient populations, such as sickle cell disease patients
Products for patients with multiple alloantibodies
RHD genotyping donors who are D-negative

Reference laboratory
Reagent RBCs for antibody detection
Genotype to determine dosage of RBC antigens
Resolution of typing discrepancies
Genotype to predict presence or absence of an antigen when no antisera exists
Determination if new antibody is an autoantibody or alloantibody
Resolution of unusual serological findings

Transfusion service
Genotype patients
Recently transfused patients
Patients with autoantibodies
D type of the patient to predict need for Rhlg or D-negative products
Providing genotyped matched products
Patients with SCD
Patients with thalassemia
Patients with AIHA
Chronically transfused patients

Prenatal testing
RHD type to predict need for Rhlg
Genotype fetal DNA to predict risk for HDFN

Reprinted with permission from Elsevier Limited.

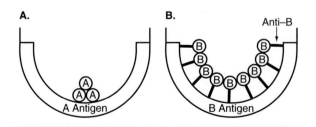

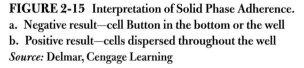

FIGURE 2-15 **Interpretation of Solid Phase Adherence.**
a. Negative result—cell Button in the bottom or the well
b. Positive result—cells dispersed throughout the well
Source: Delmar, Cengage Learning

Single Nucleotide Polymorphism (SNP)

The application of molecular techniques in the blood bank is possible due to the fact that blood groups are the result of a **single nucleotide polymorphism (SNP)** (see Figure 2-16). With the exception of ABO and Rh, these SNPs are responsible for most blood groups, and are relatively easy to detect with PCR techniques. The original PCR methods to detect SNPs were low throughput PCR methods. However, most of the current methods are high-throughput methods, such as Real-Time PCR and microarray.

Polymerase Chain Reaction (PCR)

PCR was the first molecular method for amplification of a specific DNA target sequence. Traditional PCR methods provide the basis for more advanced methods of amplification such as Real-Time PCR and microarray. PCR is an *in vivo* technique that can employ as

little as a single copy of DNA to synthesize millions of identical copies. This method permits scientists and researchers to synthesize usable amounts of a specific target sequence of DNA for further research and testing.

PCR is a relatively simple reaction, using five components (see Table 2-9). These five components are referred to as the master mix for the reaction. The master mix is subject to three steps, known as a cycle. Each PCR cycle generates a new copy of DNA from each existing copy. The cycle is repeated continuously to generate multiple copies of the DNA. The formula of X^N, where X is the starting number of DNA copies and N is the number of cycles, will determine the number of DNA copies produced through the reaction. An application of the formula X^N is

X= 5 copies of DNA at the beginning of the process
N= 6 cycles of the PCR process
$5^6 = 15,625$ copies of the original DNA

The three steps of PCR are denaturation, annealing, and extension (see Figure 2-17). In the denaturation step, the master mix is heated to about 95°C. The increase in temperature denatures the DNA by breaking the hydrogen bonds that hold the double strand together. Two single strands result from this denaturation.

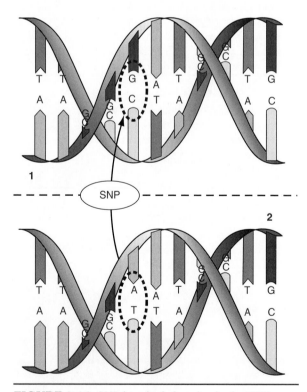

FIGURE 2-16 SNP is a single location in the DNA. A blood group determination is most often a SNP.
Source: Delmar, Cengage Learning

TABLE 2-9 PCR Components

Target DNA Sequence: Provides the template for the reaction. Can be derived from any source, such as a human, plant, or other mammal. The DNA must first be extracted from the source cells.

Primers: Pieces of single-stranded DNA complementary to the end sequences of the target. Marks initiation location of the reaction and the sequence to be amplified.

Nucleotides: Also referred to as deoxyribonucleoside triphosphates (dNTPs). They are the building blocks that are incorporated into the new piece of synthesized DNA.

Taq Polymerase: The DNA polymerase that synthesizes the new strand of DNA by incorporating the dNTPs into the template strand at the target sequence. It is isolated from the bacterium *Thermus aquaticus*, which grows in hot springs, and therefore can withstand high temperatures.

Magnesium: Cofactor required for the proper function of Taq polymerase.

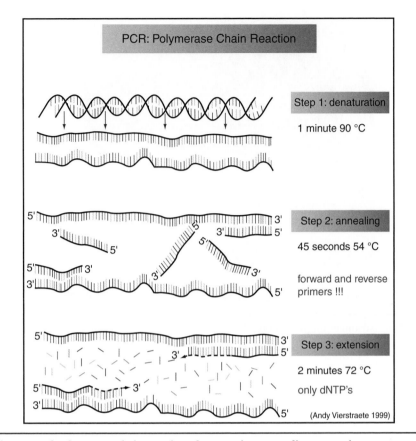

FIGURE 2-17 The steps of polymerase chain reaction: denaturation, annealing, extension
Source: Delmar, Cengage Learning

The annealing step creates a target sequence. The temperature is lowered to 50 to 60°C. This temperature adjustment will allow the sequence specific **primers** to anneal, or attach, to the target locations and mark the sequence to be replicated. The target sequence is used to create additional strands of identical DNA.

The final step is extension. In the extension step, dNTPs, the building blocks of DNA, and a DNA polymerase are used to synthesize the complementary strand. The temperature is raised to 72°C to allow the DNA polymerase to incorporate the dNTPs into the target sequence.

These three reaction steps are repeated to make multiple copies of the target sequence. The reaction sequence often takes place in a programmable instrument, called a thermocycler. The thermocycler rapidly heats and cools the reaction mixture. The TaqMan instrument by Roche Diagnostics is used to perform this type of analysis (see Figure 2-18).

In each PCR cycle, the original DNA template is copied. The copying begins at the 5' end of the primer, and a complementary strand is formed. As each cycle progresses, the number of copies of DNA increases exponentially. Typically, 20 to 40 cycles are performed, based on the quantity of DNA required. After a number of cycles, the production of new copies reaches a plateau. This is the threshold level. The initial amount of DNA, the amount of reagents in the master mix, and the efficiency of the PCR reactions determine the threshold level. In recent years, variations of PCR have been developed. These include:

- Reverse transcriptase PCR (RT-PCR)—the generation of DNA copies from an RNA template.

- Multiplex PCR—the generation of copies from multiple targets on the same DNA piece.

- Real-Time PCR—allows for DNA detection during the reaction.

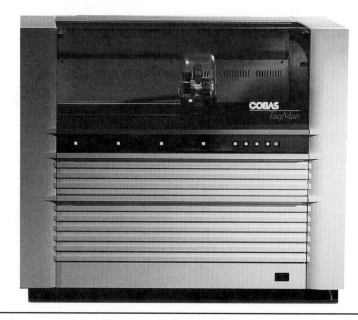

FIGURE 2-18 TaqMan instrument for performing PCR. *Reprinted with permission from Roche Diagnostics Corp., Indianapolis, IN.*

Real-Time PCR

Real-Time PCR has applications in the blood bank, since it allows for immediate detection of the target sequence. Real-Time PCR detection is accomplished with the use of a fluorescent probe. The probe binds to a specific target point on the DNA strand. The probe has a fluorescent tag that can be detected, and a quencher molecule, which inhibits the fluorescence when in close proximity. As the Taq Polymerase extends the target sequence, it removes the probe, releasing the fluorescent tag. The fluorescence allows for detection and quantitation of the target sequence. The amount of fluorescence is directly proportional to the number of copies of the target sequence present.

DNA microarray method also has applications in the blood bank. This method is used to detect specific DNA sequences. DNA microarrays, also referred to as a gene chip, allows for the simultaneous detection of thousands of different gene sequences. Microarray methods employ a solid phase, such as a glass slide, to which a probe is bound. PCR amplified DNA is labeled and applied to the surface of the solid phase, where hybridization occurs. Detection of the hybridization is typically achieved with fluorescence. Microarray methods allow for high-throughput genetic analysis. High-throughput will be essential when molecular techniques become mainstream in the blood bank laboratory.

WEB ACTIVITIES

1. Paste http://pathology2.jhu.edu into your browser.
2. Choose "Divisions" from the bar under the header.
3. Choose "Division Sites."
4. Choose "Molecular Pathology."
5. Choose "Techniques."
6. View animations "PCR" and "Real-time PCR."

SUMMARY

- Understanding equipment and reagents employed blood bank testing is imperative to application of additional concepts discussed in this text. Reagents used in testing include: Antisera for ABO, Rh, and additional red blood cell antigens.

- Red blood cells products such as reverse grouping cells, antibody screening, and identification cells and AHG indicator cells or check cells.

- Anti-human globulin sera including monospecific and polyspecific.

- Potentiating agents include bovine albumin, LISS, PEG, and Proteolytic enzymes.

- Anti-human globulin testing can be divided into indirect and direct antiglobulin methods. The final step for detecting antibody attachment to red blood cells is the same in each method. Confirmation of the viability of AHG in negative tests with Coombs control cells is utilized in all AHG testing.

- Alternates to tube testing in blood bank include:

  Automation

  Gel testing

  Microplate testing

  Solid phase adherence method.

- Molecular techniques applied to blood bank testing include PCR, Real-Time PCR, and microarray or gene chip. The applications of these molecular techniques include:

  Fetal blood grouping in pregnancies with potential risk for HDFN

  Genotyping a multi-transfused patient

  Genotyping of blood donors with potentially rare genotypes.

All of the reagents and methods discussed in this chapter will be applied throughout the remainder of this text. A thorough understanding of these basic test methods and reagents is necessary for expansion of concepts and methodologies as additional and more complex information is provided.

REVIEW QUESTIONS

1. The test that mixes unknown serum with unknown cells is:
   a. direct antiglobulin test
   b. antibody screen
   c. antibody identification
   d. compatibility test

2. Commercial antisera is used for detection of:
   a. ABO antigens
   b. BO antibodies
   c. atypical antibodies
   d. compatibility test

3. The Rh antisera that requires a parallel control is:
   a. chemically modified
   b. monoclonal
   c. high protein polyclonal
   d. monoclonal/polyclonal blend

4. A direct antiglobulin test is performed with polyspecific and anti-IgG antisera. The results are as follows:
   Polyspecific: 3+
   Anti-IgG: negative
   The most likely substance coating the red cells is:
   a. Anti-IgG
   b. Anti-D
   c. Anti-C3
   d. Anti-A,B

5. Reverse grouping cells are manufactured from:
   1. group O cells
   2. group A cells
   3. group AB cells
   4. Rh positive cells
   5. Rh negative cells

a. 1 and 4 are correct
b. 1 and 5 are correct
c. 2 and 4 are correct
d. 2 and 5 are correct
e. 3 and 4 are correct
f. 3 and 5 are correct

6. Antibody screen and antibody identification cells are group:
   a. A_1 and B
   b. A and O
   c. O only
   d. AB only
   e. Any ABO group

7. Antibody screen cells will detect the following antibodies:
   1. Anti-A_1
   2. Anti-D
   3. Anti-C
   4. Anti-Fy^a
   5. Anti-M
   a. 1, 2, and 4 are correct
   b. 2, 3, and 5 are correct
   c. 1, 2, 4, and 5 are correct
   d. 2, 3, 4, and 5 are correct

8. Anti-human globulin reagent is used for:
   a. Rh typing red cells
   b. ABO reverse grouping
   c. reducing zeta potential of red cells
   d. detecting human globulin on red cells

9. The enhancement media that affects the second stage of agglutination is:
   a. BSA
   b. LISS
   c. PEG
   d. Ficin

10. The enhancement media that may be used to suspend the red cells is:
    a. BSA
    b. LISS
    c. PEG
    d. Ficin

11. Proteolytic enzymes work by:
    a. destroying red blood cells
    b. removing negatively charged molecules from red cells
    c. coating red blood cells during the incubation process
    d. reducing zeta potential surrounding red cells

12. Coombs control cells are added:
    a. after washing the cells in the AHG test
    b. before addition of AHG sera
    c. before centrifugation with AHG sera
    d. after addition of AHG sera

13. Agglutination as seen in gel tubes is seen as:
    a. a button in the bottom of the tube
    b. a coating along the tube
    c. clumps at the top layer of the gel
    d. cells scattered throughout the gel

14. Indirect antiglobulin testing is used for:
    a. detection of *in vivo* antibody coating of red cells
    b. compatibility testing between recipient and donors
    c. reverse ABO grouping of donors
    d. typing Rh positive cells prior to transfusion

15. Solid phase testing demonstrates positive reactions with:
    a. a button in the bottom of the well
    b. a coating along the well
    c. clumps at the top layer of the well
    d. cells scattered throughout the entire well

16. The molecular technology test method that utilizes a fluorescent probe is:
    a. polymerase chain reaction
    b. single nucleotide polymorphism
    c. Real-Time polymerase chain reaction
    d. Taq Polymerase

17. The test methodology that employs generation of DNA from an RNA template is:
    a. PCR
    b. reverse transcriptase PCR Multiplex PCR—the generation of copies from
    c. Real-Time PCR—allows for DNA detection during the reaction
    d. gene chip technology

18. The component of PCR that marks the reaction initiation location and the sequence to be amplified is the:
    a. primer
    b. probe
    c. Taq Polymerase
    d. gene chip

19. The process of annealing is:
    a. breaking the hydrogen bonds of the DNA
    b. creating a target sequence
    c. replicating the DNA
    d. creating additional strands of DNA

20. The purpose of the solid phase in a microarray is to:
    a. label the DNA
    b. provide a source of fluorescence
    c. provide a solid phase
    d. denature the sample DNA

C A S E   S T U D Y

1. A technologist is assigned to the blood bank for the evening shift. Following the completion of a pre-surgical antibody screen, the check cells are negative in all tubes. The technologist attempts to resolve the problem while an additional set of tubes is washing in the automated cell washer.
   a. List five possible causes for the discrepancy.
   b. Should the test results be reported? Why or why not?
   c. What step(s) should be taken to obtain reportable results if you have decided *not* to report the results?
   The technologist recalls that the alarm on the cell washer sounded and she changed the saline. Now, upon inspection of the instrument, she notices bubbles in the reagent line. Could this have created the problem? If so, how? How can this be corrected?

2. An MLT student is doing a clinical rotation in the blood bank. The blood bank uses microplates to perform antibody screens. Tube testing is used to perform antibody identification and crossmatching. The student performs an antibody screen on the patient with the microplates. The student interprets the antibody screen as positive within both screen cells due to cell buttons found in the bottom of the microplate wells. The technologist who proceeds with the antibody identification notes no reaction within any cells at any phase. What might explain this apparent discrepancy?

REFERENCES

Anstee, David J. "Goodbye to agglutination and all that?" *Transfusion*. Vol. 45, Issue 5, 2005, pp. 652–653.

Blaney, Kathy and Howard, Paula. *Basic and Applied Concepts of Immunohematology*. Mosby, Philadelphia, 2000.

Brecher, Mark, editor. *American Association of Blood Banks Technical Manual 15th Edition*. AABB, 2005.

Coombs, RR. "Historical Note: past, present and future of the antiglobulin test." *Vox Sanguinis*. Vol. 74, 1998, pp. 67–73.

Crombach, Gerd, MD, PhD et al. "Reliability and clinical application of fetal RhD genotyping with two different fluorescent duplex polymerase chain reaction assays: Three years' experience." *American Journal of Obstetrics and Gynecology*. Vol. 180, Issue 2, 1999, pp. 435–440.

Das, Sudipta S. "A comparison of Conventional Tube Test and Gel Technique in Evaluation of Direct Antiglobulin Test." *Hematology*. Vol. 12, Issue 2, 2007, pp. 175–8.

Henry, John Bernard, *Clinical Diagnosis and Management by Laboratory Methods*. W. B. Saunders Co. 2001.

Hillyer, Christopher, Shaz, Beth H., Winkler, Anne, M., and Reid, Marion. "Integrating molecular technologies for red blood cell typing and compatibility testing into blood centers and transfusion services." *Transfusion Medicine Reviews*. Vol. 22, Issue, 2, 2008, pp. 117–132.

ID-MTS Question and Answer Guide. Ortho Clinical Diagnostics. 1996.

Issitt PD, Anstee DJ (1998). *Applied Blood Group Serology*. 4th edition, Durham, NC, USA: Montgomery Scientific Publications.

Karpasitou, Katerina et al. "Blood group genotyping for Jk(a)/Jk(b), Fy(a)/Fy(b), S/s, K/k, Kp(a)/Kp(b), Js(a)/Js(b), Co-a/Co-b, and Lu-a/Lu-b with microarray beads." *Transfusion*. Vol. 48, Issue 3, 2008, pp. 505–512.

Llopis, F., et al. "A monolayer coagglutination microplate technique for typing red cells." *Vox Sanguinis*. Vol. 72, 1997, pp. 26–30.

Llopis, F., et al. "A new method for phenotyping red blood cells using microplates." *Vox Sanguinis*. 77, 1999, pp. 143–148.

Llopis, F., et al. "A new red blood monolayer technique for screening and identification of red cell antibodies cells." *Vox Sanguinis*. 1996; 70: pp. 152–156.

Montalvo, Lani. "Clinical investigation of posttransfusion Kidd blood group typing using a rapid normalized quantitative polymerase chain reaction." *Transfusion*. Vol 44, Issue 5, 2004, pp. 694–702.

Moulds, M.K. "Review: monoclonal reagent and detection of unusual or rare phenotypes or antibodies." *Immunohematology*. 2006, Vol. 22, No. 2, pp. 52–63.

Package Insert. "Anti-Human globulin, IgG." Ortho Clinical Diagnostics, Raritan, NJ.

Package Insert. "Blood grouping reagents, Anti-A, Anti-B, Anti-A,B." Ortho Clinical Diagnostics, Raritan, NJ.

Package Insert. "Blood grouping reagents, Anti-A, Anti-B, Anti-A,B." Ortho Clinical Diagnostics, Raritan, NJ.

Package Insert. "Blood grouping reagents, Anti-D (Anti-Rh$_0$)." Ortho Clinical Diagnostics, Raritan, NJ.

Package Insert. "Blood grouping reagent, A/B/D Monoclonal and Reverse Grouping Card™, For Use with the ID-Micro Typing System™." Ortho Clinical Diagnostics, Raritan, NJ.

Package Insert. "Blood grouping reagent, Anti-A, Anti-B and Anti-A,B For Use with the ID-Micro Typing System™." Ortho Clinical Diagnostics, Raritan, NJ.

Package Insert. "Bovine serum albumin solution." Ortho Clinical Diagnostics, Raritan, NJ.

Package Insert. "Ortho antibody enhancement solution." Ortho Clinical Diagnostics, Raritan, NJ.

Package Insert. "Reagent red blood cells, (pooled cells) affirmagen." Ortho Clinical Diagnostics, Raritan, NJ.

Package Insert. "Reagent red blood cells, (pooled cells) coombs control." Ortho Clinical Diagnostics, Raritan, NJ.

Paz, N., Itzhaky, D., Ellis, M. H. "The sensitivity, specificity, and clinical relevance of gel versus tube DAT's in the clinical immunology laboratory." *Immunohematology*. Vol. 20, Issue 2, 2004, pp. 118–121.

Plapp, Fred V. and Rachel, Jane M. "Automation in blood banking, machines for clumping, sticking and gelling." *American Journal of Clinical Pathology*. October (Supplement 1) 1992, pp. 517–521.

Quill, Elizabeth. "Blood-matching goes genetic." *Science*. Vol. 319, Issue 5869, 2008, pp. 1478–1479.

Standards for Blood Banks and Transfusion Services, 25th Edition. AABB, Bethesda, MD. 2008.

Storry, Jill R. "New Technologies to replace current blood typing reagents." *Current Opinion in Hematology*. Vol. 14, Issue 6, 2007, pp. 677–681.

Uthemann, H and Poschmann, A. "Solid-phase antiglobulin test for screening and identification of red cell antibodies." *Transfusion*. Vol. 30. Issue 2, pp. 114–116.

Quality Control and Quality Assurance in the Blood Bank

LEARNING OUTCOMES

At the completion of this chapter, the reader should be able to:

- Describe general quality assurance in the blood bank laboratory.
- Outline a program for continuous quality improvement or total quality management.
- Differentiate quality assurance from quality control.
- Outline and create a procedure for quality control on reagents used in the blood bank.
- Outline temperature monitoring and preventative maintenance on blood bank equipment.
- Discuss and differentiate regulatory agencies from accrediting agencies.
- Outline personnel orientation, training, and competency assessment.
- Describe policies for validation and certification of suppliers.
- Describe error management and reporting of incidents within the blood bank.

GLOSSARY

analytical   relating to analysis or testing during the testing process of the laboratory test

audit trail   system of paper records that re-creates all steps in a process

audits   investigation of compliance with policies and procedures

continuous quality improvement (CQI)   a process for review, evaluation, and affecting change within the laboratory on an ongoing basis

external proficiency testing   specimens for evaluation of test methods distributed to laboratories by an outside agency

good manufacturing practices (GMP)   a series of procedures published in the Code of Federal Regulations (CFR) used by blood banks and transfusion services as a guideline for work practices

peer review   evaluation of a laboratory, a specific department in the laboratory, or a specific procedure performed by a group of equals

pre-analytical   time prior to the testing procedure; pre-analytical factors include specimen collection, specimen handling, interfering substances, and patient factors

post-analytical   time after the testing procedure; post-analytical factors include reporting, result delivery, and interpretation of results

quality assurance (QA)   efforts of all personnel to monitor and evaluate all aspects of laboratory testing to improve patient care

quality control   series of procedures to monitor test system

total quality management (TQM)   a strategy to create an awareness of quality in all processes in the establishment

validation   assessment that a procedure or product consistently produces the defined product or result

INTRODUCTION

Quality is at the forefront of all processes in the laboratory. Quality in the blood bank and transfusion service has all of the components of quality test performance. Its expanded focus includes the collection, testing, and issuing of blood components. Blood components will be discussed in Chapter 11. Over the past 20 years, heightened concerns regarding infectious diseases have further expanded the quality program in the blood bank and transfusion service. Donor unit screening has expanded with expanded greater need for quality assurance and documentation. Regulatory agencies have increased requirements for processing components and the use of good manufacturing practices (GMP). GMP is a series of procedures that blood banks follow as a part of quality assurance (QA) practices within the transfusion service. GMPs are published by the Food and Drug Administration (FDA) in the Code of Federal Regulations (CFR) and are summarized in Table 3-1 below. The GMPs that apply to the blood industry are found in the CFR Title 21, parts 600. The use of extensive computer technology has expanded quality services in the laboratory. Computer technology has changed documentation methods and test methods within the blood bank, while creating an internal requirement for additional validation and documentation of the electronic record systems.

Blood bank quality systems should include a global view of quality as well as daily quality control testing. The global focus should include QA systems such as continuous quality improvement (CQI) or total quality management (TQM). These total programs expand the efficiency of the QA process by looking at processes in the laboratory that are not found exclusively in the blood bank or transfusion service. The focus of global programs is the evaluation of operations, the elimination of waste, and the provision of an ongoing monitoring tool. Quality programs may seem superfluous but are vital for providing quality health care and blood products as well as reducing medical errors. The American Association of Blood Banks (AABB) has developed ten guidelines that define the minimum items required for the maintenance of a quality system in the blood bank or transfusion service. These guidelines are the Quality System Essentials (QSE). These QSEs are summarized in Table 3-2.

TABLE 3-1 General
Organization and Personnel
Buildings and Facilities
Equipment
Production and Process Controls
Finished Product Control
Laboratory Controls
Records and Reports

TABLE 3-2 AABBs Quality System Essentials (QSE)
Organization
Resources
Equipment
Supplier and Customer Issues
Process Control
Documents and Records
Deviations, Nonconformances, and Complications
Assessments: Internal and External
Process Improvement
Facilities and Safety

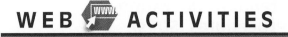

WEB ACTIVITIES

Go to the following Web site:
http://ecfr.gpoaccess.gov

Find the GMP for blood bank products in Title 21, Part 600.

Summarize in a table the guidelines listed in this section.

Share your table with a partner or the instructor.

TABLE 3-3 Components of Laboratory Quality Assurance

Personnel Requirements, Training, and Competency Assessment

Specimen and Component Collection and Labeling

Standard Operating Procedures (SOP)

Quality of Materials, Reagents, and Instruments

Record Keeping

Error Management

Process Improvement and Control

Internal Audits including Patient and Physician Satisfaction

QA is monitoring the entire testing process, beginning with the period before the sample or donor unit is collected (pre-analytical) through delivering the results or blood product to the physician or recipient (post-analytical). Discussion of QA in the transfusion service is even more extensive than the laboratory in general. Quality of transfusion service testing begins off-site, with the manufacturing of reagents. Often the collecting and processing of blood products occurs at a remote location. The **quality control** of reagents and equipment is a small portion of the overall QA in the blood bank. QA of donors and blood products will be discussed in Chapters 10 and 11.

QUALITY ASSURANCE (QA) VERSUS QUALITY CONTROL (QC)

Quality assurance is a comprehensive program that strives to monitor and evaluate all aspects of test performance. It includes three major areas of quality: **pre-analytical**, **analytical**, and **post-analytical**. A summary of QA components is found in Table 3-3.

Quality control is monitoring of test system components. It is a narrow focus within the larger scope of QA. Quality control is composed of a system that monitors test methods, reagents, instrumentation, and additional specific test items. All of these quality control monitors are included under the broad umbrella of QA.

PERSONNEL QUALIFICATIONS

A health care facility is only as good as the personnel who perform the health care procedures. In the blood bank, the medical director is responsible for determining personnel qualifications and maintaining an individual's

CRITICAL THINKING ACTIVITY

Take the items in Table 3-3 and assign the terms pre-analytical, analytical, and post-analytical to each item.

Share the results with classmates or the instructor.

competency throughout employment. Human resources may establish selection criteria with input from the blood bank personnel. Selection criteria may include education, experience, and credentials. All of the criteria must be documented and maintained in personnel records.

A written job description should exist for each position. Each job description details the tasks and responsibilities for each position. Job descriptions are updated as the tasks and responsibilities change for the position.

Performance evaluations are provided annually for all employees. A conference between the employee and supervisor should take place between the employee and supervisory staff. Evaluations should be reviewed and signed by all parties, and be included in the employee's personnel record for the duration of employment.

Training and Competency Assessment

Adequate orientation should be provided for each individual when hired. Re-training should take place when equipment and methods change. Initial orientation,

TABLE 3-4 Orientation Training Activities

Tour of all Facilities
Review of all SOP Manuals
Observation of all Procedures and Instrumentation
Practice of all Procedures and Instrumentation with Trainer Observation
Documentation of Competency for All Procedures
Observation and Training for all Quality Control/ QA Programs

training, and re-training should be documented. A training checklist signed by the trainer and the employee provides adequate documentation and should be maintained in the individual's personnel file. Sufficient time for training, practice, repetition of procedures, and inquiries by the new employee should be incorporated into the training program. Suggested items to be included in orientation training are summarized in Table 3-4.

Competency assessment is the evaluation of an employee's skills and knowledge of a skill, task, or procedure. Accrediting agencies such as AABB, College of American Pathologists (CAP), Centers for Medicare and Medicaid Services (CMS), Commission on Laboratory Accreditation (COLA) and state agencies require assessment of competency. A comprehensive competency program includes initial assessment during orientation, assessment twice annually during the first year of employment, and annually thereafter. Competency assessment programs are commercially available electronically and through agencies such as CAP. These programs are easily implemented and provide a comprehensive assessment of competency. Individual laboratories may develop internal programs that include activities from multiple sources. All activities must be documented and the documentation retained. Examples of activities that may be used as competency assessment tools are summarized in Table 3-5.

TABLE 3-5 Competency Assessment Tools

Checklists for Observation of Procedure Steps
Blind Samples
Split Samples
Proficiency Testing (Initial Testing or Repeat Testing)
Written Assessments (Quizzes, Questionnaires, etc.)

Standard Operating Procedures (SOPs)

SOPs are required by accrediting agencies and should be available for all procedures in the blood bank or the transfusion service. All procedures should be listed in a standard format. Clinical and Laboratory Standards Institute (CLSI) has devised a standard format for written procedures. This format provides a guideline for establishing a SOP manual. A compilation of procedures summarizes department activities as well as information related to external departments or suppliers. The SOP includes information necessary for daily operations such as specimen collection, quality control, record keeping, test procedures, and emergency procedures. The SOP manual is reviewed and revised on a regular basis by administrative personnel.

Historically, SOPs were kept in binders or books to provide ready access. As information technology has expanded into all aspects of laboratory testing, electronic versions are now used in many facilities.

Validation

Validation is an evaluation process intended to prove that a process or procedure results in a pre-established product or outcome. Validation is performed not only in the blood bank, but also in the industry. Through the validation process, procedures, new methods, equipment, and computer information systems are determined to be reliable and predictable prior to implementation through this process. Validation, in general, is performed as a good laboratory practice.

Qualification of Suppliers

The provision of an acceptable end product is also dependent on the quality of the component parts used in the process. Employees at blood banks maintain agreements between the facilities and suppliers. Blood banks should qualify suppliers prior to use of their products. Qualification procedures include assessments of critical products and evaluations to determine that each product performs according to its specifications. Established procedures for the qualification process should be included in the blood bank's SOP, and the performance of the procedures should be documented. A facility may document an inspection of the incoming materials, as well as audit suppliers and document these audits. All auditing and

TABLE 3-6 Product Specifications
Purity
Strength or Potency
Size
Physical Specifications such as Size or Color
Container Description
Storage Requirements (e.g. Temperature)

inspection procedures should be included in the SOP's qualification procedure. Examples of the qualification procedure's product specifications are summarized in Table 3-6.

Specimen Collection and Labeling

Quality control of specimen collection may not always be under the laboratory's control. The technician should aptly determine that the specimen originated from the patient identified on the label and that it has been properly collected. Labeling criteria for individual blood samples varies by institution. The institution may use computer-generated and bar-coded labels. Commercial banding systems are available for blood bank testing. These systems have labels that accompany the band. The labels are applied to the specimens, in addition to the institution specific labeling system. All labels should minimally include the information summarized in Table 3-7. Improperly identified samples should not be accepted for testing. SOPs contain detailed information on specimen labeling and criteria for rejection. These procedures must be available to all personnel in the blood bank and departments where specimens are collected. Additional

TABLE 3-7 Labeling Specimens for Blood Bank Tests
Patient's First and Last Names
Two Unique Identifiers; Examples Include
■ Identification Number
■ Date of Birth
Date of Collection
Phlebotomist Signature or Complete Name

CRITICAL THINKING ACTIVITY

In pairs, students should:

1. Label sample tubes using the guidelines in Table 3-7.
2. Label one tube correctly and one tube with a missing component or other error (each student should individually label two tubes).
3. Reverse roles.
4. Compare the results with the information above and point out the correct tube and identify the error in the other.
5. Summarize results with each other.

information on specimen collection and labeling is summarized in Chapter 9 in the Compatibility Testing section. Labeling of donor units and components will be discussed in conjunction with Donor Criteria and Blood Collection in Chapter 10.

Record Keeping

Good record keeping is imperative in all laboratory operations. Blood bank record keeping is complex and requires a longer paper trail than other laboratory processes. Detailed record keeping, and access to all records, is required by all government and accrediting agencies. These records may be manual (on paper) or automated (computerized). In either case, blood component records allow the tracing of blood products from collection through transfusion. Records include a thorough step-by-step analysis that can be re-created. These records are vital for investigation of errors and incidents associated with the blood bank and transfusion of blood components. All records are maintained for the period of time designated by the accrediting and licensing agencies. This detailed record keeping provides an audit trail.

Record Keeping Guidelines for Manual Records

Record keeping guidelines are provided by accreditation agencies. Manual records are maintained according to established guidelines. Basic guidelines for manual entries into written logs are outlined in Table 3-8.

TABLE 3-8 Guidelines for Written Records

1. Use indelible or permanent ink.
2. Record the information immediately.
3. Do not use ditto marks.
4. Do not use correction fluid or tape to cover the original entry. The incorrect entry should not be obliterated.
5. Corrections are made with a single line through the incorrect information. New information is recorded clearly in the proximity of the incorrect result.
6. Corrections are documented with the date and initials of individual making the correction.
7. Specific information should be recorded when indicated.

Computer Record Keeping Guidelines

As information technology continues to develop, guidelines for computer systems and computerized records have been developed by accrediting agencies. According to the *AABB Standards for Blood Banks and Transfusion Services, 25th edition*, all computer systems must have the procedure to implement, modify, and validate both software and hardware. Table 3-9 summarizes specific records required by the AABB.

Corrections of electronic records are made in the same manner as paper records. The corrections must be documented in the electronic record. Back-up methods for retrieval of computer records in the event of system failure must be in place for all computer systems. An abbreviated compilation of times for records retention is summarized in Table 3-10.

TABLE 3-9 Computer Systems Records

1. Validation of system software, hardware, databases, user-defined tables, electronic data transfer, and/or electronic data receipt.
2. Fulfillment of applicable life-cycle requirements for internally developed software.
3. Numerical designation of system versions, if applicable, with inclusive dates for use.
4. Monitoring of data integrity for critical data elements.

TABLE 3-10 Retention Intervals for Blood Bank Records

Indefinite Retention

- Donors placed on permanent deferral, indefinite deferral, and on surveillance for protection of the recipient.
- Difficulty in typing, clinically significant antibodies, significant adverse event to transfusions, and special transfusion requirements.

Minimum of 10 years

- All records with the exception of those listed as "indefinite retention," minimum of five years or minimum or two years. Some examples of ten year retention are listed below:

  1. Identification of individuals performing each significant step in collection, processing, compatibility testing, and transportation of blood and components.
  2. Donor information, including address, medical history, physical examination, health history, or other conditions thought to compromise suitability of blood or component.
  3. Cytapheresis record.
  4. Adverse events related to donation.
  5. Look-back investigation.
  6. Patient test results including ABO, Rh, and antibodies to unexpected antibodies.
  7. Signed statement from physician indicating that the clinical situation was sufficiently urgent to require the release of blood before completion of compatibility testing or infectious disease testing.

Minimum of five years: Some examples of five-year retention are listed below:

1. Requests for blood and components.
2. Comparison of patient's previous test results for ABO and Rh type in last 12 months.
3. Verification of patient identification before transfusion.
4. Patient's medical record.
5. Records of suspected transfusion reactions.
6. Quality control records including test methods, temperatures, equipment validations, personnel training, and competency.

Source: Adapted from *AABB Standards for Blood Banks and Transfusion Services, 25th edition.*

Error Management

Errors in blood banks and transfusion services can lead to serious consequences including bodily harm, and possible death. All errors and incidents must be thoroughly investigated and recorded. As a part of routine QA, protocols must be in place for handling the detection, management, and the resulting outcomes from errors. A systematic approach to the investigation should be part of the QA program in any blood bank. Once the possible cause or root of the problem has been identified (root cause analysis), a plan for proposed changes for prevention of future incidents should be drafted. After implementation of the proposed changes, a re-evaluation should take place. Each step requires documentation and retention of records for the prescribed time interval. Possible errors that may require this approach are summarized in Table 3-11.

Sentinel Events

Hospital-wide accrediting agencies such as The Joint Commission require an existing policy for the investigation of sentinel events. The purpose is to investigate alleged incidents where bodily harm or death may have occurred. Transfusion-related incidents fall under this umbrella. Personnel should be advised of the institution's sentinel-event procedure follow that protocol when required, and document the investigation.

FDA Reporting

The FDA requires that licensed facilities report any error or accident that compromises the safety of a donor or patient. This notification is required under 21 CFR 600.14. The FDA also requires the "reporting of any event associated with the manufacturing, to

include testing, processing, packing, labeling, or storage, or with the holding or distribution of a licensed biological product or a blood or a blood component, in which the safety, purity, or potency of a distributed product may be affected." This reporting is required under 21 CFR 606.171. If the incident reveals an implication of the faulty equipment, a method exists for reporting faulty devices. An individual (or group of individuals) should be assigned the task of reporting these deviations. Within an organization, the correct chain of command for reporting these issues should be outlined in the SOP.

Reagent Quality Control Procedures

Quality control is the actual quality testing or monitoring performed on reagents or equipment used in test procedures. These quality control procedures were discussed briefly in the Chapter 2 section, Reagents and Methods Used for Immunohematology Testing. Some reagents used in routine tests require daily quality control procedures. Some reagents may require no quality control testing, but visual examination must be performed and documented each day of use. Reagents used infrequently may only require quality control testing each day of use. All quality control is documented and the records are maintained for

TABLE 3-11 Errors Requiring Investigation in the Transfusion Service

- Failure to identify the patient.
- Phlebotomy error.
- Blood issued for incorrect patients and not detected at bedside.
- Incorrect sample used for testing.
- ABO typing error.

the appropriate time period. If multiple work shifts are employed in the institution, control procedures are performed at the beginning of each shift. Commercial quality control kits are available. The purchase of a kit is not necessary, but the use of a detailed procedure for the process should be available in the standard operating procedure.

Antisera Controls

Antisera are tested with two separate controls. Their routine testing is comprised of one cell that is positive and one cell that is negative for the antigen being assessed. For anti-A, anti-B, anti-A,B and anti-RhD, the control procedure uses a 1:1 ratio of antisera and cells. Potent antisera such as anti-A and anti-B may be diluted to ensure that the antisera will detect weak antigens. Whenever possible, heterozygous cells should be chosen as the positive control. This will help determine that the antisera will detect antigens in a state of weakened expression.

Antisera that are not used on a daily basis should be tested each day of use. These antisera are also tested with positive and negative controls using the previously described guidelines.

Quality Control of Anti-Human Globulin (AHG) Sera

Quality control of anti-human globulin (AHG) sera is performed using cells that are coated with an antibody. Combination of AHG sera with check cells serves this purpose.

CRITICAL THINKING ACTIVITY

1. In pairs or small groups, examine an antibody identification panel antigram provided by the instructor.
2. Choose cells that are appropriate for use as positive and negative controls for the following antisera:

   Anti–C
   Anti–K
   Anti–Jk^a
   Anti–Fy^b
3. Share these results with other pairs or groups or the instructor.

Quality Control of Cell Products

Quality control of cell products begins with a visual examination of the supernatant. Cells that exhibit hemolysis may not be acceptable for use. If the hemolysis can be removed with one wash, the cells may be used on that day.

Additionally, reverse grouping cells, antibody screen cells, and check cells should be tested each day of use. Reverse grouping cells are tested with one positive and one negative antisera. Antibody screen cells are tested with a weak saline reactive antibody and a weak AHG reactive antibody. Check cells are tested with AHG sera, serving as a positive control. A negative control is performed using a solution that is not expected to produce a positive result.

Cells comprising an antibody identification panel do not require quality control. Visual examination and careful observation for testing discrepancies serve as an acceptable quality control.

Records of Reagent Quality Control

Records of daily reagent quality control should be maintained for review by accrediting agencies. These records include the information summarized in Table 3-12. A sample procedure for daily reagent quality control is found in Sample Procedure 3-1.

Facilities and Equipment

Facilities

The blood bank must address the adequacy of the department facility. GMPs require a clean and well-kept environment. A schedule for a regular housekeeping regimen should be available. Not only is the visual appearance of the facility important to all of the stakeholders (patients, donors, employees, and hospital personnel), but a clean physical plant is imperative to ensure the reduction of contamination and equipment malfunction.

TABLE 3-12 Records of Daily Reagent Controls
Date of Testing
Source of Reagent Used
Expiration Dates
Lot Numbers of Reagents
Visual Inspection of Reagents
Identification of Person Performing Testing

SAMPLE PROCEDURE 3-1

DAILY REAGENT QUALITY CONTROL

ABO Antiseras

1. Label two sets of tubes for forward ABO grouping. Label one set "positive" and the second "negative."
2. Place one drop of the appropriate antisera into each of the six tubes.
3. Into each tube of the positive set, place one drop of cells that will produce a positive result with that antisera. For example, place one drop of A cells into the anti-A and anti-A,B tubes.
4. Into the negative set, add one drop of group O cells to each tube (screen cells may be used).
5. Centrifuge for 15 seconds. Examine using an agglutination viewer and record results. Record and correct any discrepancies noted.

Rh Antisera

1. Label two tubes for Rh typing. Label one "positive" and the second "negative."
2. Place one drop of anti-D into each tube.
3. Into the tube labeled "positive," place one drop of Rh positive cells.
4. Into the tube labeled "negative," place one drop of Rh negative cells.
5. Centrifuge for 15 to 30 seconds as designated for the type of antisera being used. Examine using an agglutination viewer and record results. Record and correct any discrepancies noted

AHG Sera and Check Cells

1. Label two tubes "AHG." Label one "positive" and one "negative." Note that the positive tube serves as a positive control for both AHG and check cells.
2. Label one tube "saline." This will serve as a negative tube for check cells.
3. Place two drops of AHG sera into both "AHG" tubes.
4. Place two drops of saline into "saline" tube.
5. Place one drop of check cells into the positive tube and the saline tube. Note that the positive tube serves as a positive control for the AHG sera and the check cells. The saline tube serves as a negative control for the check cells.
6. Into the negative tube, place one drop of antibody screen cells.
7. Centrifuge for 15 seconds. Examine using an agglutination viewer and record results. Record and correct any discrepancies noted.

ABO Reverse Grouping Cells

1. Label two sets of tubes for reverse grouping. Label one set "positive" and the second set "negative."
2. Place two drops of anti-A into the A tube and two drops of anti-B into the B tube of the "positive" set.

(continued)

SAMPLE PROCEDURE 3-1 (CONTINUED)

3. Into the "negative" set place two drops of anti-B into the A tube and two drops of anti-A into the B tube.
4. Place one drop of the appropriate reverse group cell into the correct tube.
5. Centrifuge for 15 seconds. Examine using an agglutination viewer, and record results. Record and correct any discrepancies noted.

Antibody Screen Cells

1. Label two sets of tubes for antibody screen. Label one set "positive" and the second set "negative."
2. Using an antigram for the screen cells, choose antisera that will produce a positive result in the saline phase and will react with one of the cells. Choose a second antisera that will react with the other cell at the AHG phase. Using the positive set of tubes, place two drops of the appropriate antisera into the correct tube. It is best to choose antisera that will react with an antigen set that has a heterozygous presentation on the screening cell.
3. Into each tube of the "negative" set place two drops of 6% albumin.
4. Place one drop of the appropriate cell into each tube.
5. Centrifuge for 15 seconds, examine with an agglutination viewer and record results.
6. Add two drops of LISS (or other enhancement media) to each tube.
7. Centrifuge for 20 seconds, examine with an agglutination viewer and record results.
8. Incubate for 5 to 15 minutes (incubation time is dependent on the media being used) in a 37°C heat block.
9. Centrifuge for 20 seconds. Examine using an agglutination viewer and record results.
10. Wash three or four times and add two drops of AHG sera to each tube.
11. Centrifuge for 15 seconds and examine using an agglutination viewer. Record and correct any discrepancies noted.
12. Add one drop of check cells to each tube. Centrifuge, examine, and record results.
13. Interpret all results to determine discrepancies. Note all discrepancies and determine the cause.

CRITICAL THINKING ACTIVITY

1. Each student should prepare a record sheet for quality control.
2. The guidelines in Table 3-12 should be used as a reference. The reagents included should be those summarized in the sections above.
3. Results should be reviewed by instructor.

Equipment Quality Control and Preventative Maintenance

Equipment and instruments must have quality control procedures and preventive maintenance performed in accordance with a designated schedule. Preventive maintenance on equipment should include routine inspection and cleaning. The schedule is published in the SOP manual. Documentation of maintenance should be kept for review. Routine quality control on temperature-dependent equipment includes daily temperature monitoring. This particular equipment is summarized in Table 3-13.

TABLE 3-13 Equipment Requiring Temperature Records
Heat Blocks
Water Baths
Refrigerators
Freezers
Refrigerated Centrifuges
Rh Viewing Boxes
Platelet Incubators

TABLE 3-14 Required Features and Quality Control for Refrigerators and Freezers
Circulating Air Fan
Audible Alarm
Alarm to Sound Where Readily Heard
Temperature Recording Device
Temperatures Monitored Minimally Every Four Hours
Emergency Power System Connected
Daily Temperature Checks
Alarms Periodically Checked

Centrifuges and Cell Washers.
Small centrifuges, more commonly known as serofuges, are vital equipment in the blood bank. These serofuges have several purposes, the most critical being the ability to pack red blood cells into a well-defined button. Proper packing is vital to the interpretation of serological testing. Additional equipment maintenance includes checking the speed with a tachometer at least every six months. The timers should be periodically checked with a stopwatch. Quality control on these instruments includes calibration for determination of proper spin times to obtain a correct cell button and adequate washing of cells. Additionally, internal quality control checks may be required. Frequency and proper procedures for quality control checks are outlined in the operator's manual.

Automated cell washers require quality control related to the specific function of the instrument. The operating manual may be consulted for these specific requirements. Additional quality control includes a check of proper saline filling and adequate button formation. If the cell washer adds AHG sera, proper addition of this reagent should also be verified.

Water Baths and Heat Blocks.
Water baths and heat blocks are used for incubation for detection of warm reacting antibodies. Water baths are used for thawing fresh frozen plasma, as well. The temperature is usually maintained at 37°C with a temperature range of 30 to 37°C. When checking daily temperatures of heat blocks, a system of rotating the thermometer to all wells may be established and documented. In addition, water in water baths must be routinely changed and cultured for pathogens.

Refrigerators and Freezers.
Refrigerators and freezers are used for multiple purposes in the blood bank.

Refrigerators are used for storage of reagents, specimens, and blood components. Freezers are used for storage of frozen reagents and specimens as well as frozen components for transfusion. Required features and quality control for refrigerators and freezers is summarized in Table 3-14.

Rh View Boxes and Platelet Incubators.
Rh view boxes and platelet incubators also require temperature monitoring. Rh view boxes must heat slides to 37°C on their surface. In order to achieve this, the glass surface of the view box must be 45 to 50°C. The surface must be monitored with a thermometer.

Platelet incubators, with the ability to rotate, are required for storage of platelets. The temperature range should be 20 to 24°C continuously and the temperature should be monitored at least every four hours. If the platelets are stored at ambient temperature, the ambient temperature must be monitored every four hours. RPMs of the rotator must be checked periodically as designated by the operator's manual.

External QA

Procedures and guidelines described in previous sections reflect the internal quality control in the blood bank laboratory. External quality assurance is provided from outside agencies. Regulatory agencies such as the FDA and state agencies issue licenses that permit the laboratories to operate. Other agencies such as AABB are utilized for voluntary review.

Proficiency Testing

External proficiency testing is required as a part of a laboratory's QA program. The laboratory personnel perform

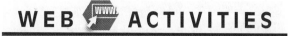

WEB ACTIVITIES

A source of agencies that provide proficiency testing may be obtained by accessing the following web site:

1. Type www.cms.hhs.gov into your browser.
2. Choose "Regulations and Guidance."
3. Under the column labeled "Legislation" choose "Clinical Laboratory Improvement Amendments (CLIA).
4. In the column marked "Overview," choose "Proficiency Testing Providers."

WEB ACTIVITIES

1. Type www.aabb.org into your browser.
2. In the left column choose "Newsletters and Jou rnal."
3. Choose "AABB Smartbrief."
4. Register to receive the daily e-mail publication.

this testing on samples that are provided by an outside agency. Agencies such as CAP operate proficiency testing programs that provide samples on a regular schedule. The samples are evaluated following established procedures and treated like patient samples. Results are submitted to the originating agency for evaluation. The outcome of testing is forwarded to the performing laboratory. These results are retained as a part of the institution's QA programs.

Accrediting and Regulatory Agencies

Regulatory agencies such as the FDA, CMS, and state agencies by law require mandatory compliance with their standards. These agencies enforce regulations by mandatory inspections, often unannounced. Failure to comply with regulations may result in revocation of the laboratory's license. The CFR provides guidance for FDA requirements. State agencies publish their own guidelines.

Agencies such as AABB and CAP are utilized for voluntary peer review. These agencies are invited to review the practices of the blood bank or transfusion service. Guidelines for the AABB are published in *Standards for Blood Banks and Transfusion Services, Technical Manual,* and *Accreditation Requirements Manual.* Agencies seeking accreditation should follow the guidelines in these publications. These organizations provide accreditation and their approval is not required for blood

bank operation. That is in contrast to the FDA and state agencies whose approval is imperative to blood bank operation.

International Standards Organization (ISO) 9000

The International Standards Organization (ISO) is an organization that has developed a set of standards for quality management. ISO 9000 Quality Systems Standards is a series of five international standards that provide guidance for the development of a quality system. ISO quality systems have gained recognition with blood bank organizations. Blood banks must register to comply with two documents ISO-9000-1 is the umbrella document and ISO 9002 is a broad standard that follows the development and implementation of the quality system within a specific organization.

QA Department Functions

As an overall monitoring device, laboratories and blood banks should have a QA department or, minimally, a QA officer. The function of this department or individual is to organize and monitor activities that fall under the QA umbrella. QA department functions are summarized in Table 3-15.

Audits are tools used to explore compliance with established policies and procedures. Audits are usually internal reviews of selected areas performed on a rotating basis. The results of these audits may be used in the laboratory's continuous quality improvement or total quality improvement programs. Satisfaction surveys or polls are useful tools for employees (internal stakeholders), patients, donors, physicians, and other hospital

TABLE 3-15 Functions of the QA Department

1. Organization, review, and approval of all SOPs.
2. Validation procedures.
3. Compliance officers for GMPs and accreditation standards.
4. Training programs and documentation.
5. Internal reviews, audits, and surveys.
6. Investigation and reporting (as needed) for incidents, errors, product recalls, and complaints.

stakeholders (external). Information gathered from these surveys provides valuable insight into the effectiveness of the quality assurance program.

Transfusion Committee

As part of QA both internal to the blood bank and within the hospital or clinic, there is often a transfusion committee. This committee is comprised of personnel from appropriate departments within the hospital. The committee members will include the medical director of the blood bank, the blood bank supervisor, other laboratory administrators, as well as representatives from departments such as surgery and the emergency department. These individuals meet as a committee on a regular basis to discuss the disposition of blood products and specific issues related to this process and its outcomes. This committee may suggest changes or recommend additions or deletions to the products and processes of the blood bank operations.

SUMMARY

QA is a broad concept that monitors all aspects of testing. Quality control is a part of the QA system that includes a set of procedures performed daily or on an established schedule. A broader application of quality principles is encompassed in global programs such as CQI or TQM. These programs examine components throughout the laboratory for the effectiveness and efficiency of the total laboratory operation. All aspects of QA and quality control are important for provision of appropriate patient care. Following established procedures determines that test methods, reagents, and equipment are accurate and appropriate within the limits of the procedures.

- GMPs guide the quality of all blood bank processes.

- All inclusive QA programs should include pre-analytical, analytical, and post-analytical components of laboratory testing. All of these components should be incorporated into the overall QA program of the blood bank.

- Qualified personnel should be hired, oriented, and trained when appropriate and tested for competence on a regular basis.

- A compilation of SOPs should be available to all personnel within the blood bank.

- All processes and products should be validated on-site and the validations documented.

- Specimen collection should be performed with established criteria. Labeling of specimens must take place as outlined in the organization's SOP.

- Quality control begins with the off-site manufacturing of all reagents, equipment, and supplies used in the blood bank.

- Quality control procedures require that most reagents be tested on the day of use to determine that achieved results will be accurate.

- Quality control and preventative maintenance of equipment must be performed to determine that the temperatures and basic functions are appropriate for the tests being performed.

- Results of all quality control procedures must be recorded and maintained. These records may be manual or computerized records.

- All errors and deviations should be investigated with the results recorded and reported to the FDA, if indicated.

- External agencies provide either mandatory or voluntary review to ascertain that operations follow established practices. Some of the voluntary agencies also provide test samples to be analyzed.

- A QA department or officer may be established to monitor all processes within the laboratory.

REVIEW QUESTIONS

1. Quality control for antibody screen cells consists of testing each cell with a:
   a. antisera reactive with each cell
   b. albumin diluted to 6%
   c. Anti-A_1
   d. pooled human serum

2. Daily quality control does *not* include:
   a. temperature monitoring
   b. controls for antibody screen cells
   c. examination of suspension fluid on cell products
   d. external proficiency testing

3. Cells in antibody identification panels require quality control testing:
   a. daily regardless of use
   b. daily regardless of use
   c. with each use
   d. at no time

4. Corrective steps taken for discrepancies found in daily quality control:
   a. are not important
   b. must be recorded
   c. do not require documentation
   d. follow specific guidelines

5. Specimen collection requires proper labeling. The item that is *not* required on the label is:
   a. patient's name
   b. identification number
   c. anticoagulant
   d. date

6. Quality control of centrifuges includes:
   a. measurement of saline volume
   b. balance check
   c. examination of supernatant fluid
   d. check of timer accuracy

7. Controls of antisera not used on a daily basis are performed:
   a. daily
   b. monthly
   c. day of use
   d. at no time

8. A positive control for Anti-D would consist of:
   a. Group O cells
   b. Rh positive cells
   c. Rh negative cells
   d. heterozygous C cells

9. Anti-human globulin sera and check cells are combined to form a positive control for:
   a. only AHG sera
   b. only check cells
   c. both AHG sera and check cells
   d. neither AHG sera nor check cells

10. ABO reagents used for forward and reverse grouping have quality control assessment:
    a. daily
    b. weekly
    c. monthly
    d. at no time

11. GMPs were described by:
    a. AABB
    b. FDA
    c. CAP
    d. CLSI

12. A technician is assigned a blind sample to test. The results are compared to actual results. The results do not correspond to the original result.

    The supervisor should:
    a. allow the technician to repeat the testing until the results are correct
    b. provide the technician with an additional sample and the expected results
    c. retrain the technician on the procedure and provide an additional sample for testing
    d. discuss the discrepancy with the technician and not document the original results

13. A new employee is practicing procedures after a demonstration by the supervisor. She needs some review of the testing steps. When she inquires, she is told that there is no procedure manual. The lack of procedure manual is:
    a. satisfactory since the employee was given demonstrations of the procedures
    b. a deficiency to be reported to the FDA and an on-site inspection requested
    c. unacceptable by good manufacturing practices
    d. not necessary for laboratory operation

14. The blood bank supervisor is searching for a new supplier for LISS. When the new reagent is located, it should be qualified by considering:
    1. purity
    2. potency
    3. size
    4. storage requirements
    5. expiration date
    a. all are correct
    b. 1, 3, 4, and 5 are correct
    c. 1, 2, 3, and 4 are correct
    d. 2, 3, 4, and 5 are correct

15. The blood bank record that is kept indefinitely is:
    a. compatibility testing
    b. look-back investigation
    c. patient's medical record
    d. donor for permanent deferral

16. An error that requires reporting to the FDA:
    a. label on patient sample does not have phlebotomist identification
    b. unit of blood is returned to blood bank after 30 minutes
    c. blood transfusion started on incorrect patient
    d. ABO group not indicated on blood tag

17. Calibration should be performed on the following:
    a. centrifuge
    b. agglutination viewer
    c. reagent refrigerator
    d. platelet incubator

18–20. Identify each of the following organizations as:
    a. voluntary accreditation
    b. mandatory licensure
    _____ 18. AABB
    _____ 19. FDA
    _____ 20. CAP

CASE STUDY

A blood bank supervisor performs weekly quality control review. The supervisor was off-site the previous week. She notices the following discrepancies:

1. Temperature out of range on well #7 of the #2 incubator. Documentation of temperature adjustment and repeat reading one hour later with a result that was in range.
2. Tuesday: Quality control on the day shift recorded a result with the AHG sera that was negative in the positive control. No additional documentation was provided.
3. Antibody identification panel had no quality control performed other than visual observation of vials and notation of no hemolysis in the supernatant of the vials.
4. Visual inspection of RhD antisera revealed a cloudy solution. The technologist discarded the vial, documented the discarding, and replaced the vial with a new vial that was marked with the date and initials of the technologist that opened the vial.
A. Which of the previously described quality control discrepancies was handled properly. Explain why.
B. Which of the discrepancies was NOT handled properly. Why? Expand by providing specifics on how each of these situations SHOULD have been handled.

REFERENCES

Blaney, Kathy and Howard, Paula. *Basic and Applied Concepts of Immunohematology*. Mosby, Philadelphia, 2000.

Brecher, Mark, editor. *American Association of Blood Banks Technical Manual 15th edition*. AABB, 2005.

Code of Federal Regulations 21 CFR Part 606 Current Good Manufacturing Practice for Blood and Blood Components. August 2007.

McCullough, Jeffrey. *Transfusion Medicine 2nd edition*. Elsevier. 2005.

Ooley, Patrick. "Quality systems 101: Overview and introduction." Presentation notes, AABB Spring Meeting 2008.

Slopecki, A. "The value of good manufacturing practice to a blood service in managing the delivery of quality." *Vox Sanguinis*. Vol. 92, Issue 3, 2007, pp. 187–96.

Standards for Blood Banks and Transfusion Services, 25th Edition. AABB, Bethesda, MD. 2008.

UNIT 2

Blood Group Systems

4

Genetics and Inheritance of Blood Group System Antigens

LEARNING OUTCOMES

Upon completion of this chapter, the student should be able to:

- Outline the basic concepts of Mendelian genetics as they relate to antigen inheritance.
- Define and differentiate genotype and phenotype.
- Define and differentiate homozygous and heterozygous inheritance.
- Define and differentiate recessive, dominant, and codominant.
- Describe the structure of DNA.
- Describe the structure and relationship of chromosomes and genes.
- Outline and diagram the concepts of crossing over, cis, and trans.
- Explain and differentiate cis and trans gene interactions.
- Explain independent assortment and provide examples related to blood groups.
- Explain independent segregation and provide examples related to blood groups.
- Define the term haplotype and relate it to inheritance.
- Diagram and interpret the possible genotypes and phenotypes of offspring using a Punnett Square and pedigree charts.

GLOSSARY

amorph   a gene that does not code express any detectable product

autosomes   chromosomes other than sex chromosomes; humans have 22 pairs

chromosome   nuclear structures composed of DNA; carriers of genetic information

cis   two or more genes on the same chromosome of a homologous pair

codominant   two inherited alleles that are expressed equally

crossing over   physical exchange of genetic material between two chromosomes

DNA   deoxyribonucleic acid; chromosomes are made of this substance

dominant   an allele that is expressed over another gene

dosage   a situation where an antibody reacts more strongly with red cells with a double dose of an antigen (homozygous) than with those that have a single dose of an antigen (heterozygous)

gene   basic unit of inheritance on a chromosome; an area of DNA that controls a trait or characteristic

genetic locus   the location of a specific gene on the chromosome

genetics   a discipline of biology that is the science of heredity

genotype   the genetic constitution of a cell, an organism, or an individual

haplotype   set of genes inherited together because of their proximity to one another on a chromosome

heterozygous   two different alleles for a single trait inherited on homologous chromosomes

homozygous   two identical alleles for a single trait on homologous chromosomes

independent assortment   traits are inherited separately and expressed discretely from one another

independent segregation   transmission of a trait from one generation to the next in a predictable fashion

linkage disequilibrium   genes inherited as a set occur more frequently than would be expected by chance

molecular diagnostics   tests for nucleic acid targets found in various settings in medicine. Three areas of testing are genetics, hematopathology, and infectious disease

pedigree chart   schematic illustration of an inheritance pattern of a specific trait within a family

phenotype   outward expression of inherited characteristics

polymorphism   the expression of more than one phenotype

Punnett Square   a diagram used to determine the probability of frequencies of genotypes and phenotypes in offspring having a particular genotype when two parents are crossed

recessive   an allele that is not expressed when inherited in combination with another allele that is expressed

trans   alleles found on different chromosomes of a homologous pair

zygosity   the similarity or dissimilarity of genes at an allelic position on two homologous chromosomes

INTRODUCTION

The study of Immunohematology focuses on specific antigens and antibodies related to blood group systems. The antigens are related to the red blood cell membrane. The antigens are inherited characteristics. Each individual receives a combination of antigens from his or her parents. The antibodies are created by an immune response to the specific antigen.

The antigens on the red cells may be detected by direct testing methods. Historically, serologic test results were interpreted and genetic information extrapolated from these results. Molecular diagnostics has expanded the knowledge of inheritance and structure of blood group antigens. This knowledge and the development of molecular methodology has provided specific information that has been applied to testing methods as well as providing additional insight into the classification of red cell antigens. Molecular diagnostic test methods and applications were discussed in Chapter 2.

The basic concepts of genetics will be considered in this chapter. An understanding of these genetic concepts will provide a technologist with a basic understanding of the inheritance pattern of red blood cell antigens. Chapters on individual blood group systems will incorporate these basic genetic concepts and apply them to specific blood group systems.

BASIC GENETIC COMPONENTS

DNA

The main building block of genetic material is DNA. DNA, or deoxyribonucleic acid, is composed of four building blocks: adenine, guanine, cytosine, and thymine. These building blocks are bases. Each base attaches to a sugar molecule and a phosphate molecule. These building blocks form strings (like a string of pearls). Following the "stringing" of a single strand, there is a "pairing" process where the partner for each building block attaches and forms a double strand. The pairing that occurs is specific: adenine is partnered with guanine and thymine is partnered with cytosine. Through the process of binding, the strands twist and form a double helix (see Figure 4-1).

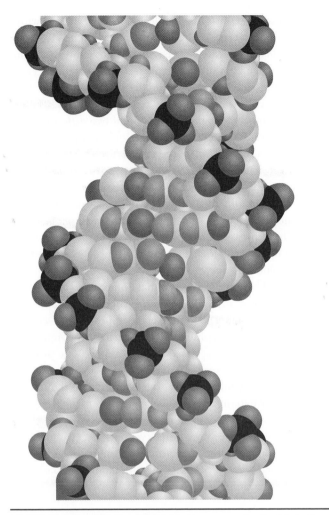

A diagram of a short chain of DNA and its double helical structure

S = Deoxyribose, P = Phosphate, C = Cytosine, G = Guanine, A = Adenine, T = Thymine

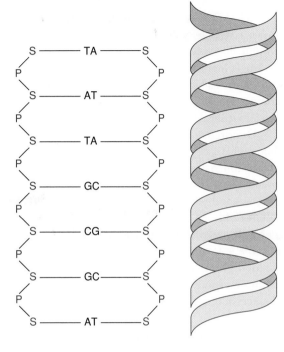

FIGURE 4-1 DNA Double Helix Structure; the double helix structure of DNA is two strands of bases that twist into a helix as the bases pair with one another.
Source: Delmar, Cengage Learning

WEB 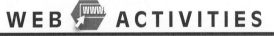 ACTIVITIES

1. Proceed to the Web site http://en.wikipedia.org/wiki/DNA
2. Scroll down to the rotating DNA double helix to visualize the three dimensional aspect of the molecule.

WEB 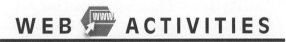 ACTIVITIES

1. Proceed to the Web site http://learn.genetics.utah.edu
2. Choose Basics and Beyond.
3. Choose Build a DNA Molecule.
4. Work through an exercise.
5. Discuss the outcome with the class or your instructor.

Genes and Chromosomes

The double helix DNA forms an actual unit of inheritance, a gene. The gene is an area of DNA that controls a trait or characteristic. The product of the gene is usually a protein or RNA. The location of a specific gene on the chromosome is known as its genetic locus. The alternate gene forms for a specific locus are known as alleles. For example, eye color might be determined by allele: blue, brown, hazel, or green. A single allele for eye color would be inherited from each parent. This simple pattern of inheritance of a single allele from each parent will be applicable for blood group antigen inheritance discussed in later chapters.

When multiple alleles exist at a single locus, this is known as polymorphism. Some systems are more polymorphic than others. A trait that has ten possible alleles at a single locus will be more polymorphic than a trait with four possible alleles. Polymorphism of a locus determines the likelihood that two individuals will be found with an identical allelic composition.

Hundreds of genes comprise each chromosome. Humans have 23 pairs of chromosomes. Each individual inherits one half of his or her chromosomes from each parent. The pairs consist of 22 pairs of autosomal chromosomes and one pair of sex chromosomes. With rare exception, genes that code for blood group antigens are found on the autosomal chromosomes. As outlined in Table 4-1, the genes that code for the production of blood group antigens are found on several different chromosomes. These antigens will be discussed in Chapters 5, 6, and 7.

GENE EXPRESSION

With inherited physical traits, there are certain patterns of expression. Gene expression of simple physical traits typically follows one of three patterns. If one gene is always expressed when found in combination with a second gene, the expressed gene is said to be dominant. In this case, there is a gene that is not expressed. This silent gene can only be expressed if two identical genes are present. This gene is said to be recessive.

A third level of gene expression is codominant. Codominance is the expression of two *different* genes that are inherited at the same loci on a pair of chromosomes. With rare exceptions, blood group systems that will be discussed in the appropriate chapters are expressed as codominant characteristics. For example, when an individual inherits an A gene from one parent and a B gene from the other parent, the genotype is AB. The expressed blood type, or phenotype, will be AB. In this case, neither the A nor B gene is expressed in a dominant manner.

There are also genes that do not code for the production of any detectable product. These genes are labeled an amorph. These genes appear to be recessive. When the amorphic gene is inherited in conjunction with an allele that does produce a detectable product, the detectable product of that allele is expressed. This allele is not dominant over the amorph nor is the amorph recessive to the expressed allele. A common example of an amorph is the gene that codes for the O blood group. When inherited in a homozygous state, two O genes, there is no detectable product. Amorphic genes will be discussed in conjunction with blood group systems where appropriate.

Patterns of Inheritance

Descriptive terms can be combined to produce an expanded terminology for patterns of inheritance. These terms describe the inheritance pattern of a specific trait by the type of chromosome: autosome or sex chromosome. The gene expression is dominant or recessive. For a summary of these terms, refer to Table 4-2.

Zygosity

Zygosity describes the similarity or dissimilarity of genes at an allelic position on two homologous chromosomes. When the genes are identical, they are said to be homozygous. Conversely, when the genes are different, they are said to be heterozygous. Examples using eye color would include an individual with the genotype of brown/blue (heterozygous) and a second individual with the genotype of blue/blue (homozygous).

TABLE 4-1 Chromosome Location for the Most Common Blood Group Antigen Genes	
SYSTEM	CHROMOSOME
ABO	9
MNS	4
P	22
Rh	1
Lutheran	19
Kell	7
Lewis	19
Duffy	1
Kidd	18
H	19
I	6

TABLE 4-2 Patterns of Inheritance

autosomal—inherited on one of the 22 pairs of autosomal chromosomes

sex-linked—inherited on the X chromosome

autosomal dominant—the trait will be expressed whenever the allele is present; found in males and females with the same frequency

autosomal recessive—the trait will only be expressed when the allele is present in the homozygous state; parents may be carriers and not express the trait

sex-linked dominant—trait that will be expressed when it is passed from father to daughter; no father to son transmission

sex-linked recessive—trait is expressed almost exclusively in males; males will inherit this trait from their female parent; hemophilia A is inherited in this manner

The concept of zygosity can be related to antigen strength. There are some gene products that exhibit dosage. When genes are inherited as homozygous (i.e. two identical alleles coding for the same product), the individual is said to have a "double dose" of this product. The expression of the trait or product is stronger when present in the homozygous state. In comparison, an individual that inherits a heterozygous set of genes (i.e. two different alleles coding for two different products) is said to have a "single dose" of each gene since only one gene for each product has been inherited. In this case, the expression of each trait or product is weaker than when two identical genes are inherited.

Dosage is exhibited with some blood group systems. Red cells that are heterozygous for a specific antigen will demonstrate a weaker reaction than the homozygous cells when they react with the specific antisera. This is an important concept in blood group testing. Blood group

systems displaying dosage are summarized in Box 4-1. Dosage will be discussed in relationship to blood groups, as appropriate.

Gene Interactions

Interactions may occur between two genes. Interactions are dependent on location of the inherited genes (see Figure 4-2). The likelihood of an interaction occurring is determined by the proximity of the genes on the autosomal chromosomes. When two genes are inherited on the same chromosomes, their relationship to each other is cis. The genes are describe as trans when inherited on different chromosomes. The steric arrangement of two genes may create a weakened expression of one of the gene products. This is a position effect or steric hindrance of that particular gene product.

An example of gene interaction exists within the Rh blood group system. D and C are specific genes in this system. All genes in the Rh system are inherited on the same chromosome. When C and D genes are inherited trans to each other (C on one chromosome and D on the opposite homologous chromosome), the steric effect will weaken the expression of the D antigen. When the genetic relationship is cis (D and C on the same homologous chromosome), there is no effect on the antigen expression. This will be discussed further in Chapter 6 on the Rh blood group system.

Box 4-1

Red Blood Cell Antigen Systems Displaying Dosage

Rh
Lewis
MNS
Kidd (Jk)
Duffy (Fy)

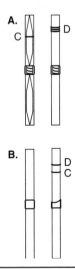

FIGURE 4-2 The concept of cis and trans as related to the Rh blood group system; when C is trans (on the opposite chromosome) to the D gene, the amount of D antigen produced will be depressed.
Source: Delmar, Cengage Learning

GENOTYPE AND PHENOTYPE

For each genetic characteristic, an individual receives a gene from each of his or her parents. The sum total of both genes is known as the individual's genotype. For example, the inheritance of a "blue" gene from the mother and a "blue" gene from the father produces a genotype of "blue/blue." This individual is homozygous for the "blue" allele. An individual that inherits a P gene from his or her mother and a Q gene from his or her father has a genotype of P/Q and is heterozygous for the P/Q alleles. The frequency of each genotype is reflective of the degree of polymorphism within that system. Systems that display a greater degree of polymorphism (i.e. more alleles at each locus) will have a lower frequency for each allele than those that are less polymorphic.

The phenotype is a function of gene expression. The product of a recessive gene will not be expressed in a phenotype. The dominant gene will produce a detectable product, whether in the homozygous or heterozygous state. If the alleles are codominant, both will be expressed in the phenotype. In a system where the alleles are codominant, an individual with a genotype of Z/Y will have a phenotype of ZY while an individual with the genotype Z/Z will have a phenotype of Z. See Figure 4-3 for an example of genotypes and phenotypes.

Example 1: Trait X and Y are codominant

Genotype: XX Phenotype: X

Genotype: XY Phenotype: XY

Genotype: YY Phenotype: Y

Example 2: Trait X is dominant over its allele x

Genotype: XX Phenotype: X

Genotype: Xx Phenotype: X

Genotype: xx Phenotype: x

FIGURE 4-3 Example 1 Demonstrates Phenotypes and Genotypes of Codominant Traits Z and Y.
Example 2 Demonstrates Phenotypes and Genotypes of Trait Z with a recessive allele z.
Source: Delmar, Cengage Learning

PUNNETT SQUARES AND PEDIGREE CHARTS
Punnett Squares

Prediction of possible genotypes and phenotypes in an offspring can be performed using a **Punnett Square**. In order to use the Punnett Square as a predictive tool, the user must know the exact genotype or inferred genotype of both parents. Using this information, a Punnett Square can be set up to predict the likelihood of the genotype and phenotype of the offspring. See Figure 4-4 to see the probabilities of phenotypes and genotypes for offspring when utilizing different genotypes for parents.

Pedigree Charts

A method for tracking family history and inheritance patterns is a **pedigree chart**. This pedigree chart is a

	B	b
B	BB	Bb
b	Bb	bb

Allele B is dominant over allele b

Genotype of both parents: Bb Phenotype of both parents: B

Genotype of offspring: BB = 25%
Bb = 50%
bb = 25%

Phenotype of offspring: B = 75%
b = 25%

FIGURE 4-4 Punnett Square using trait = B with recessive allele = b; genotypes and phenotypes that are produced with two heterozygous parents.
Source: Delmar, Cengage Learning

CRITICAL THINKING ACTIVITY

Create a Punnett Square that represents percentages of genotypes and phenotypes for a trait that is codominant. One parent must be homozygous for the trait. The other parent must be heterozygous for the trait.

visual representation of the parents and the possible genotypes and phenotypes for the offspring. This chart illustrates the inheritance patterns of all the family members and can be used for visualization of inherited traits, including blood group systems. The pedigree chart is useful since it is more detailed than the Punnett Square. See Figure 4-5 for a key for symbols used in the pedigree chart. Figures 4-6 and 4-7 illustrate some samples of pedigree charts.

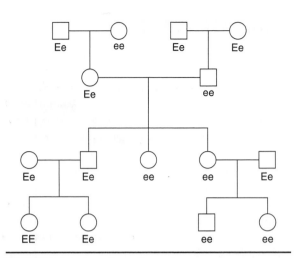

FIGURE 4-6 Sample pedigree chart
Source: Delmar, Cengage Learning

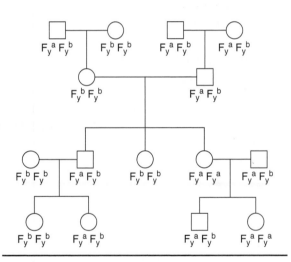

FIGURE 4-7 Sample pedigree chart
Source: Delmar, Cengage Learning

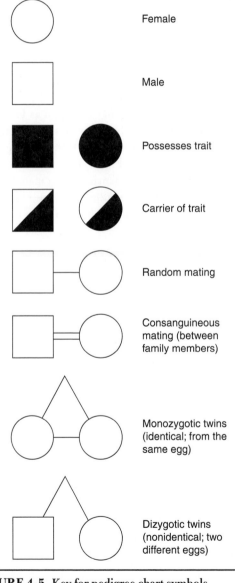

Female	
Male	
Possesses trait	
Carrier of trait	
Random mating	
Consanguineous mating (between family members)	
Monozygotic twins (identical; from the same egg)	
Dizygotic twins (nonidentical; two different eggs)	

FIGURE 4-5 Key for pedigree chart symbols
Source: Delmar, Cengage Learning

WEB ACTIVITIES

1. Proceed to Web site www.dnai.org
2. Choose Applications.
3. Choose Genes in Medicine.
4. Choose Gene Testing.
5. Choose Make a Pedigree.
6. Proceed with the activity.
7. Discuss with your partner or the class.

MENDELIAN GENETICS

Gregor Mendel is recognized as the father of genetics. The results of his genetic research can be directly applied to the inheritance of blood group antigens. He first described the law known as **independent segregation**, which refers to the transmission of a trait between generations in a predictable fashion. Blood group antigens are inherited in this fashion with only rare variations. The outcome of this type of inheritance can be predicted by a Punnett Square (see Figure 4-8).

A second concept of Mendelian genetics is **independent assortment**. Genes located on different chromosomes are inherited separately and expressed discreetly from one another. In most cases, this applies to the blood group antigens. Even blood groups that are inherited on the same **chromosome,** such as Rh and Duffy (Chromosome #1), are inherited as separate entities. One is not dependent on the other for inheritance or expression.

Linkage and Linkage Disequilibrium

Separate **genes** account for the inheritance of blood group system antigens. When genes are in very close proximity, they may be linked. When linkage occurs, the genes are inherited as a unit rather than as separate entities. Some blood group systems have multiple antigens: a separate gene on the same chromosome codes for each antigen. Independent assortment does not occur with antigens that are linked. For example, the two genes that code for M/N and S/s antigen pairs are very close to one another. They are inherited as a "package" from each parent. This "package" is known as a **haplotype.** Linkage can be determined by examining the frequency of the antigen or product in the general population. Two genes are linked if the products appear with greater frequency than expected if inherited independently. This deviance from anticipated frequencies is termed linkage disequilibrium.

A more complex example of linkage disequilibrium occurs within the HLA antigen system. The HLA-A and HLA-B antigens are more closely linked than the M/N and S/s genes. As discussed with the previous example, an individual's haplotype is the set of HLA antigens inherited from one parent. For example, the mother of an offspring may be typed as HLA-A3, A69; B7, B45. This mother may pass along to her progeny the haplotype A3, B7, *or* A69, B45 but never A3, B45, or A69, B7. See Figure 4-10 for an example of this mother's possible offspring when mated with a father with HLA-A1, B27; A28, B35. See Figure 4-9 for an example of linkage disequilibrium using the HLA antigen system.

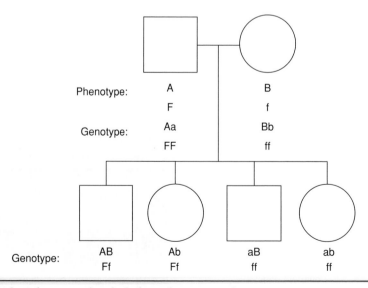

FIGURE 4-8 Pedigree chart demonstrating the independent segregation
Source: Delmar, Cengage Learning

Father	Mother	
	HLA-A3, B7	HLA-A69, B45
HLA-A1, B8	HLA-A3, B7; A1, B8	HLA-A69, B45; A1, B8
HLA-A28, B45	HLA-A3, B7; A28, B45	HLA-A69, B45; A28, B45

FIGURE 4-9 Examples of HLA genotypes of parents and potential offspring
Source: Delmar, Cengage Learning

CRITICAL THINKING ACTIVITY

Diagram the HLA chromosomes of a mother and father who are expecting an offspring. List all of the possible HLA genotypes for the offspring. Using a Punnett Square, predict the possible percentages for each genotype.

One exception to this inheritance pattern would include the occurrence of genetic crossing over. Crossing over is the physical exchange of genetic material between two autosomal chromosomes. See Figure 4-10 for an example.

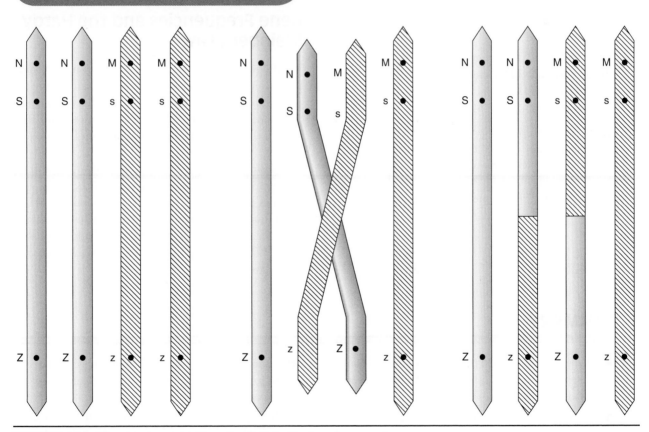

FIGURE 4-10 The crossing over of two closely linked loci on the same chromosome:
1. Original Chromosomes
2. Cross Over of Two Chromosomes Exchanging Genetic Material
3. Final Result after Exchange of Genetic Material
Source: Delmar, Cengage Learning

POPULATION GENETICS

Population genetics is a set of statistical analyses that provides information on genotype and phenotype frequency. The calculations are dependent on the frequency of each of the genes. Calculations of combined phenotype frequency are useful in the blood bank for determining the likelihood of finding units of red cells that are negative for a combination of antigens.

Calculating Phenotype Frequencies

Multiplying the frequency of each of the traits provides a calculation of the combined phenotypic frequency. The likelihood of the chosen traits appearing concurrently is obtained by converting the combined frequency calculation to a ratio.

    Example: Frequency of blond hair and blue eyes occurring together

20% of individuals have blond hair
15% of individuals have blue eyes
0.20 x 0.15 = .030 = 3% or
3/100 individuals will have blond hair and blue eyes

    This same principle is applied to determine the percentage of units of red blood cells that will be negative for a combination of antigens. Two units of blood are required, which are negative, for the Kell (K) and E antigens. The frequencies of these antigens are known.

9% K positive	91% K negative
30% E positive	70% E negative

The calculation is performed using the percentage of donors that would be negative for each of these antigens:

x 0.70 = 0.64
64% of units would be negative for both of these antigens
Theoretically, 6/10 units will be negative for both of these antigens.

Gene Frequencies and the Hardy-Weinberg Law

The frequency of each gene in a population is a known parameter. These populations have been studied and the overall frequency of individual genes determined and published. The Hardy-Weinberg law states that the sum total of the frequency of alleles at a given loci is equal to one.

    Using the simple example of alleles A, B, and O, the approximate gene frequencies of the A, B, and O genes are 28%, 6%, and 66%, consecutively. When the frequencies of these are added together they must equal one. The values of .28, .06, and .66 added together equal 1.0. Therefore, the ABO alleles conform to the Hardy-Weinberg law.

SUMMARY

- Deoxyribonucleic acid (DNA) is the composition of genes. Genes are the basic unit of inheritance and are located on chromosomes.

- DNA is constructed of four bases: adenine, guanine, cytosine, and thymine. These building blocks form strings (like a string of pearls). When two strands of DNA line up next to each other, the bases pair and the strands twist into a double helix.

- Humans have 23 pairs of chromosomes: 22 pairs of autologous chromosomes and one pair of sex chromosomes.

- Inherited traits come from parents. One half of each individual's chromosomes comes from the father and one half from the mother.

- Genes inherited on the same chromosome of a homologous pair are "cis" to each other while those inherited on opposite chromosomes are "trans."

- Inherited genes are an individual's genotype. The expressed characteristics are the individual's phenotype.

- Two or more possible blood group genes may exist at a single locus. Each of these possible genes is labeled an allele.

- The number of possible alleles at each genetic locus determines the polymorphism of the trait. Characteristics with many possible alleles are more polymorphic than those with only a few possible alleles.

- The inheritance of blood group antigens follows the laws of genetics as defined by Gregor Mendel.

- Some genetic traits display dosage. The number of identical genes inherited determines variable

expression of strength of a trait. Homozygous inheritance of the gene results in stronger expression of the trait. Heterozygous inheritance will result in weaker expression. There are blood group antigen systems that exhibit dosage.

- Gene expression may occur as dominant, recessive, or codominant.

- Prediction of possible genotypes and phenotypes can be determined using a Punnett Square.

- Pedigree charts may be used to trace the inheritance of single or multiple traits through descendents of a family.

- Population genetics is used to statistically predict the occurrence of a trait or the absence of that trait.

REVIEW QUESTIONS

1. With regard to inheritance, the relationship of "cis" and "trans" is:
   a. "cis" is when two genes are on the same chromosome; "trans" is when two genes are on different chromosomes
   b. "cis" is when two genes are on different chromosomes; "trans" is when two genes are on the same chromosome
   c. "cis" is when the same allelic gene is present on both chromosomes in a pair; "trans" is when the different allelic genes are present on the two chromosomes in a pair
   d. "cis" is when the different allelic genes are present on the two chromosomes in a pair; "trans" is when the same allelic gene is present on both chromosomes in a pair

2. The genotype of parents of a newborn for characteristic B: Mother Bb and Father Bb. B is dominant and b is recessive. The probability of traits B and b in this newborn is:
   a. 100% B
   b. 25% b; 75% B
   c. 50% b; 50% B
   d. 75% b; 25% B

3. A blood group that is polymorphic has:
   a. multiple possible alleles for antigen production
   b. more than one locus for antigen production

   c. one allele at each locus required for antigen production
   d. multiple antigenic products produced

4. Two genes are close to each other and are inherited together as a unit. The combination of the two genes that are inherited together is known as a:
   a. genotype
   b. haplotype
   c. phenotype
   d. amorph

5. A patient awaiting open heart surgery has three atypical antibodies in his or her serum. In order to obtain compatible blood for transfusion, the technologist must estimate how many units of type specific blood to test. The method for doing this is to:
   a. add the frequencies of each antigen and test that number of units
   b. add the frequencies of each antigen and the ABO frequency and test that number of units
   c. multiply the frequencies of each antigen and use the obtained value to determine how many units to test
   d. multiply the negative frequency for each antigen and use the obtained value to determine how many units to test

6. The Mendelian law that refers to the transmission of a trait from one generation to the next in a predictable fashion is:
   a. genetic crossing over
   b. independent assortment
   c. independent segregation
   d. linkage disequilibrium

7. A new blood group has been discovered with multiple antigens. As the discovering lab is researching the inheritance with familial studies, the technologists discover that some antigens are found together with greater frequency than was predicted based on Mendelian principles. This phenomenon is known as:
   a. genetic crossing over
   b. independent assortment
   c. independent segregation
   d. linkage disequilibrium

8. A mother's HLA genotype is HLA A1, B7; A10, B15. The father's genotype is HLA A3, B12; A11, B17. Choose the possible genotype for an offspring.
   a. HLA A3, B17; HLA A1, B7
   b. HLA A3, B12; HLA A10, B15
   c. HLA A11, B17; HLA A10, B7
   d. HLA A11; B12; A10 B15

9. A blood group system conforms to the Hardy-Weinberg Law. This statement can be interpreted as:
   a. phenotype frequencies are incremental
   b. phenotype frequencies total 1.0 when added
   c. genotype frequencies total 1.0 when added
   d. genotype frequencies equal 100%

10. A trait that is passed from father to daughter is:
    a. autosomal dominant
    b. autosomal recessive

c. sex-linked dominant
d. sex-linked recessive

11. Using the Punnett Square below, choose the correct representation of phenotypes of the offspring. The gene expression is codominant:

	A	B
A	AA	AB
B	AB	BB

    a. 33% AB; 33% A; 33% B
    b. 25% AB; 25% A; 50% B
    c. 50% AB; 25% A; 25% B
    d. 25% AB; 50% A; 25% B

12. Genes located close to each other on the same chromosome are likely to be:
    a. an amorph
    b. linked
    c. subject to crossing over
    d. suppressed

13. In a pedigree, an open circle is the standard symbol for:
    a. male
    b. female
    c. carrier of a trait
    d. twins

14. An individual's genotype is homozygous for a trait while the sibling is heterozygous for the trait. The homozygous individual exhibits a strong expression of the trait while the expression is weakened in the heterozygous sibling. This trait is:
    a. codominant
    b. expressing linkage
    c. displaying dosage
    d. exhibiting position effect

CASE STUDY

1. Two parents have genotypes Dd and Dd. D is a dominant trait and d represents a recessive trait. The parents wish to determine the likelihood that the offspring will be phenotypically "D." Predict the percentage of offspring that will have a phenotype: d.
2. Alleles R and G are codominant. Both alleles produce detectable products. The allele O is an amorph. Parents have genotypes:

RO

GO

a. Determine the percentage of genotypes of each possible combination in the mating of these parents.

b. Determine the percentage of phenotypes of each possible combination in the mating of these parents.

c. What is the percentage of phenotypes that produce a detectable product?

d. What is the percentage of phenotypes that do not produce a detectable product?

REFERENCES

Blaney, Kathy and Howard, Paula. *Basic and Applied Concepts of Immunohematology.* Mosby, Philadelphia, 2000.

Brecher, Mark, editor. *American Association of Blood Banks Technical Manual 15th edition.* AABB, 2005.

Henry, John Bernard, *Clinical Diagnosis and Management by Laboratory Methods.* W. B. Saunders Co. 2001.

Harmening, Denise. *Modern Blood Banking and Transfusion Practices.* F. A. Davis, Philadelphia, 2005.

Issitt PD, Anstee DJ (1998). *Applied Blood Group Serology 4th edition,* Durham, NC, USA: Montgomery Scientific Publications.

McCullough, Jeffrey. *Transfusion Medicine 2nd edition.* Elsevier. 2005.

Reid, Marion E. and Lomas-Francis, Christine. *The Blood Group Antigen: Facts Book.* Elsevier, 2004.

Reid, Marion E, McManus and Zelinski, Teresa. "Chromosome Location of Genes Encoding Human Blood Groups." *Transfusion Medicine Reviews.* Vol. 12, Issue 3. July 1998, pp. 151–161.

Schenkel-Brunner, Helmut. *Human Blood Groups: Chemical and Biochemical Basis of Antigen Specificity.* Springer Wien, 2000.

Turgeon, Mary Louise. *Fundamentals of Immunohematology.* Williams and Wilkins, Media, PA, 1995.

Sheehan, Catherine. *Clinical Immunology, Principles and Laboratory Diagnosis.* Lippincott, Philadelphia, 1997.

ABO Blood Group System

LEARNING OUTCOMES

Upon completion of this chapter, the student should be able to:

- Outline the history of the discovery of the ABO blood group.
- List all antigens and antibodies associated with the ABO and H blood group systems.
- Describe the development of A, B, and H antigens.
- Diagram the chemical structure of A, B, and H antigens.
- State frequency of occurrence of the ABO blood groups.
- Explain the relationship of the H antigen to the ABO blood group system.
- Outline the genetics and biochemistry of the Bombay phenotype.
- Describe forward and reverse ABO blood grouping.
- State test results for ABO forward and reverse grouping for each of the four major ABO groups.
- Describe the antisera and lectins for detection of the A, B, and H antigens.
- List subgroups of A and B.
- Outline the characteristics A, B, and H antibodies.
- Explain the clinical significance of ABH antibodies.
- Describe and categorize ABO discrepancies.
- Create situations where ABO discrepancies can be illustrated.

GLOSSARY

agammaglobulinemia   the absence of gamma globulins in the plasma

Bombay phenotype   phenotype in an individual who does not possess the gene to produce the H antigen; designated O_h

hypogammaglobulinemia   decreased production of gamma globulins; results in decreased quantities in the plasma

isoagglutinin   an antibody present in the plasma of an individual that may cause agglutination of the red blood cells of another individual of the same species

lectin   protein originating from a seed extract; the protein has antibody specificity

monoclonal   originating from a single clone of cells; antibody that will have increased specificity for an antigen as a result of the use of a single clone

nonsecretor   individual who does not produce soluble antigens to be released into the body fluids

oligosaccharide   a polymer composed of simple saccharides (sugars)

secretors   individuals who have a gene causing soluble forms of antigens to be released into the body fluids

transferase   enzyme that catalyzes the transfer of atoms from one chemical compound to another chemical compound

universal donor   group O individual who provides red blood cells that may be transfused to a recipient of any ABO blood group

universal recipient   group AB individual who may receive red blood cells of any ABO blood group

INTRODUCTION

The major blood group systems are the primary focus of blood banking and transfusion therapy. Blood group systems and antibodies form the basis for pretransfusion testing. Antigens and antibodies are the etiologies of hemolytic disease of the fetus and newborn and hemolytic transfusion reactions. Some antigens play a primary role in transplant therapy. Pretransfusion testing focuses on ABO and Rh antigen testing, as well as screening for antibodies in the plasma. Major characteristics of other blood group systems will be outlined in Chapter 7.

INTERNATIONAL SOCIETY OF BLOOD TRANSFUSION (ISBT)

Historically, all blood group antigens have been assigned a name and an abbreviation. The International Society of Blood Transfusion (ISBT) examined this identification system, and a committee was developed in 1980 to standardize blood group terminology. This committee, the Working Party on Terminology for Red Cell Antigens, was originally established to create a terminology system suitable for computer software. This "new" system intended to standardize the original terminology. The committee's criteria required genetic studies and serologic testing prior to an antigen's assignment to a blood group system. The committee's work resulted in the development of 23 blood group systems based on genetics. This text uses the traditional blood group terminology, but will relate the ISBT symbols and numbers to each system as appropriate. See Table 5-1 for a summary of the ISBT Blood Group System.

TABLE 5-1 Summary of ISBT Nomenclature

BLOOD GROUP	ISBT ABBREVIATION	ISBT NUMBER
ABO	ABO	001
MNSs	MNS	002
P	P1	003
Rh	RH	004
Lutheran	LU	005
Kell	KEL	006
Lewis	LE	007
Duffy	FY	008
Kidd	JK	009
Diego	DI	010
Cartwright	YT	011
Xg	XG	012
Scianna	SC	013
Dombrock	DO	014
Colton	CO	015
Landsteiner-Wiener	LW	016
Chido/Rogers	CH/RG	017
Hh	H	018
Kx	XK	019
Gerbich	GE	020
Cromer	CROMER	021
Knops	KN	022
Indian	IN	023
Ok	OK	024
Raph	RAPH	025
JMH	JMH	026

WEB ACTIVITIES

1. Proceed to the Web site http://ibgrl.blood.co.uk
2. Choose ISBT Terminology and Workshops.
3. Choose the link: ISBT Committee on Terminology for Red Cell Surface Antigens.
4. Read the included materials.
5. Discuss the findings with classmates or the instructor.

Box 5-1 Applications of ABO Grouping

Pre-transfusion Testing
Prenatal Testing
Presurgical Testing
Paternity Determination
Transplant Matching
Donor Testing

HISTORICAL PERSPECTIVE OF THE ABO BLOOD GROUP SYSTEM

Karl Landsteiner discovered the ABO blood group system in 1900, which incited the beginning of modern blood banking and transfusion medicine. Landsteiner performed a series of experiments demonstrating serological incompatibilities between individuals. In 1901, using his blood and the blood of his colleagues, he mixed the serum of some individuals with other people's cells. Inadvertently, he was the first person to perform forward and reverse grouping. This series of experiments led him to discover three of the four ABO groups: A, B, and O.

Shortly after Landsteiner's initial discovery, his associates, Alfred von Decastello and Adriano Sturli, discovered the fourth blood group, AB. In later studies, Landsteiner correlated the presence of the ABO antigens on red cells and the reciprocal agglutinating antibodies in the serum of the same individual (e.g. A antigens on red blood cells and anti-B in the serum). This discovery was labeled Landsteiner's Law or Landsteiner's Rule. This rule is the basis for all transfusion therapy as well as a guideline for determining the compatibility of donor and recipients. ABO grouping is one of the primary tests performed in the blood bank. Applications of ABO grouping are summarized in Box 5-1.

Felix Bernstein discovered the group inheritance pattern of multiple alleles at one locus in 1924. This discovery explained the inheritance of ABO blood groups. Additionally, it was established that an individual inherits one ABO gene from each parent. These genes produce the antigens present on the surface of an individual's red cells. Like Landsteiner's discoveries, Bernstein's determination of inheritance patterns of the ABO group has played a major role in the knowledge base for all blood group systems.

In 1930, O. Thompson postulated a four-allele system of inheritance. This proposed system was based on the discovery of Emil Frieherr von Dungern and Ludwig Hirtzfeld in 1911—that the group A antigen can be divided into two subgroups, A_1 and A_2. Thompson expanded this premise and proposed the four allelic genes: A^1, A^2, B, and O. His expansion of Landsteiner's original findings enhanced the ability to provide safe blood for transfusion.

ABO AND H SYSTEM ANTIGENS

ABO Antigens

Antigens detected in blood bank testing, including ABO antigens, are located on the surface of the red blood cell. ABO antigens are also present on lymphocytes, thrombocytes, organs, endothelial cells, and epithelial cells. When Landsteiner performed his mixing tests, he detected the ABO antigens. The biochemistry and structure of ABO antigens are well-established.

Antigens of the ABO system are well-developed in adults. They are detectable at 5 to 6 weeks of gestation. Newborns demonstrate weaker antigens, but ABO antigens are fully developed by two to four years of age. One factor contributing to the difference in ABO antigen strength between newborns and adults is the number of branched oligosaccharides. Adults demonstrate greater numbers of branched chains compared to newborns, who have more linear chains. The branched chains permit attachment of more molecules to determine H antigen specificity. Following H antigen development, the A and/or B specific molecule may be attached.

TABLE 5-2 Comparison of Amount of A Antigen on Adult vs. Cord Cells

PHENOTYPE	NUMBER OF ANTIGEN SITES*
A_1 Adult	810,000 to 1,170,000
A_1 Cord	250,000 to 370,000

*Numbers from Issitt PD, Anstee DJ (1998). Applied Blood Group Serology. 4th edition, Durham, NC, USA: Montgomery Scientific Publications.

Adults have more branched chains and, hence, the ability to add on more terminal sugars and produce more antigens. Newborns and infants have fewer antigen sites on their red cells. See Table 5-2 for a summary of the number of ABO antigens on the surface of the red cells of adults and newborns.

Inheritance of A, B, and H Antigens

As Bernstein discovered, ABO antigens are inherited in a simple Mendelian fashion from an individual's parents. Each individual possesses a pair of genes. Each gene occupies an identical locus on chromosome 9. There are three possible genes that can be inherited. The three genes are: A, B, and O. A and B genes produce a detectable product while the O gene is an amorph that does *not* produce a detectable product. The expression of the A and B genes is codominant. Table 5-3 provides a summary of gene combinations (genotypes) and their expression as blood groups (phenotypes).

The H antigen is required to produce A and/or B antigens. The H gene is also inherited in Mendelian

TABLE 5-3 Summary of ABO Gene Combinations and Phenotypes

GENE COMBINATION	PHENOTYPE
AO	A
AA	A
BO	B
BB	B
AB	AB
OO	O

fashion and occupies a locus on chromosome 19. Each parent contributes one gene, either H or h. The possible genetic combinations are HH, Hh, or hh. Individuals who are genetically either HH or Hh will produce the H antigen, and it can be detected on their red cells. The frequency of occurrence of the H antigen in the Caucasian population is greater than 99.99%. Individuals inheriting an hh genotype do not produce the H antigen and have the **Bombay phenotype,** O_h. The plasma of an individual with a Bombay phenotype frequently demonstrates an anti-H.

Biochemical and Structural Development of A, B, and H Antigens

Expression of A, B, and H genes does not result in the direct production of antigens. Rather, each gene codes for the production of an enzyme known as a **transferase**.

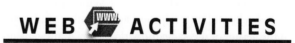

WEB ACTIVITIES

TABLE 5-4 Summary of Transferase Enzymes for ABH Antigen Production	
GENE	**TRANSFERASE**
H	α-L-fucosyltransferase
A	α-3-N-acetyl-D-galactosaminyl Transferase
B	α-3-D-acetyl-D-galactosyl Transferase
O	No Transferase Produced

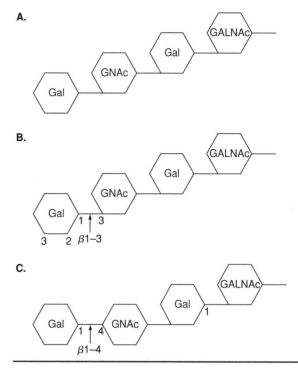

FIGURE 5-1 The structural differences of common oligosaccharide chains that serve as precursors for ABH antigens.
a. Common Precursor Chain.
b. Type 1 Oligosaccharide Chain—β 1–3 linked of D-galactose.
c. Type 2 Oligosaccharide Chain—β 1–4 linked of D-galactose.
(Key: Gal = D Galactose; GALNAc = N-acetyl-glucosamine)
Adapted from Turgeon, M. Fundamentals of Immunohematology. *1995.*

Each transferase catalyzes the transfer of a carbohydrate molecule to an oligosaccharide chain. The attached carbohydrate provides antigenic specificity. The O gene codes for an enzymatically inactive protein and, hence, no antigen is produced. A summary of these transferase molecules is found in Table 5-4.

Common Blood Group Structure

The common structure of A, B, and H antigens is an oligosaccharide chain attached to either a protein or a lipid molecule. This common structure is utilized as the basic structural component for multiple antigens. Multiple antigen systems built from a common structure implies that the related systems will impact each other. The impacts and interactions of these systems will be discussed, as appropriate, in the text. The antigens incorporating this basic structure are summarized in Box 5-2.

The structure of the common oligosaccharide is carbohydrate molecules linked either in simple linear forms or in a complex structure with a high degree of branching. There are two variations of oligosaccharide chains. The structural difference is in the attachment of the terminal sugar molecules (see Figure 5-1).

Type 1 and type 2 chains are differentiated by the attachment of the terminal sugars. This is illustrated in Figure 5-2. A type 1 chain is formed by β 1→3

Box 5-2 Antigens with a Common Basic Structure	
ABH	Lewis
P	I/i

linkage of the number 1 carbon of D-galactose to the number 3 carbon of the *N*-acetylglucosamine. A type 2 chain is formed by a β 1→4 linkage of the number 1 carbon of D-galactose to the number 4 carbon of the *N*-acetylglucosamine. Type 1 chains are found in body fluids and secretions, while type 2 chains are found on the red blood cell membrane.

Development of H Antigen

The H allele codes for the transferase, L-fucosyltransferase. This enzyme catalyzes the formation of the H antigen by transfer of L-fucose to either type

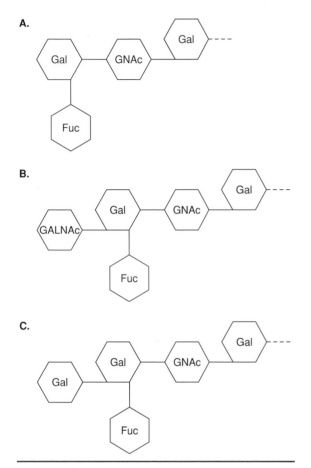

A.

B.

C.

FIGURE 5-2
a. The H antigen confers its specificity with the attachment of L-fucose as the terminal sugar.
b. Group specificity is conferred by the attachment of N-acetyl-D-galactosamine to the H antigen oligosaccharide chain.
c. Group B specificity is conferred by the attachment of D-galactose to the H antigen oligosaccharide chain. (Key: Fuc = L Fucose; Gal = D Galactose; GALNAc = N-acetyl-glucosamine)
Adapted from Turgeon, M. Fundamentals of Immunohematology. 1995.

one or type two oligosaccharide chains. The L-fucose is the immunodominant sugar for the H antigen. It is the sugar that confers antigenic specificity to the H antigen. The H antigen serves as a precursor for A and B antigens. The h allele is an amorph and does not produce a detectable product. See Figure 5-2 for the H antigen structure.

Development of A and B Antigens

The H antigen oligosaccharide chain serves as a precursor for both the A and B antigens. The A and B alleles each code for a transferase that attaches a sugar molecule to the terminal end of the H antigen oligosaccharide chain, which forms either the A or B antigen. The A allele codes for N-acetylgalactosamine transferase. This transferase attaches N-acetyl-D-galactosamine to the H antigen forming the A antigen. The B allele codes for D-galactosyltransferase. This transferase attaches D-galactose to the H antigen forming the B antigen. Structures of A and B antigens are presented in Figure 5-3. The product of the O allele is an enzymatically inactive protein. Hence, this allele produces no detectable antigen. Conversely, group O cells contain the most H antigen. This results from no conversion of H antigen to A and/or B antigens. In comparison, group A_1B cells have the least amount of H antigen since quantitatively the most H is converted to A_1 and B antigens. See Figure 5-3 for a continuum of the amount of H antigen found on the cells of various ABO groups.

Secretor Status

Soluble forms of A, B, and H antigens may be found in body secretions. The ability of a person to secrete water-soluble substances is controlled by independently inherited genes. The secretor gene is the or FUT2 (α 1,2 fucosyltransferase) gene on chromosome 19. The allele, se, is amorphic. At least one Se gene is required for the secretory property to be expressed. Persons with soluble ABH antigen (SeSe or Sese) in their secretions are **secretors**. While those with no A or B antigens in secretions (sese) are **nonsecretors**.

Continuum of H Antigen in the Common Blood Groups		
Most H	$O>A_2>A_2B>B>A_1>A_1B$	LEAST H

FIGURE 5-3 A continuum of H antigen on the red cells of the common blood groups. This continuum begins with no conversion of H antigen in group O individuals. Each blood group listed in the continuum contains less of the H antigen. The blood group with the least amount H antigen detectable on the cells is group A_1B in which the most H antigen conversion occurs. A_1B red cells have the least amount of H antigen on the cell surface.
Source: Delmar, Cengage Learning

CHAPTER 5 ABO Blood Group System

Approximately 78% of the population possesses at least one Se gene. An individual that possesses a Se gene will secrete A, B, and/or H antigen(s) dependent on possession of the corresponding ABH gene(s). The enzyme produced by Se acts predominantly on Type 1 chains and almost exclusively in the secretory glands. This contrasts with the enzyme produced by the H gene that acts almost entirely on Type 2 chains and predominantly on the red cell membranes.

The Se gene codes for the production of the transferase, L-fucosyltransferase. This enzyme promotes the transfer of L-fucose to the terminal galactose of type 1 chains and forms H substance in the secreted fluids. The A and B transferase enzymes are found in the secretions of A and B persons regardless of their secretor status. Therefore, when the H substance is found in secretions, A and/or B antigens will be formed if the corresponding transferase enzymes are present. Examples of fluids where A, B, and H substances can be detected are summarized in Table 5-5.

TABLE 5-5 Summary of Fluids in Which ABH Substances Can Be Found

Saliva
Sweat
Tears
Semen
Serum
Amniotic Fluid

CRITICAL THINKING ACTIVITY

Research additional body fluids (e.g. pleural fluid, etc.). Determine if ABH antigens are present in each of these fluids. Determine which body fluids will never contain secreted antigens. Explain *why* secreted antigens will never be in the previously listed body fluid(s).

A and B Subgroups

A_1 and A_2 Subgroups

Group A antigens can be differentiated into multiple subgroups. The two major subgroups are A_1, 80% of Group A individuals, and A_2, 20% of group A individuals. Persons typing as AB can be divided into the same percentages of A antigen presentation. A_1B make up approximately 80% and A_2B are 20% of all AB individuals. The remaining group A individuals fall into one of many minor subgroups.

A_1 and A_2 antigens have qualitative and quantitative differences. These differences are summarized in Table 5-6. When red cells are qualitatively tested for antigens, A_1 and A_2 red cells have differing amounts of antigens on the cell surface (see Table 5-6). The A^1 gene produces a transferase that has a greater ability to convert H antigen to A antigen than the A^2 gene. This quantitative difference results from the kinetics of the reaction catalyzed by each of the transferases.

TABLE 5-6 Quantitative and Qualitative Differences in A_1 and A_2 Red Cells*

	GROUP A_1	GROUP A_2
Qualitative Differences		
Reaction with Anti-A in Forward Grouping	4+	4+
Number of Antigen Sites-Adults	1,000,000	250,000
Number of Antigen Sites-Newborn	300,000	140,000
Quantitative Differences		
Reaction with Anti-A_1	Positive	Negative
Anti-A_1 in Serum	Absent	May Be Present
α-3-N-acetyl-D-galactosaminyl Transferase Activity	Normal Level	Diminished Activity

*Adapted from Henry, John Bernard, Clinical Diagnosis and Management by Laboratory Methods. W. B. Saunders Co. 2001.

There are also differences in the quantity of transferase produced. Individuals exhibiting the A_1 phenotype have five to ten times more transferase than those with an A_2 phenotype. Two mutations have been detected that produce this A_2 phenotype. These are: a Pro-156Leu substitution and a single nucleotide deletion (nucleotide 1060). These substitutions are responsible for the decreased enzyme activity that differentiates A_2 from A_1 cells.

The antigens also differ qualitatively. A_2 antigens are composed mainly of linear oligosaccharide chains while the A_1 cells have a greater number of branched chains. In routine testing, this qualitative difference is not detectable but can be determined biochemically.

Typing of A_1 and A_2 cells is unremarkable with routine antisera. Both A_1 and A_2 cells will react equally with anti-A and anti-A,B. The lectin, *Dolichos biflorus*, is used to obtain an extract with anti-A_1 specificity. *Dolichos biflorus* will react specifically with A_1 cells and will be negative with A_2 cells. ABO grouping will be discussed, in detail, later in this chapter.

A_2 individuals can develop antibodies to the A_1 antigens. The typical reaction pattern of reverse grouping in a group A individual is no agglutination with the A cells (no anti-A) and agglutination with B cells (anti-B present). In A_2 persons with an anti-A_1, the A cells will also be agglutinated in the reverse grouping. This discrepancy should be confirmed by testing the red cells with the *Dolichos biflorus* lectin. See Table 5-7 for a summary of forward and reverse grouping results of A_1 and A_2 subgroups.

Additional A subgroups

Occurring subgroups of A exist less frequently. These subgroups are also genetically controlled. Subgroups of A include A_{intr}, A_3, A_x, A_m, A_{end}, A_{el}, and A_{bantu}. These subgroups follow the patterns of A_1 and A_2 with regard to quantitative and qualitative antigenic differences.

The cells of these subgroups exhibit fewer antigen sites on their surface while many demonstrate an anti-A_1 in the plasma. Adsorption and elution techniques may be necessary for detection of antigens on the surface of red cells. These techniques will be discussed in detail in Chapter 8.

The classification of subgroups is based on reactions of the patient's red cells with anti-A, anti-B, anti-A,B, and anti-A_1 antisera as well as A_1, A_2, and B reverse grouping cells. While testing for subgroups of A, a mixed field agglutination reaction may be noted. A_3 cells will demonstrate this pattern of agglutination with anti-A and anti-A,B. A summary of test reactions for subgroups of A can be found in Table 5-8.

Subgroups of B

Subgroups of B are very rare and encountered less frequently than subgroups of A. The methods of detection and classification are similar to those used for the subgroups of A. The major subgroups of B are summarized in Table 5-9.

ABO ANTIBODIES

"Antibodies directed against ABO antigens are the most important antibodies in transfusion medicine." This is a profound, but true statement. For this reason, ABO antibodies require detailed description.

The ABO blood group presents a unique situation in Immunohematology. It is the only example of a blood group where *each* individual produces antibodies to antigens not present on the red cells. These ABO antibodies were originally thought to be natural antibodies formed with no apparent antigenic stimulus. Since the antibodies are not stimulated by exposure to red cells, they may also be considered non-red cell stimulated antibodies. However, some form of an antigenic stimulus must exist. The proposed mechanism is

TABLE 5-7 Reaction Patterns for Forward Grouping of A_1 and A_2 Cells

BLOOD GROUP	ANTI-A	ANTI-B	ANTI-A,B	ANTI-A$_1$
A_1	4+	Negative	4+	4+
A_2	4+	Negative	4+	Negative

TABLE 5-8 Serological Reactions of Subgroups of A

BLOOD GROUP	ANTI-A	ANTI-B	ANTI-A,B	ANTI-A$_1$	ANTI-A$_1$ IN SERUM	ANTI-A IN SERUM
A$_1$	4+	Negative	4+	4+	negative	Negative
A$_2$	4+	Negative	2+	Negative	+/−	Negative
A$_3$	2+ mf*	Negative	2+ mf*	Negative	+/−	Negative
A$_{int}$	4+	Negative	4+	2+	Negative	Negative
A$_x$	Negative	Negative	1-2+	Negative	−/+	−/+
A$_m$	+/−	Negative	+	Negative	Negative	Negative
A$_{end}$	+ mf	Negative	+mf	Negative	+/−	Negative

*mf = mixed field

TABLE 5-9 Subgroups of B

BLOOD GROUP	ANTI-B	ANTI-A,B	ANTI-A$_1$ IN SERUM	ANTI-A IN SERUM	ANTI-B IN SERUM
B	4+	4+	+	+	Negative
B$_3$	2+ mf*	2+ mf*	+	+	Negative
B$_x$	+	+	+	+	+/−
B$_m$	Negative	Negative	+	+	Negative
B$_{el}$	Negative	Negative	+	+	+/−

*mf = mixed field

environmental. These "naturally occurring" substances resemble A and B antigens and stimulate the production of complementary antibodies to the antigens that are not present on the red cell surface. For a summary of the antigens and antibodies found in each blood group, refer to Table 5-10.

Newborns have no ABO antibodies. When newborns are tested, only a forward group is performed. Newborns may exhibit passive ABO antibodies that have crossed the placental barrier. Reverse grouping of a newborn or umbilical cord serum indicates the blood group of the mother. The child will begin antibody production, and have a detectable titer, at three to six months of age. ABO antibody production peaks at age five to ten years of age and continues in immunocompetent individuals throughout life. Titers

TABLE 5-10 Antigens and Antibodies in ABO Blood Groups

BLOOD GROUP	ANTIGENS	ANTIBODIES
A	A	Anti-B
B	B	Anti-A
O	Neither A or B	Anti-A, anti-B, and anti-A,B
AB	A and B	Neither anti-A or anti-B

begin to wane in the elderly. Additional situations that exhibit reduced ABO antibody titers are summarized in Table 5-11.

TABLE 5-11 Conditions with Decreased Levels of ABO Antibodies

- Age related
  - Newborns and young infants
  - Elderly individuals
- Immunodeficient individuals
  - Congenital conditions
    - Congenital hypogammaglobulinemia
    - Congenital agammaglobulinemia
- Immunosuppressed patients
  - Immunosuppressive therapy
  - Chronic lymphocytic leukemia
  - Bone marrow transplant
  - Multiple myeloma
  - Acquired hypogammaglobulinemia
  - Acquired agammaglobulinemia

Immunoglobulin Class

ABO antibodies are typically isoagglutinins. They are saline agglutinins with optimal reactivity at 4°C. These naturally occurring antibodies are mostly IgM isotype, but IgG and IgA classes of ABO antibodies have been detected. The development of IgG antibodies occurs without apparent antigen exposure via transfusion of incompatible red cells or fetal maternal incompatibility.

Anti-A,B

Group O individuals do not have A or B antigens on their cells. Consequently, they produce anti-A, anti-B, and anti-A,B. Anti-A,B is an antibody that has cross-reactivity with A and B cells. This cross-reactive antibody detects a common molecular structure in both antigens. Although the antibody reacts with both antigens, it cannot be divided into individual components (i.e. anti-A plus anti-B). Anti-A,B is used as a third antisera in forward grouping. Anti-A,B is not required in forward grouping. Since it is a valuable reagent for determining subgroups of A and B, anti-A,B is often included as a routine part of forward grouping. Monoclonal anti-A,B have replaced the use of human anti-A, B in forward grouping (see Tables 5-8 and 5-9).

Anti-A₁

As per Landsteiner's Law, group B and O individuals produce anti-A. This anti-A can be separated by absorption procedures. These absorption procedures can produce two components of the antibody found in group B and O individuals. These components are anti-A and anti-A$_1$. The anti-A$_1$ antibody reacts specifically with A$_1$ cells and not with A$_2$ cells or cells from other subgroups of A. Like other ABO antibodies, this antibody reacts optimally at room temperature or colder. Anti-A$_1$ is not considered clinically significant as it relates to transfusion. It is, however, significant when it causes incompatible crossmatches at the immediate spin phase. Antibodies to other A subgroups, such as A$_2$, are not produced. As discussed previously, these subgroups have the A antigen but in reduced amounts. Therefore, transfusion of A$_1$ individuals with A$_2$ cells will not stimulate the production of anti-A$_2$ since both A$_1$ and A$_2$ individuals have the A antigen in common.

Clinical Significance of ABO Antibodies

ABO antibodies are capable of causing both Hemolytic Disease of the Fetus and Newborn (HDFN) and Hemolytic Transfusion Reactions (HTR). These issues explain the clinical significance of "naturally occurring" antibodies.

HDFN usually presents itself with a maternal antibody of an IgG isotype that corresponds to an antigen on the surface of the baby's red cells. The most common scenario is a group O mother and a group A baby. ABO hemolytic disease may affect a woman's first pregnancy. This is in contrast to Rh HDFN where the antigenic stimulation usually occurs in the first pregnancy and subsequent antigen-positive newborns are affected.

Hemolytic transfusion reaction occurs when a recipient is transfused with red cells that are an ABO group incompatible with the antibodies in his or her serum. Because of the complement-binding ability of the ABO antibodies, this is always a life-threatening situation. As the recipient antibodies react with the incompatible red cells, complement is activated and *in vivo* hemolysis, agglutination, and red blood cell destruction occurs. The mechanisms and outcomes of hemolytic transfusion reactions will be discussed further in Chapter 12.

ABO compatibility is also significant in solid organ transplantation. For most organs, an ideal scenario for transplant is an ABO compatible solid organ. Post-transfusion antibody titer, and pheresis to reduce the titer of the incompatible antibody, will assist in achieving a positive outcome when an ABO incompatible organ is transplanted.

FORWARD AND REVERSE GROUPING

ABO Forward Grouping

As previously described, ABO antigens are present on the surface of red cells, while the antibodies are found in plasma or serum. Routine testing for antigens and antibodies is performed as a forward and reverse grouping, respectively.

The forward grouping is a test performed for antigens using known antisera with patient's cells that may contain unknown antigens. Test methods for forward grouping include tube typing, gel technology, automation, and solid phase technology. Refer to Chapter 2 for an overview of these methods.

ABO forward grouping with tube typing uses a saline suspension of 3 to 5% washed patient red cells. These cells are combined in a 1:1 ratio with commercial antisera. See Sample Procedure 5-1 for an overview of ABO forward grouping. When utilizing gel technology, the cell suspension consists of a 0.8% suspension of washed patient cells in the manufacturer's recommended diluent. These cells are applied to the anti-A and anti-B

SAMPLE PROCEDURE 5-1

ABO FORWARD GROUPING: TUBE TYPING METHOD

Procedure

1. Prepare a 3 to 5% suspension of patient's red cells.
2. Label three small test tubes with the patient's name and identification number.
3. Each of these tubes should then be labeled as follows:
   First tube: "Anti-A"
   Second tube: "Anti-B"
   Third tube: "Anti-A,B"
   NOTE: Labeling should be done with care since clerical errors are the most frequent errors in the blood bank.
4. Check clarity and expiration date on antisera; record information.
5. To each of these tubes, add one drop of the corresponding antisera.
   NOTE: Use a free floating drop.
        Do not touch the dropper to the side of the tube.
        Always add antisera before cells.
6. Using a transfer pipet, add one drop of the well-mixed 5% cell suspension to each of these three tubes.
   NOTE: Use a free floating drop.
        Do not touch the pipet to the side of the tube.
7. Gently mix all tubes.
8. Serofuge all three test tubes for 15 seconds.
   NOTE: Time may vary with each serofuge. Check the calibration information for each individual serofuge.
9. Remove each tube and examine for hemolysis.
10. Using an agglutination viewer, gently resuspend each cell button, and examine for agglutination.
11. Grade each reaction and record the results.

SAMPLE PROCEDURE 5-2

1. Prepare a 0.8% suspension of test cells in the appropriate diluent.
2. Choose a gel card for ABO forward grouping and label with patient identification.
3. Add 10µl of cell suspension of test cells to each microtube on the card.
4. Centrifuge the card.
5. Evaluate each microtube for agglutination. Record and interpret results.

CRITICAL THINKING ACTIVITY

Research the manufacturing process for ABO antisera. Write a procedure for making a substitute as if you were doing missionary work in a remote area and had run out of the commercial sera.

tubes of the gel card. In both methods, centrifugation is applied and results interpreted. See Sample Procedure 5-2 for an example of forward grouping using gel testing.

Antisera

When performing tube typing, three antiseras are available for ABO forward grouping. These antiseras are summarized in Table 5-12. Forward grouping may be performed using all three, or in the case of patients or transfusion recipients anti-A and anti-B are used. Antisera are combined in a 1:1 ratio with the patient's cell suspension. The reaction patterns are summarized in Table 5-12. When evaluating reaction patterns, the antigens on the cells are reacting with the specific antibodies in the antisera. Upon examination of Table 5-12 it is clear that a group A individual has the A antigen and reacts with both anti-A and anti-A,B while a group O will react with no antisera since these cells have neither A nor B antigens.

TABLE 5-12   Reaction Patterns for ABO Groups

BLOOD GROUP	ANTI-A	ANTI-B	ANTI-A,B
A	Positive	Negative	Positive
B	Negative	Positive	Positive
AB	Positive	Positive	Positive
O	Negative	Negative	Negative

The inclusion of anti-A,B antisera in forward grouping is significant. It is not a mixture of anti-A and anti-B, but rather a separate antibody that will react with both the A and B antigens. It is included in forward grouping and serves two purposes:

1. To confirm the results of the anti-A and anti-B (see Table 5-12).
2. To detect weak subgroups of A and B. These subgroups may demonstrate a positive reaction with anti-A,B but not with anti-A and anti-B.

Molecular Testing

As molecular diagnostic testing continues to develop, applications to ABO forward grouping may become commonplace in the laboratory. Molecular testing has the potential to solve typing discrepancy in recently or chronically transfused patients. These patients present unique challenges to the blood bank, since typing through traditional methods frequently produces discrepant or erroneous results. Polymerase chain reaction (PCR) methods have been proven to be more reliable then traditional serological methods in resolution of typing discrepancies in recipients that have been transfused within the last 30 days. As PCR test results are available within several hours, this testing method presents a promising future for resolution of discrepancies that were previously major compatibility challenges.

Reverse Grouping

ABO reverse grouping uses patient plasma combined in a 2:1 ratio with commercially prepared cells. The cells are packaged in sets of two (A_1 and B) or three (A_1, A_2, and B). The cells are used to detect unknown antibodies in the plasma. The result is evaluated by examining the tubes for hemolysis and agglutination. Agglutination reactions are graded according to the criteria outlined in Chapter 1.

SAMPLE PROCEDURE 5-3

1. Label two 10 × 75 test tubes with the patient's name and identification number.

2. Label one of the tubes A and one of them B.
   NOTE: Labeling is a crucial step in the blood typing procedure. Fatal errors are made when clerical errors occur.

3. Add two drops of serum to each tube.

4. To the appropriate tube, add one drop of well-mixed reagent red cells.
   NOTE: Before adding reagent red cells, be certain they are well-mixed and that all of the cells are resuspended from the bottom of the vial.

5. Gently mix the two tubes.

6. Serofuge for 15 seconds.
   NOTE: The time for centrifugation may vary with each serofuge. Check the calibration on the serofuge being used for testing.

7. Remove each tube and examine for hemolysis.

8. Using an agglutination viewer, gently resuspend each cell button and examine for agglutination.

9. Grade and record each reaction.

See Sample Procedure 5-3 for a sample procedure for reverse grouping. Interpretations of reverse grouping in the four major blood groups are summarized in Table 5-13.

Recall that antibodies present in the test plasma correspond to antigens missing on the red cell surface. For example, group A has the A antigen and the B antigen is not present. The corresponding B antibody is demonstrated in the group A individual's plasma. When the plasma reacts with the reagent red blood cells, the B antibody reacts with specific antigens on the B cells, but not antigens on the A cells. Therefore, a positive reaction will be seen in the B tube, but not in the A tube (see Table 5-13).

TABLE 5-13 Interpretation of Reverse Grouping Test Results

BLOOD GROUP	A₁ CELLS	B CELLS
A	Negative	Positive
B	Positive	Negative
O	Positive	Positive
AB	Negative	Negative

WEB ACTIVITIES

1. Proceed to the Web site http://interactivehuman.blogspot.com

2. Search for Blood Typing.

3. Using each of the four major ABO groups, perform typing.

SELECTION OF ABO GROUP FOR TRANSFUSION OF BLOOD AND BLOOD PRODUCTS

Selection of ABO group for transfusion of blood or blood components is often simple, but may prove difficult when blood supply is low or the patient is serologically complicated. Therefore, it is imperative for technologists to be knowledgeable in ABO substitution.

The ideal scenario is to transfuse ABO identical blood components to any recipient. When ABO specific components are not available, or when the recipient presents with atypical antibodies in his or her plasma,

ABO substitution may be required. Guidelines for ABO substitution will follow in this section. The discussion of atypical antibodies in the recipient's plasma and matching antigen appropriate units will take place in later chapters.

Group O individuals are labeled **universal donors**. Group O red cells lack A and B antigens; these cells may be transfused to a recipient of any ABO group. Note, however, that the plasma may only be transfused to a group O individual. This plasma contains both anti-A and -B and would cause a hemolytic transfusion reaction in any recipient with these antigens. Group O individuals may, however, receive plasma products from *any* ABO group since they have no A or B antigens. Group A or B recipients may receive ABO specific *or* group O cells. Conversely, they may only receive plasma products of their own type *or* group AB, since it has no anti-A or -B.

In contrast, group AB individuals are **universal recipients** for red cells. Group AB recipients may receive red cells of any ABO group because they lack A and B antibodies. However, AB individuals may only receive plasma from an AB donor since it contains neither A nor B antibodies. If A and B antibodies were present, a reaction would occur between A and B antigens on the recipient's red blood cells. Table 5-14 summarizes possible red cell and plasma substitutions for each blood group.

ABO DISCREPANCIES

ABO discrepancies are infrequent but present a technical issue for testing personnel. Discrepancies are detected by comparing the forward and reverse grouping. If forward and reverse grouping do not produce the anticipated matched results, further investigation is warranted.

Resolution of an ABO discrepancy begins with a review of all technical and clerical steps. Careful observation and detailed recording of all serological reactions is imperative to resolve any ABO discrepancies. Careful review of past typing and transfusion history, as well as past and current diagnosis, may provide clues to the origin of the problem. See Table 5-15 for a summary of technical and clerical issues that may result in an ABO discrepancy. Once clerical steps have been reviewed, and test results confirmed by repeat testing, if appropriate, the technologist may classify a discrepancy as plasma or cell related. Plasma or antibody related discrepancies are more common than those that are red cell associated.

TABLE 5-15 Possible Technical and Clerical Issues for Potential ABO Typing Errors

Clerical Issues
Mislabeled specimen or testing tubes
Improper recording of test results
Improper recording of test reactions
Deleted procedural step

Technical Issues
Not following manufacturer's instructions
Missed or underinterpreted weak reactions
Incorrect interpretation of serological reactions
Missing or incorrect reagents in test samples
Equipment malfunction; centrifuge time or RPMs not correct
Contaminated antisera or cells
Incorrect cell suspension

TABLE 5-14 Red Cell and Plasma Substitution for ABO Blood Groups

BLOOD GROUP	RED CELL PRODUCTS FOR SUBSTITUTION	PLASMA PRODUCTS FOR SUBSTITUTION
A	O	AB
B	O	AB
AB	A, B, or O	None
O	None	A, B, or AB

ABO Discrepancies Associated with the Forward Grouping

Forward grouping discrepancies may be divided into the three categories summarized in Table 5-16. Each of these categories will be reviewed in the following sections.

Examples of ABO Discrepancies
Weak or Missing Antigens

Subgroups of A or B may initially present themselves as an ABO discrepancy. Forward and reverse grouping results do not "match." Discrepant forward and reverse grouping seen in a subgroup of A may appear as:

Anti-A	Anti-B	Anti-A,B	A_1 Cells	B Cells
0	0	1+	0	3+

TABLE 5-16 Forward Grouping Discrepancies

1. Clinical conditions with a weak or missing antigen:
   A or B subgroup
   Leukemias and other related disease states
   Presence of excess blood group soluble substances
2. Clinical conditions with an unexpected antigen:
   Acquired B antigen
   B (A) phenotype
   Altered antigens
   Antibody coated red cells
   Rouleaux
3. Mixed cell populations
   Post transfusion with non-type specific blood
   Bone marrow transplant
   A_3 genotype

Evaluation:

1. The forward grouping does not present with the usual reaction patterns.
   a. Reactions are weaker than typically observed with ABO forward and reverse grouping.
   b. No reactions in either anti-A or anti-B while anti-A,B presents with a weak reaction.

2. Reverse grouping presents as a group A, although B cells present with a weaker reaction than typically observed in reverse grouping.

Additional Testing:

1. Adsorption and elution studies may be performed to determine the presence of anti-A attached to the patient's cells.

2. Prolonged incubation of the forward grouping may present with stronger and more consistent reactions.

Presence of Unexpected Antigens

Unexpected antigens serve as a rare and confusing ABO typing discrepancy. The acquired B phenomenon is encountered in association with specific clinical conditions. Diseases of the gastrointestinal tract, cancer of the colon or bowel, and gram-negative sepsis are clinical conditions that classically produce this phenomenon. The biochemical mechanism is deacetylation of N-acetylgalactosamine, the group A specific sugar, to produce galactosamine which resembles galactose, the group B specific sugar. Cross-reaction with anti-B occurs.

Anti-A	Anti-B	Anti-A,B	A_1 Cells	B Cells
4+	1+	4+	0	4+

Evaluation:

1. The forward grouping does not present with the usual pattern.
   a. Reactions of the ABO forward and reverse grouping do not match.
   b. Strength of the patient's cells with anti-B is weak in comparison to reactions with of anti-A and anti-A,B.

2. Reverse grouping presents as a group A in spite of the reaction of the patient's cells with anti-B.

Additional Testing and Clinical History:

1. Check clinical and medical history. Conditions such as colon cancer may produce the acquired B.

2. Test the patient's cells with autologous serum. The acquired B antigen will not react with the patient's own anti-B.

3. Use of polyclonal antisera may provide more consistent results.

A similar situation exists with a B(A) phenotype. This is a scenario that has been observed more frequently since the introduction of monoclonal typing sera. Monoclonal anti-B may detect small quantities of A antigens on the cells of group B individuals. This situation represents the reverse of the acquired B. Sample reactions are demonstrated below:

Anti-A	Anti-B	Anti-A,B	A_1 Cells	B Cells
1+	4+	4+	4+	0

Evaluation:

1. The forward grouping does not present with the typical pattern.
   a. Reactions of the ABO forward and reverse grouping do not match.
   b. Strength of the patient's cells with anti-A is weak as compared to those of anti-B and anti-A,B.
2. Reverse grouping presents as a group B in spite of the reaction of the patient's cells with anti-A.

Additional Testing and Clinical History:

1. Review the patient's diagnosis and past transfusion history.
2. Determine if the reagents used were monoclonal or polyclonal.
3. Retest the patient's cells with an alternate monoclonal antisera to achieve more consistent results.

Mixed Field Reactions

Mixed field reactions are characteristically observed when two distinct populations of cells are detected in a single individual. Clinical situations exhibiting this phenomenon include:

- Recipient of non-ABO specific transfusion (e.g. group A, B, or AB who received group O red cells).
- Mother with a large fetal-maternal hemorrhage.
- Recent bone marrow or stem cell transplant.
- A_3 or B_3 blood group.

Anti-A	Anti-B	Anti-A,B	A_1 Cells	B Cells
2+mf	0	2+mf	0	3+

Evaluation:

1. The forward grouping does not present with the usual pattern.
   a. Reactions of the ABO forward grouping present with a mixed field pattern.
   b. Reaction strength of the patient's cells with anti-A and anti-A,B is weak when compared to the expected results.
2. Reverse grouping presents as a group A.

Additional Testing and Clinical History:

Review the patient's diagnosis and past transfusion history. This is most likely a group A patient who was transfused with group O red cells.

ABO Discrepancies Associated with Reverse Grouping

Discrepancies associated with ABO reverse grouping parallel those encountered in forward grouping. Two broad categories of reverse grouping discrepancies include missing antibodies and the presence of unexpected antibodies. Specific examples are summarized in Table 5-17.

Weak or Absent Antibodies

Newborns and the elderly are the populations that most frequently present with reduced antibody titers. Newborns are not routinely tested for ABO antibodies. Antibody detected in the plasma of a neonate is maternal in origin. Until a child has developed his or her own antibodies, reverse grouping is not routinely performed.

The fact that waning antibody titers as an individual ages provides an explanation for reduced reverse grouping reactions in elderly individuals. This discrepancy is easily researched and resolved without incident. See the following example:

Anti-A	Anti-B	Anti-A,B	A_1 Cells	B Cells
4+	0	4+	0	0

TABLE 5-17 Weak or Absent Antibodies

Elderly Patients
Newborns
Acquired or Inherited Hypogammaglobulinemia
Acquired or Inherited Agammaglobulinemia
Unexpected Antibodies
Anti-A_1 in Subgroups of A
Cold Reacting Antibodies

Evaluation:

The forward and reverse groupings do not match. The patient forward groups as a group A and reverse groups as an AB.

Additional Testing and Clinical History:

1. Review medical and transfusion history. If the patient has been successfully typed in the past, check on age and current clinical condition.

2. Incubate the reverse group at room temperature for 15 to 30 minutes. Centrifuge and examine tube for agglutination. Weak ABO antibodies may appear after incubation. The incubation time allows for antigen-antibody binding.

   Hypogammaglobulinemia or **agammaglobulinemia**, whether acquired or inherited, results in reduced levels or absence of gamma globulins, respectively. Either of these conditions can result in reverse grouping that does not produce the expected results. Again, the resolution to this situation is careful research into the recipient's medical and clinical history. Correction of the underlying condition is the ideal resolution for this discrepancy. In the interim, the patient is typed by forward grouping with confirmation of established blood type by comparison with previous records.

Presence of Unexpected Antibodies

Unexpected antibodies may present in the reverse grouping. The antibody must have its specificity verified. The two most common scenarios for unexpected antibodies in ABO grouping are the presence of an anti-A_1 in a subgroup of A and cold reacting antibodies. View the following example:

Anti-A	Anti-B	Anti-A,B	A_1 Cells	B Cells
4+	0	4+	4+	4+

Evaluation:

The patient forward groups as a group A. The reverse grouping appears to be group O. It does not match the forward grouping.

Additional Testing and Clinical History:

1. Review medical and transfusion history. If the patient has been successfully typed in the past, check the current clinical condition.

2. Type the patient's cells with the lectin *Dolichos biflorus*. If the result is negative, the patient is not phenotypically A_1. Therefore, an anti-A_1 may be present in the patient's plasma. All donor units should be typed for the A_1 antigen. As a recipient, this individual should receive only A_2 cells.

3. Perform an antibody screen and direct antiglobulin test. If either test is positive, the presence of a cold reacting antibody should be considered. A cold alloantibody will demonstrate positive reactions in the immediate spin phase of the antibody screen. If agglutination is no longer present after incubation of the antibody screen test at 37°C, the presence of a cold alloantibody is confirmed. All testing, including compatibility testing, should be performed at 37°C. If the direct antiglobulin test is positive, the presence of a cold autoantibody is confirmed. Again, all testing should be performed at 37°C. Cold adsorption may be performed and the plasma reevaluated to rule out the presence of alloantibodies that may have been masked by the strong cold autoantibody. These testing techniques will be discussed in Chapter 8.

SUMMARY

- The ABO antigens were first discovered by Landsteiner and play a prominent role in pretransfusion, prenatal, and presurgical testing.

- ISBT has classified 23 antigen systems. ABO is the most significant of these systems.

- There are four ABO groups: A, B, AB, and O.

- The ABO antigens are carbohydrate in nature. Structurally, they are oligosaccharide chains.

- The H antigen is also an oligosaccharide and serves as a precursor to the A and B antigens.

- Individuals may also secrete a soluble form of the A, B, and H antigens into the body fluids. Secretor status may be determined by testing saliva.

- Group A antigens may be divided into subgroups with A_1 being the most common. The A_1 antigen may be detected using a specific antisera. This test is significant since an individual with another subgroup may develop an antibody to the A_1 antigen.

- Subgroups of B also exist but are less common.

- Decreased levels of ABO antibodies are found in the very young, the elderly, as well as inherited and acquired clinical conditions.

- ABO antibodies are formed without apparent antigen stimulation. They are IgM, cold reacting, complement binding antibodies, which can cause HDFN when encountered in the IgG form.

- ABO incompatibility poses a significant risk of HTR.

- Routine testing involves the forward grouping that tests the donor or recipient red cells with commercial antisera. Reverse grouping tests the unknown plasma with commercial red cells of group A and B.

- Group O individuals are universal donors of red cells. Group AB individuals are universal recipients of red cells.

- Group O individuals are universal recipients of plasma products. Group AB individuals are universal donors of plasma.

- Discrepancies are created by a variety of clinical conditions. The well-versed technologist must be able to resolve these discrepancies in order to provide appropriate blood products.

REVIEW QUESTIONS

1. The oligosaccharide molecule that creates the active A antigen is:
   a. fucose
   b. galactose
   c. N-acetylgalactosamine
   d. paragloboside

2. The Bombay phenotype is comprised of a genetic combination of:
   a. O_h
   b. HH
   c. Hh
   d. hh

3. The notation of AO represents a (an):
   a. Bombay phenotype
   b. genotype
   c. phenotype
   d. transferase

4. An individual presents with the following typing results:

Anti-A	Anti-B	Anti-A,B	A_1 cells	B cells
4+	0	4+	1+	4+

   This individual is:
   a. group AB
   b. group A_2 with anti-A_1
   c. group A_1 with anti-A
   d. unable to determine

5. Anti-H is found in the sera of individuals of group:
   a. A
   b. B
   c. O
   d. O_h

6. Parents of group A and AB can *not* produce offspring of group:
   a. A
   b. B
   c. AB
   d. O

7. If a group A individual reacts 3+ with A_1 lectin, this person is a (an):
   a. A_1
   b. A_2
   c. AB
   d. Bombay

8. An individual presents with the following ABO grouping results:

Anti-A	Anti-B	Anti-A,B	A_1 cells	B cells
0	4+	4+	4+	0

This individual is blood group:
a. A
b. B
c. AB
d. O

9. Of the following choices, the individual with a potential for a reduced amount of ABO antibody are a (an):
1. blood donor
2. elderly patient
3. recently immunized adult
4. newborn
5. post-surgical patient
a. 1 and 3 are correct
b. 1 and 5 are correct
c. 2 and 3 are correct
d. 2 and 4 are correct
e. 1 and 2 are correct

10. Anti-A antisera comes from an individual who is group:
a. A
b. B
c. AB
d. O

11. According to Landsteiner's Law, if an individual's red cells have negative reactions with anti-A and anti-B, what antibodies will one find in his/her serum:
a. Anti-A
b. Anti-B
c. anti-A and anti-B
d. Neither anti-A nor anti-B

12. If a mother is genetically AO and the father is genetically AA, the frequencies of phenotypes for potential offspring are:
a. all Group A
b. 50% Group A; 50% Group O
c. 75% Group A; 25% Group O
d. 25% Group A; 75% Group O

13. Using the diagrams below, choose the one that represents the group A antigenic determinant:

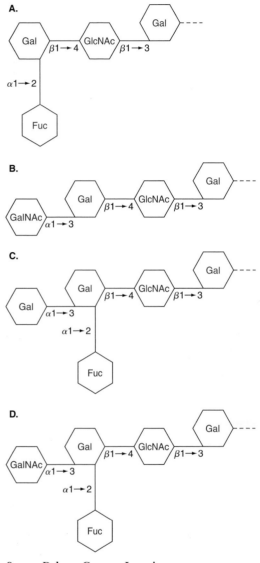

Source: Delmar, Cengage Learning

14. A clinical condition where one may see an acquired B antigen is:
a. hemolytic disease of the newborn
b. colon cancer
c. *E. coli* pyelonephritis
d. hypogammaglobulinemia

15. A presurgical patient has been tested to determine the blood group in case a transfusion is necessary

during surgery. The results of the ABO grouping is as follows:

Anti-A	Anti-B	Anti-A,B	A cells	B cells
4+	0	4+	2+	4+

What is the cause of this "discrepancy?"
a. B(A) phenomenon
b. hypogammaglobulinemia
c. Anti-A_1 in A_2 individual
d. sepsis resulting in acquired antigen

16. The blood group with the most H antigen is:
a. A_2B
b. O
c. A_1
d. B

17. ABO antibodies display which of the following characteristics:
1. IgM
2. IgA
3. Complement Binding
4. 4°C reactive
5. 37°C reactive
a. 1, 3, and 4 are correct
b. 2, 3, and 5 are correct
c. 1 and 4 are correct
d. 2 and 5 are correct

18. Choose the correct statement regarding ABO antigens:
a. newborns have fewer ABO antigens than adults
b. adults have fewer ABO antigens than newborns
c. newborns have the same number of ABO antigens as adults
d. newborns have only the ABO antigens that they have acquired from the maternal serum

19. An individual who is genetically AO/Sese will have which soluble antigens in their saliva:
a. none
b. group A only
c. group H only
d. group A and H
e. group A, B, and H

20. Group A red cells may be transfused to which of the following blood groups:
1. group O
2. group B
3. group AB

a. 1, 2, and 3 are correct
b. only 1 is correct
c. only 2 is correct
d. only 3 is correct
e. none of the above

21. Red cells that are used for reverse grouping are:
a. enzyme treated
b. saline suspended
c. suspended in gel
d. lectins

22. Choose the set of reactions that is most likely to result in an individual with agammaglobulinemia:

	Anti-A	Anti-B	Anti-A,B	A cells	B cells
a.	4+	0	4+	1+	4+
b.	0	0	0	0	0
c.	4+	4+	4+	4+	4+
d.	0	4+	4+	0	4+

23. A technologist encounters a set of typing sera that are hand labeled and visually appear as follows:
Anti-A—clear
Anti-B—yellow
Anti-A,B—blue
Do these correspond to what one would expect to see? If not, what is expected?
a. all are correct
b. Anti-A is correct, anti-B should be blue and anti-A,B should be yellow
c. Anti-A should be blue, anti-B is correct, and anti-A,B should be clear
d. Anti-A is correct, anti-B should be yellow, and anti-A,B should be blue
e. none are correct

24. The laboratory is very hot due to a malfunction in the heating system. How will this affect the ABO forward and reverse grouping?
a. no affect
b. both forward and reverse may have decreased reactions due to warm temperatures
c. both forward and reverse may have increased reactions due to warm temperatures
d. only reverse grouping may be affected but it is unclear how the temperature will impact the testing

25. Choose the correct statement regarding the subgroups of A:
    a. always exhibit anti-A$_1$ in the serum
    b. always react with Anti-A in the forward group
    c. sometimes react with anti-A,B but not with anti-A in the forward group
    d. never react with any forward grouping sera

C A S E   S T U D Y

1. A patient was seen in the emergency room and a crossmatch was ordered. The ABO forward and reverse grouping results are as follows:

Anti-A	Anti-B	Anti-A,B	A1 Cells	B Cells
0	0	1+	1+	4+

   a. Are these test results consistent? Why or why not?
   b. What steps should be taken to resolve any existing discrepancies?
   c. What blood group should be transfused to the patient?

2. An 85 year old cancer patient requires a transfusion. The typing results are as follows:

Anti-A	Anti-B	Anti-A,B	A1 Cells	B Cells
4+	0	4+	0	0

   a. Are these test results consistent? Why or why not?
   b. What steps should be taken to resolve any existing discrepancies?
   c. What blood group should be transfused to the patient?

REFERENCES

Bird, GWG. "Lectins: A Hundred Years." *Immunohematology*. Vol. 4, No. 3, pp. 45–48. 1988.

Blaney, Kathy and Howard, Paula. *Basic and Applied Concepts of Immunohematology*. Mosby, Philadelphia, 2000.

Brecher, Mark, editor. *American Association of Blood Banks Technical Manual 15th edition*. AABB, 2005.

Eonomidous, J, Hughes-Jones, NC and Gardner, B. "Quantitative Measurements Concerning A and B Antigen Sites." *Vox Sanguinis*. Vol. 12, Issue 321, 1967, pp. 321–28.

Garraty, G, Glynn, SA, McEntire, R. "ABO and RhD phenotype frequencies of different racial/ethnic groups in the United States." *Transfusion*, Vol. 44, pp. 703–706. 2004.

Gottlieb, A. Matthew. "Karl Landsteiner, the Melancholy Genius: His Time and His Colleagues," 1868–1943. *Transfusion Medicine Reviews*. Vol. 12, No. 1, pp. 18–27. 1998.

Hackomori, Sen-itiroh. "Blood Group ABH and Ii Antigens of Human Erythrocytes: Chemistry, Polymorphism, and Their Developmental Change." *Seminars in Hematology*. Vol. 18, No. 1, pp. 39–58. 1981.

Harmening, Denise. *Modern Blood Banking and Transfusion Practices*. F. A. Davis, Philadelphia, 2005.

Henry, John Bernard, *Clinical Diagnosis and Management by Laboratory Methods*. W. B. Saunders Co. 2001.

Issitt PD, Anstee DJ (1998). *Applied Blood Group Serology. 4th edition*, Durham, NC, USA: Montgomery Scientific Publications.

Langston, MM. "Evaluation of the Gel System for ABO Grouping and D Typing." *Transfusion*. Vol. 39, Issue 3, pp. 300–305.

Montalvo, Lani. "Clinical investigation of posttransfusion Kidd blood group typing using a rapid normalized quantitative polymerase chain reaction." *Transfusion*. Vol. 44, Issue 5, 2004, pp. 694–702.

Package Insert. "Anti-A, Anti-B, Anti-A,B" Seroclone®. Biotest.

Package Insert. "Anti-A$_1$, Anti-H Seroclone®." Biotest.

Package Insert. "Anti-A, Anti-B, Anti-A,B Seroclone®." Biotest.

Package Insert. "Biotestcell®- A$_1$, A$_2$, B and O. Biotest."

Package Insert. "Erytypecell®- A$_1$, A$_2$, B and O. Biotest."

Package Insert. "Blood Group Reagent, A/B/D Monoclonal and Reverse Grouping Card™." Microtyping systems, Pompano Florida, 2001.

Package Insert. "Blood Grouping Reagent, Anti-A, Anti-B, Anti-A,B (Murine Monoclonal)." For use with the ID-Micro Typing System™. Microtyping systems, Pompano Florida, 2001.

Package Insert. "Blood Group Reagents, Anti-A, Anti-B, Anti-A,B (Murine Monoclonal Blend) Bioclone®," For use with the ID-Micro Typing System. Ortho Clinical Diagnostics, Raritan, NJ. 2004.

Package Insert. "Reagent Red Blood Cells (Pooled Cells) Affirmagen®," For use with the ID-Micro Typing System. Ortho Clinical Diagnostics, Raritan, NJ. 2004.

Poole, Joyce and Daniels, Geoff. "Blood group Antibodies and Their Significance in Transfusion Medicine." *Transfusion Medicine Reviews*. Vol. 21, No. 1. January 2007, pp. 58–71.

Reid, Marion E. and Lomas-Francis, Christine. *The Blood Group Antigen: Facts Book*. Elsevier, 2004.

Schenkel-Brunner, Helmut. *Human Blood Groups: Chemical and Biochemical Basis of Antigen Specificity*. 2nd ed. Springer Wein, New York. 2000, pp. 54–150.

Turgeon, Mary Louise. *Fundamentals of Immunohematology*. Williams and Wilkins, Media, PA, 1995.

Yu, Lung-Chih, et al. "A Newly Identified Nonsecretor Allele of the Human Histo-Blood Group $\alpha(1,2)$ Fucosyltransferase Gene (FUT2)." *Vox Sanguinis*, 1999; 76; 115–119.

Rh Blood Group System

LEARNING OUTCOMES

At the completion of this chapter, the student should be able to:

- List the major Rh antigens.
- Describe the biochemistry of the Rh system.
- Compare the theories of inheritance of Rh antigens described by Fisher-Race and Weiner.
- Describe the Rh system terminologies as defined by Rosenfield and International Society for Blood Transfusion.
- Perform conversion of Rh terminology between Fisher-Race, Weiner, Rosenfield, and ISBT.
- Outline the characteristics of antibodies to the Rh antigens.
- Discuss the weak D antigen and the genetic basis for each category of weak D.
- Describe the reagents and testing for Rh antigens.
- Describe the procedure for testing for the D and weak D antigen.
- Define and discuss compound antigens of the Rh system.
- Discuss diminished and undetectable Rh antigens and the antibodies associated with these phenotypes.
- Define dosage and apply the concept to the Rh blood group system.
- Determine the most probable Rh genotype given red cell typing results.

GLOSSARY

agglutinogen   group of antigens or factors in the Weiner inheritance theory

antithetical   opposite allele

autoagglutinins   antibodies that agglutinate an individual's own cells

compound or *cis*-product antigens   antigens found as a result of two genes being found on the same chromosome

epitope   single antigenic determinate; physically the part of the antigen that combines with the antibody

locus   location of a gene on a chromosome

partial D   phenotype of the D antigen that is missing a part of the antigenic determinant or epitope of the D antigen

recipient   individual receiving a transfusion of blood or its components

Rh null   phenotype with a lack of Rh antigens on the surface of the red cells

steric   related to the spatial arrangement of the molecules

sublocus   location within the gene locus

INTRODUCTION

The Rh blood group system is the second most-recognized system. It is a highly complex, polymorphic system with more than 50 recognized antigens. The designation of Rh positive refers only to the presence of the D antigen, while Rh negative refers to its absence. Karl Landsteiner and Alexander Weiner discovered the D antigen in 1940. Philip Levine and R. E. Stetson discovered the first anti-D in 1939 from a stillborn fetus of a mother who had been transfused with her husband's blood during her pregnancy.

The Rh notation accompanies the ABO group in blood type designation. Donors and recipients are identified by ABO and Rh antigen status. Blood components for transfusion are also labeled with ABO and Rh. The major Rh antigen, D, plays a vital role in hemolytic disease of the fetus and newborn (HDFN) and will be discussed in that role in Chapter 13.

The D, Cc, and Ee antigens will be the primary focus of this chapter. These antigens and corresponding antibodies compose the major constituents of the Rh system. The discussion of specific antigens will include biochemical composition, inheritance theories, antibody characteristics, clinical significance of the antibodies, and transfusion-related issues.

RH ANTIGENS
Biochemical Composition of Rh Antigens

As with the ABO system, Rh antigens are located on the surface of red blood cells. In contrast to the ABO system, the major Rh antigens are found exclusively on red cells and not on tissue cells or in body fluids in soluble form.

The biochemical nature of RhD and RhCE antigens is protein. Protein relies on lipids in the red cell

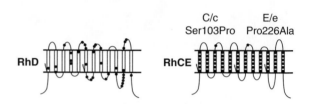

FIGURE 6-1 Rh proteins within the RBC membrane. *Reproduced with permission from* Seminars in Hematology, *Westhoff, C.M. "Structure and function of the Rh Antigen." pp. 43–73, copyright, Elsevier, 2007.*

membrane for physical support. Each of the antigens is constructed of 416 amino acids. The string of amino acids loops through the red cell membrane and displays short loops on the exterior (see Figure 6-1). The active amino acids vary with an individual's genetic coding. As demonstrated in Figure 6-1, Rh antigens are integral to the red cell membrane. This theory is supported by the fact that cells without any Rh antigens, **Rh null**, present an altered physical appearance and decreased red cell survival. Rh null will be discussed later in this chapter.

Glycoproteins that are associated with the biochemical structure of the Rh system have been identified. These glycoproteins are not related to antigenic properties of any blood group system but rather are associated with the red cell membrane. These glycoproteins play a role in association of the RhD and RhCE with the red cell membrane. The glycoprotein associated with the red cell membrane is RhAG. Mutation or absence of these glycoproteins results in lack of expression of any Rh antigens (Rh_{null}).

There have been comparable glycoproteins identified in the brain, the liver, the kidney, and the skin. These glycoproteins have been labeled RhBG and RhCG. They have not been associated with any specific blood group antigens but research indicates involvement with ammonia transport.

Genetics of the Rh Blood Group System

The genes for the Rh system reside on Chromosome 1. The genetic composition of the Rh system includes two genes (RhD and RhCE) located in close proximity. These genes encode for the proteins RhD and RhCE. The RhD protein carries the D antigen while the latter carries C and E antigens. C and E can present in various combinations (e.g. CE, ce, Ce, cE). There is no **antithetical** component for the RhD antigen. Therefore, a "d" does not exist. If the D antigen is not present, there is a total absence or deletion in this location. This corresponds to the Rh negative or D negative phenotype. The lack of any antigenic material is the result of absence of the RhD gene.

The RhD and RhCE genes each have ten exons, are 97% identical, and most likely arose from gene duplication. RhD and RhCE differ by 32 to 35 of their 416 amino acid composition. The difference in antithetical antigens (e.g. C and c are antithetical) results from a difference of fewer amino acids than the comparison of antigens from alternate blood groups. This fact also explains the large degree of foreignness when the RhD antigen is introduced into an RhD negative individual. The highly antigenic nature of the RhD antigen is in contrast to other antigen systems.

Terminology of the Rh Blood Group System

Historically, two major theories of inheritance were proposed. These proposals were based on serological testing results combined with inheritance information available through family studies. From this research, two theories were designated: Fisher-Race and Weiner.

The development of molecular genetic techniques has resolved the dichotomy and clarified the true genetic nature of the Rh blood group system.

Two additional theories have been developed to provide a system to adapt the Rh terminology to computer technology. The original system, developed by Rosenfield, was used as a basis for development of the International Society of Blood Transfusion (ISBT) system. Each of these four terminologies are outlined in the following sections.

Fisher-Race Theory of Inheritance

The Fisher-Race theory proposed that the Rh antigens were inherited as a gene complex or haplotype.

Each parent contributes one haplotype. A haplotype codes for three closely linked sets of alleles. The proximity of the alleles makes it impossible for crossing-over to occur and alter the strict Mendelian inheritance of these genes. Each gene originates at a separate **locus** or location. The three loci are labeled: *D, Cc, Ee*. The D is inherited at one locus. C or c is inherited at the second locus and E or e at the third locus. Less commonly encountered alleles may occupy the C and E loci. The D loci does not have an alternate allele. Originally, the theory proposed that "d" was inherited when D was absent. The "d" notation may be used to denote the absence of the D antigen. The physical sequence of the genes on the chromosome is DCE. When written, the genes are often listed in alphabetical order, CDE. All of the major antigens can be detected on the red cell surface with the corresponding antisera.

The individual genes are not inherited singly. For example, a parent with the genotype DCe/DcE will contribute either DCe or DcE to an offspring. Other combinations, such as Dce, could not possibly be inherited from this parent. This parent's offspring could be DCe/dce, with DCe coming from one parent and dce contributed by the other. The population frequencies of the various gene combinations are summarized in Table 6-1. The frequencies will, again, vary in different racial and ethnic populations.

Weiner Theory of Inheritance

Weiner and his colleagues proposed that Rh antigens were inherited from a *single* locus, or gene. This theory has been proven to be an inaccurate representation of inheritance, but will be presented here as a significant historical progression of inheritance theories. Each of the individual antigens represents a **sublocus** within that single locus. Therefore, two or three antigens are inherited as a single unit rather than as two or three closely linked units, as was proposed by Fisher-Race.

CRITICAL THINKING ACTIVITY

For the following sets of parents, determine the possible genotypes of offspring.

1. CDe/dce and cDE/cDe
2. CDE/dce and CDe/cDE
3. dce/dce and cDe/cDE

TABLE 6-1 Fisher-Race Weiner

GENE COMBINATIONS	SHORTHAND NOTATION	% IN WHITES	% IN AFRICAN-AMERICANS
CDe	R^1	0.42	0.17
cDE	R^2	0.14	0.11
cDe	R^0	0.04	0.44
CDE	R^z	Rare	Rare
cde	r	0.37	0.26
Cde	r'	0.02	0.02
cdE	r"	<0.01	Rare
CdE	r^y	Rare	Rare

The created gene product is termed an **agglutinogen**. Each factor of the agglutinogen can be identified with the same antiseras used to test for antigens listed in the Fisher-Race discussion.

According to Weiner, eight possible alleles may exist at the Rh locus. The shorthand for these alleles are: R^0, R^1, R^2, R^z, r, r', r", and r^y. Each allele codes for either two or three factors. A summary of the factors in each of these alleles is presented in the first two columns of Table 6-1. These factors correspond to the antigens defined by Fisher-Race. See Table 6-2 for a summary of Fisher-Race and Weiner terminology. Weiner nomenclature is not routinely used, but at times it is easier to use a single factor than to list individual alleles as designated by the Fisher-Race terminology.

Conversion of Fisher-Race and Weiner Terminologies.
It is important to understand the relationship between Fisher-Race and Weiner

terminologies and to capably use the two systems interchangeably. A few simple guidelines are outlined below:

1. A capital R always denotes Rh positive or D.
2. A lower case r always denotes Rh negative.
3. The number 1 and ' always denote C.
4. The number 2 and " always denote E.
5. The letters Z and Y each denote a combination of C and E.
6. A zero or blank indicates ce.

For a summary of these conversions see Table 6-2.

Rosenfield Numeric System
The Rosenfield system is not based on the genetic concepts from which Fisher-Race and Weiner developed their inheritance theories, but rather is a numeric

TABLE 6-2 Conversions between Fisher-Race and Weiner Nomenclatures

FISHER-RACE		WEINER	
Gene Combinations	**Antigens**	**Gene**	**Factors**
DCe	D, C, e	R^1	Rh_o, rh', hr"
DcE	D, c, E	R^2	Rh_o, hr', rh"
Dce	D, c, e,	R^0	Rh_o, hr', hr"
DCE	D, C, E	R^z	Rh_o, rh', rh"
dce	c, e	r	hr', hr"
dCe	C, e	r'	rh', hr"
dcE	c, E	r"	hr', rh"
dCE	C, E	r^y	rh', rh"

TABLE 6-3 Summary of Nomenclature for the Rh Blood Group System

NUMERIC	FISHER-RACE	WIENER	ISBT NUMBER
Rh:1	D	Rh_0	004001
Rh:2	C	rh'	004002
Rh:3	E	rh"	004003
Rh:4	c	hr'	004004
Rh:5	e	hr"	004005
Rh:6	ce	hr	004006
Rh:7	Ce	rh_i	004007
Rh:8	C^w	rh^{w1}	004008
Rh:9	C^x	rh^x	004009
Rh:10	ce^s	hr^v	004010
Rh:12	G	rh^G	004012

system developed for use in software applications. Each individual antigen is phenotypically designated by "Rh" followed by a colon and the number assigned to that antigen. If the antigen is absent, a negative sign is placed in front of the number. The full Rh phenotype for a donor or recipient's red cells is detailed by listing each antigen followed by a comma. For example, a cell that types as D+, C-, E-, c+, e+ will be denoted as Rh:1,-2,-3,4,5. Table 6-3 provides a summary of Fisher-Race, Weiner, Rosenfield, and ISBT terminologies.

ISBT Standardized Terminology

ISBT has standardized blood group system nomenclature. A six-digit number has been assigned to each blood group specific antigen. The first three digits of the number represent the blood group system, (e.g. Rh, Lewis, Duffy, etc.). Rh has been designated as 004. The remaining three numbers use the Rosenfield number for that antigen. For example, the ISBT number for the D antigen is 004001. ISBT also designates a system for providing an alphanumeric identifier for each antigen. This system includes the designation for the system, in capital letters, followed by the specific number for the antigen: RH1 represents the D antigen. Refer to Table 6-3 for a summary of these designations.

CRITICAL THINKING ACTIVITY

For each of the following sets of typing results, state the Rosenfield terminology.

1. Anti-D = negative; Anti-C = negative; Anti-E = negative; Anti-c = positive; Anti-e = positive.
2. Anti-D = positive; Anti-C = negative; Anti-E = positive; Anti-c = positive; Anti-e = positive.
3. Anti-D = positive; Anti-C = positive; Anti-E = negative; Anti-c = positive; Anti-e = positive.
4. Anti-D = positive; Anti-C = positive; Anti-E = positive; Anti-c = positive; Anti-e = positive.

WEB ACTIVITIES

1. Type http://ibgrl.blood.co.uk/ into your browser.
2. Choose "ISBT Terminology and Workshops."
3. Click on the location that states: "*Click Here* for the **ISBT Committee on Terminology for Red Cell Surface Antigens** pages."
4. Choose "Table of blood group antigens within systems."
5. Find the Rh antigens and document the corresponding ISBT numbers for each.

D Antigen

The D antigen is the primary antigen in the Rh system. When present on red cells, the individual is designated as "Rh positive." An individual may inherit one D gene from each parent. The inheritance of either one or two D genes will designate that person as "Rh positive." The incidence of Rh positive individuals is 85% in the Caucasian population and 92% in the African-American population. Conversely when no D gene is inherited from either parent, the individual is designated as "Rh negative." Rh negative individuals comprise about 15% in the Caucasian population and 8% in the African-American population.

The D antigen is very antigenic. More than 80% of Rh negative (D negative) individuals transfused with Rh positive blood will develop an anti-D on initial exposure. Rh positive individuals may be transfused with either Rh positive or Rh negative blood. Rh negative individuals, however, should always be transfused with Rh negative blood unless the situation is life threatening and only Rh positive blood is available. Exclusive administration of Rh negative blood is crucial for women of child-bearing age. Rh negative women who develop anti-D are likely to develop Hemolytic Disease of the Fetus and Newborn (HDFN) if an Rh positive infant is born to an Rh negative mother. HDFN will be discussed, in detail, in Chapter 13.

The amount of D antigen present on the red cells varies with an individual's genotype. There is a quantitative continuum for the D antigen presented in Figure 6-2. Genetically determined weak expressions of the D antigen may also be detected.

Weakened Expression of D

Testing for the presence of the D antigen on the red cell surface is performed using specific antisera. Detection of weak D antigens has been enhanced by the development of monoclonal antisera. However, when monoclonal antisera presents with a negative result in anti-D, it may be necessary to perform further testing using the indirect antiglobulin test (IAT). See Chapter 2 for a summary of the IAT method.

$$D\text{--} > R_2R_2 > R_1R_1 > R_1r \quad \text{or} \quad R_0r > R_1r' > R_0r'$$

FIGURE 6-2 A continuum of the amount of D antigen on red blood cells by genotype
Source: Delmar, Cengage Learning

The weakened D antigen is produced through multiple genetic mechanisms. Most of these mechanisms are genetic point mutations. Any detection of D antigen, whether in initial testing or with IAT enhancement, classifies a donor unit as Rh positive. On the other hand, **recipients** (in particular, women of child bearing age) who type with a weakened D antigen may be classified as Rh negative for purposes of transfusion. This policy varies by institution.

Genetic Suppression of the D Antigen. As discussed in Chapter 4, positional effect or **steric** suppression may occur when genes are present on different chromosomes or trans to one another. Weakened D occurs when the C antigen is inherited trans to the D antigen. See Figure 6-2 for an illustration of this concept. Specifically, this weakened expression occurs when the r' (Cde) is paired with either R^1 (CDe) or R^0 (cDe). Using monoclonal antisera, this weakened expression of the D antigen does not require IAT testing.

Partial D Antigen. There are individuals that type as D positive, but demonstrate an anti-D in the plasma. Antibody development follows exposure to the D antigen via pregnancy or transfusion. Historically, the D antigen structure was believed to be a mosaic. If one or more mosaic pieces were missing, the antigen was called a "Mosaic D." This terminology was abandoned when molecular methods determined that these antigens are actually missing one or more **epitopes**. The antibody is developed to the missing epitope(s).

Molecular diagnostics has provided accurate information on the partial D phenotypes. "Up to 50 weak RHD alleles have been described and are due to missense mutations exclusively located in the transmembranous or intracellular parts of the RhD protein." All **partial D** individuals do not produce an anti-D when exposed to the D antigen via pregnancy or transfusion. Weak D phenotypes produced in association with haplotypes CDe and cDE do not produce an anti-D when exposed to the D positive cells. Individuals with alternate forms of the partial D will produce anti-D when immunized.

Daily blood bank operations strive to accomplish two goals related to partial D phenotypes: avoiding alloimmunization and wastage of D negative red cells. Development of affordable and readily available molecular techniques will provide sufficient information to routinely achieve these goals.

When tested with monoclonal antisera, partial D antigens may give varying reactions with different monoclonal antisera. Some of these antisera may produce reactions with the partial D as strong those encountered with complete D antigens. A positive result with one antisera and a negative result with another may be the result of one of the clones not detecting all of the epitopes. Reactions of partial D antigens with monoclonal antisera should be researched. The scope of reactivity of the antisera provided by different manufacturers is significant for detection of partial D antigens. The blood bank may choose specific antisera based on this research. For example, the VI category of partial D reacts with fewer monoclonal antisera than some other categories. Selection of an antiserum may be made using this information.

Test Methods for D Antigen and Weak D

Antisera containing antibodies specific for the D antigen is used to test for the D antigen. The antisera is designated "anti-D." As discussed in Chapter 2, anti-D antisera are monoclonal. The antibody contained in the antisera will attach to the D antigen on red cells and agglutinate if the cells possess the antigen. Comparison of D testing results to the ABO test is utilized to detect interference from **autoagglutinins**. The tube tests and gel tests are similar to those described for the ABO antigens in Chapter 5. Testing methodologies have also been automated for high volume testing. See Chapter 2 for information on gel tests and automated methods. All reagents, however, do vary in methodology and users should refer to the manufacturers package insert for detailed directions.

When an individual types as an Rh negative on immediate spin testing, an extended test is performed on donors and some recipients. This testing proceeds

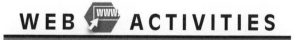

WEB ACTIVITIES

1. Go to www.nobelprize.org
2. Go to "Educational Games."
3. Choose "Blood Typing Game."
4. Determine blood types: ABO and Rh, of all three patients.

to the IAT and final interpretations are made at the end of this phase. This testing methodology is discussed in Chapter 2.

AABB requirements for D antigen testing include mandatory weak D testing for all donors. As discussed previously, individuals who have a weak D are considered Rh positive for the purposes of blood donation. Conversely, recipients considered Rh positive will receive Rh positive blood.

CcEe Antigens

The Rh system contains numerous additional antigens. The most significant ones are the two pairs of alleles: Cc and Ee. Frequency of occurrence for these antigens is summarized in Table 6-4. Additional antigens may be present at this locus. They are less frequently encountered, but may produce atypical antibodies when transfused into antigen-negative individuals. Some of these less common antigens, and their antibody characteristics, are summarized in Table 6-5.

Most Probable Genotypes

In the laboratory, the technician will perform Rh phenotyping by testing the patient's red cells for antigens with antisera specific for each antigen. Included are tests for the D, C, c, E, and e antigens. The phenotype of the patient is reflected in these results. Determination of the genotype is not possible without testing parents and other family members. For this reason, most probable genotype is determined using a table such as Table 6-6.

TABLE 6-4 Frequencies of Fisher-Race Gene Combinations

Gene Combinations	FISHER-RACE % in Whites	% in African-Americans
CDe	0.42	0.17
cDE	0.14	0.11
cDe	0.04	0.44
CDE	Rare	Rare
cde	0.37	0.26
Cde	0.02	0.02
cdE	<0.01	Rare
CdE	Rare	Rare

TABLE 6-5 Less Common Antigens of the Rh System and Corresponding Antibody Characteristics

ANTIGEN	CHARACTERISTICS OF ANTIGEN	ANTIBODY
C^w	Low frequency antigen; most cells positive for C^w are also C positive	Immune antibody that may cause HDFN or HTR
C^x	Very low frequency antigen (<0.1 %) Most cells positive for C^x are also C positive	Immune antibody; very rare; can cause mild HDFN or HTR
V (also Ce^s)	Observed in 30% of blacks; <1% of whites	Causes HTR; not HDFN; may be found in combination with other antibodies
G (also rh^G)	On all C+ cells and most D+ cells	Antibody appears like anti-C and anti-D but cannot be separated into two antibodies; causes HDFN and HTR
f (also ce)	Found when c and e are inherited on the same chromosome (*cis*); in the same haplotype	Rare antibody; causes HDFN and HTR

TABLE 6-6 Summary of Most Probable Rh Genotypes

ANTIGEN TYPING RESULTS AND DETERMINATION OF MOST PROBABLE GENOTYPES

Typing Results					Possibilities in Order of Frequency
D	C	E	c	e	
+	+	0	+	+	CDe/cde, CDe/Dce, Cde/cDe
+	+	0	0	+	CDe/CDe, CDe/Cde
+	+	+	+	+	cDE/CDe, CDe/cdE, CDE/cde, CDE/cDe, CdE/cDe
+	0	+	+	0	cDE/cDE, cDE/cdE
+	0	0	+	+	cDe/cde, cDe/cDe
0	0	0	+	+	cde/cde
0	+	0	+	+	Cde/cde
0	0	+	+	+	cdE/cde
0	+	+	+	+	Cde/cdE, CdE/cde
0	+	0	0	+	Cde/Cde
0	0	+	+	0	cdE/cdE
+	+	+	0	+	CDE/CDe, CDE/Cde
+	+	+	+	0	CDE/cDE, CDE/cdE
+	+	+	0	0	CDE/CDE, CDE/CdE
0	+	+	0	+	CdE/Cde
0	+	+	+	0	CdE/cdE
0	+	+	0	0	CdE/CdE

Antigen typing results are recorded and compared to the table. The most probable genotype is the one having the highest percentage of incidence for the antigens present. For example, consider the following antigen typing results:

Anti-D = positive
Anti-C = positive
Anti-E = negative
Anti-c = positive
Anti-e = positive

CRITICAL THINKING ACTIVITY

For the following phenotypes, list all of the possible genotypes and determine the most probable genotype using Table 6-6.

a. Anti-D = positive
   Anti-C = positive
   Anti-E = positive
   Anti-c = positive
   Anti-e = positive

b. Anti-D = negative
   Anti-C = positive
   Anti-E = negative
   Anti-c = positive
   Anti-e = positive

c. Anti-D = positive
   Anti-C = positive
   Anti-E = negative
   Anti-c = negative
   Anti-e = positive

Comparing these results to the table, the possible genotypes in order of frequency are: CDe/cde, CDe/cDe, Cde/cDe. Therefore the *most probable* genotype is CDe/cde.

Compound Antigens

The Rh blood group system exhibits an unusual antigen presence when combinations of specific genes are inherited as a haplotype and hence are present on the same chromosome or *cis* to each other. These are labeled **compound** or *cis-product antigens.* For example when one parent contributes cde, the antigen f will also be found on the red cells. If this same patient typed positive for both c and e, but genotype is cdE/Cde, the f antigen will not be present. Examples of this phenomenon include:

- Rh6 (*cis* ce or f)
- Rh7 (*cis* Ce or rh$_i$)
- Rh27 (*cis* cE)
- Rh22 (*cis* CE).

The antigens are inherited as a haplotype and will be present on the same chromosome. Antibodies to these compound antigens are encountered infrequently. When encountered, the resulting antibodies cannot be separated into individual components. For example; anti-f does not equal anti-c plus anti-e.

G antigen

The G antigen is an antigen that is present on any red cells where C or D are found. This is not a compound antigen. Both C and D antigens do not have to be inherited for the G antigen to be present. Anti-G may be encountered in persons who have either of these antigens. Hence, the antibody formed will appear to be reactive with BOTH C and D antigens even if only one of the antigens is present on the red cells: e.g. an Rh positive individual who appears to have anti-D. Anti-G should be differentiated from anti-C plus anti-D by adsorption and elution. These techniques are discussed in Chapter 8.

Rh Phenotypes with Diminished or Undetectable Rh Antigens

The complexity of the Rh blood group system allows for existent phenotyes to be either decreased in the levels of detectable Rh antigens or completely absent in these antigens. These phenotypes have arisen as mutations. The most common of these phenotypes is Rh null.

Rh Null. Very rarely, an individual will present with a total lack of Rh antigens on the surface of the red cells. These individuals are known as Rh$_{null}$. These Rh$_{null}$ red cells also lack Fy and LW, which are high-frequency antigens and demonstrate weakened expression of S/s and U antigens.

The most common cause of the Rh$_{null}$ phenotype results from mutations in the RHAG gene. This gene is required for the expression of the Rh antigens on the red cell. Mutations in the RHAG gene will affect the expression of all the Rh antigens. Historically, this Rh$_{null}$ expression was called the "regulator-type" of Rh$_{null}$. It was believed that this expression was the result of homozygous inheritance of an inactive form of a regulator gene. The second form of Rh$_{null}$ was believed to result from homozygous inheritance of an Rh$_{null}$ amorph. This "amorph" form actually results from mutations in the RhCE gene in D negative individuals.

The clinical significance of Rh_{null} phenotype consists of two major issues:

- Difficulty finding compatible blood for Rh_{null} individuals who have developed multiple, complex, antibodies.

- Decreased life span of the red cells due to an abnormal red cell membrane. The cells demonstrate an increased osmotic fragility, a shortened half-life, and a mild hemolytic anemia.

Rh_{mod} Phenotype.

The Rh_{mod} phenotype is similar to Rh_{null} except that Rh antigens are present in greatly reduced amounts as opposed to being entirely missing. The cells have decreased amounts of RHAG and Rh antigen expression is detectable only by adsorption and elution. The Rh_{mod} phenotype appears to be the result of a mutation in the RHAG gene. These individuals also display a hemolytic anemia due to a defective red cell membrane.

D Deletion Phenotypes.

Rare Rh phenotypes exist with complete lack of C, c, E, and e antigens. The notation for this phenotype is written either as -D- or D--. These cells may exhibit increased amounts of the D antigen. These individuals can develop complex antibodies to the antigens that are not present on the red cell surface.

Rh Antibodies

Compared to the ABO system, individuals who lack any of the Rh antigens rarely develop antibodies to those antigens without red cell stimulation via pregnancy or transfusion. Antibodies to all of the Rh antigens may cause both HDFN and Hemolytic Transfusion Reaction (HTR).

TABLE 6-7 Characteristics of Rh Antibodies

Immunoglobulin Class	IgG
Optimal Temperature of Reactivity	37°C
Optimal Media of Reactivity	AHG
Effect of Enzymes	Enhanced
Display dosage	Yes
Capable of crossing the placenta	Yes
Capable of causing HDFN	Yes
Capable of causing HTR	Yes

The characteristics of all Rh antibodies are the same regardless of the corresponding antigen. They are IgG antibodies that bind to their respective antigens at 37°C. They may display agglutination at 37°C and in the AHG testing phase. They do not bind complement and are enhanced by enzymes. Characteristics of each of the antibodies in the Rh blood group are summarized in Table 6-7.

CRITICAL THINKING ACTIVITY

Refer to Figure 6-2. Answer the following question related to anti-c.

a. Which cell(s) will react with this antibody?

b. Provide reactions that will show this antibody demonstrating dosage.

c. Provide reactions that will show the effect on enzymes on this antibody.

SUMMARY

- The Rh blood group is the second most recognized blood group.

- Genes for Rh system are on chromosome 1.

- The Rh blood group consists of two major loci RHD and RHCE. Five major antigens are possible: D, Cc, and Ee. There is no antithetical component for D.

- The biochemical nature of the Rh antigens is protein.

- Rh antigens are an integral part of the red cell membrane.

- Additional membrane glycoproteins that are not related to blood group antigenic properties are labeled RhAG. Mutation of these glycoproteins result in lack of expression of the Rh antigens.

- Four terminologies have been developed for labeling the Rh blood group systems: Fisher-Race, Weiner, Rosenfield, and ISBT.

- Fisher-Race theory described Rh inheritance as resulting from three loci. Molecular techniques have identified this theory as the one that most closely describes the true inheritance of the Rh system.

- Historically, Weiner proposed one gene with either two or three factors.

- A system for conversion from Fisher-Race to Weiner exists and can readily be accomplished by referring to a summarizing chart.

- Rosenfield nomenclature is numerical and was developed to aid in the conversion of terminologies to use with computer software. ISBT is an expansion of the Rosenfield nomenclature.

- The D antigen is present in 85% of the Caucasian population. It is very antigenic and stimulates antibody production in 80% of antigen negative individuals on their first exposure.

- A weakened expression of D exists. This weakened expression may result from steric effects or absence of epitopes. The absence of one or more epitopes is a partial D.

- Compound antigens exist. These compound antigens are found when two antigens exist on the same chromosome.

- Rh_{null} phenotype is the complete absence of Rh antigens on the red cell surface. These individuals present with unique challenges to the blood banking community.

- There are also Rh deletion phenotypes. These phenotypes exhibit missing antigens or reduced levels of Rh antigens. They, too, present challenges when the individuals develop atypical antibodies.

- Rh antibodies are most often IgG, 37°C, enzyme enhanced, AHG reactive antibodies that do not bind complement.

REVIEW QUESTIONS

1. The approximate percentage of persons in the Caucasian population who are Rh negative is:
   a. 15
   b. 25
   c. 50
   d. 85

2. The antigen missing in the Rh negative individual is:
   a. C
   b. c
   c. D
   d. d

3. The Weiner notation R_1R_2 translates to Fisher-Race as:
   a. CDe/cDE
   b. CDe/CDE
   c. CDE/cDE
   d. CDe/cDe

4. For the Rosenfield nomenclature RH1, the ISBT notation would be:
   a. 004001
   b. 001004
   c. 001400
   d. 004100

5. The following test results are obtained:

Anti-D	Anti-C	Anti-c	Anti-E	Anti-e
0	+	+	0	+

   The most probable genotype is:
   a. R_1r
   b. R_0r
   c. r'r
   d. rr

6. Formation of Rh antibodies may be stimulated by:
   a. environmental substances
   b. proteins

c. ABO antibodies

d. transfusions

7. The some forms of weak D antigen may be:

a. identical to the D antigen

b. missing part of the D antigen

c. an Rh negative antigen

d. not at all related to the D antigen

8. The weak D may be created when the D antigen is:

a. absent on both chromosomes

b. inherited from only one parent

c. in the trans position to the C gene

d. received in an Rh positive transfusion

9. Fisher-Race describes the inheritance of the Rh antigens as resulting from:

a. one locus with three subloci

b. a single complete unit

c. three separate closely linked loci

d. linkage to the ABO genes

10. Choose the correct statements regarding the weak D test:

1. donors must always have a weak D test performed

2. recipients must always have a weak D test performed

3. donors do not require a weak D test performed

4. recipients do not require a weak D test performed

a. 1 and 2 are correct

b. 1 and 4 are correct

c. 2 and 3 are correct

d. 3 and 4 are correct

11. RhAG is associated with

a. the production of RhD antigen

b. only red cell Rh antigens

c. organs such as brain and liver

d. ion transport across the red cell membrane

12. Monoclonal an anti-D serum is being used in the blood bank of the local hospital. This blood bank also performs weak D testing on all donors and recipients. Choose the correct statement regarding the frequency that this lab will have to perform the weak D test compared to a lab that uses antisera that are not monoclonal. This lab will perform:

a. more weak D tests

b. fewer weak D tests

c. the same number of weak D tests

d. unable to determine

13. Rh antibodies are:

1. IgG

2. IgM

3. complement binding

4. non-complement binding

5. cold-reaction

6. warm-reacting

a. 1, 3, and 5 are correct

b. 1, 4, and 6 are correct

c. 2, 3, and 6 are correct

d. 2, 4, and 5 are correct

14. Choose the genotype that is heterozygous for E antigen:

a. rr

b. r"r^y

c. R^{1}R^2

d. rR^Z

15. Parents who are heterozygous for D antigen will have what likelihood of producing an Rh negative child?

a. 25%

b. 50%

c. 75%

d. no Rh negative children can be produced

Matching:

Choose the Weiner notation from the right column that matches the Fisher-Race notation in the left column.

_____ 16. CDe	a. R^1	
_____ 17. cde	b. R^2	
_____ 18. cDE	c. R^Z	
_____ 19. CDE	d. R^0	
_____ 20. CdE	e. r'	
	f. r"	
	g. r	
	h. r^y	

C A S E   S T U D Y

1. You are working in a donor facility. A request has arrived from a local hospital for 4 units of A positive R_2R_2 blood. The inventory shows low stock of A positive blood. You are going to request a shipment of blood from a sister blood bank. How many units should you request to be "statistically" certain that the number of antigen correct units will be in that shipment? Explain your answer.

2. You are screening donor units for a patient who has antibody and is an R_1r_y. Donors with an identical genotype have been requested from the consulting hematologist. Describe the anticipated antisera reactions when testing each donor's cells with the 5 major Rh antisera. If you cannot find cells with an identical genetic make-up, what alternative genotypes may be safely substituted.

REFERENCES

Avent, Neil, et al. "Molecular biology of Rh proteins and Relevance to Molecular Medicine." *Expert Reviews in Molecular Medicine*, Vol. 8, Issue 13. pp. 1–20, 2006.

Avent, Neil and Reid, Marion. "The Rh Blood Group System: a Review." *Blood*. Vol. 95, Issue 2. pp. 375–378, 2000.

Blaney, Kathy and Howard, Paula. *Basic and Applied Concepts of Immunohematology*. Mosby, Philadelphia, 2000.

Brecher, Mark, editor. *American Association of Blood Banks Technical Manual 15th edition*. AABB, 2005.

Conroy, MJ, et al. "Modeling the Human Rhesus Proteins: Implications for Structure and Function." *Transfusion*. pp. 543–551, 2005.

Denomme, Gregory A., et al. "Rh Discrepancies Caused by variable Reactivity of Partial and Weak D Types with Different Serological Techniques." *Immunohematology*. Vol. 48, 2008, pp. 473–476.

Flegel, W. "Honing in on D Antigen Antigenicity." *Transfusion*. pp. 466–468, 2005.

Flegel, W. and Wagner Franz F. "Molecular Genetics of RH." *Vox Sanguinis*. Vol. 78 (Supplement 2); 2000, pp. 109–115.

Harmening, Denise. *Modern Blood Banking and Transfusion Practices*. F. A. Davis, Philadelphia, 2005.

Henry, John Bernard, *Clinical Diagnosis and Management by Laboratory Methods*. W. B. Saunders Co. 2001.

Hughes-Jones, NC, et al. "Observations of the Number of Available c, D, e, and E Antigen Sites on Red Cells." *Vox Sanguinis*. 1971.

Issitt PD. "Review: the Rh Blood Group System: An Historical Calendar." *Transfusion*, Vol. 21, Issue 4. pp. 141–5, 2005.

Issitt PD, Anstee DJ (1998). Applied Blood Group Serology. 4th edition, Durham, NC, USA: Montgomery Scientific Publications.

Lai, Marco, et al. "Detection of weak D with a Fully Automated Solid-Phase Red Cell Adherence System." Vol. 45, 2005, pp. 689–692.

McCullough, Jeffrey. *Transfusion Medicine 2nd edition*. Elsevier. 2005.

Noizat-Pirenne, France, et al. "Weak D Phenotypes and Transfusion Safety: Where do We Stand in Daily Practice." Vol. 47, 2007, pp. 1616–1620.

Package Insert. "Blood Group Reagent, Anti-D (Anti-Rh$_0$) Bioclone®." Ortho Clinical Diagnostics, Raritan, NJ. 2006.

Package Insert. "Blood Group Reagent, Anti-D (Monoclonal) (IgM). For use with the ID-Micro Typing System." Ortho Clinical Diagnostics, Raritan, NJ. 2000.

Package Insert. "Blood Group Reagent, Anti-C (Anti-RH2), Anti-E (Anti-RH3), Anti-c (Anti-RH4), Anti-C (Anti-RH5) Bioclone®." Ortho Clinical Diagnostics, Raritan, NJ. 1999.

Poole, Joyce and Daniels, Geoff. "Blood Group Antibodies and Their Significance in Transfusion Medicine." *Transfusion Medicine Reviews*. Vol. 21, Number 1. January 2007, pp. 58–71.

Reid, Marion E. and Lomas-Francis, Christine. *The Blood Group Antigen: Facts Book*. Elsevier, 2004.

Schenkel-Brunner, Helmut. *Human Blood Groups: Chemical and Biochemical Basis of Antigen Specificity*. Springer Wien, 2000.

Standards for Blood Banks and Transfusion Services, 25th Edition. AABB, Bethesda, MD, 2008.

Turgeon, Mary Louise. *Fundamentals of Immunohematology*. Williams and Wilkins, Media, PA, 1995.

Westhoff, Connie M. "The Rh Blood Group D Antigen: Dominant, divers and difficult." *Immunohematology*, 2005. pp. 155–163.

Westhoff, Connie M. "The Structure and Function of the Rh Antigen Complex." *Seminars in Hematology*. Elsevier. 2007.

Other Blood Group Systems

LEARNING OUTCOMES

After studying this unit, it is the responsibility of the student to know the following objectives:

- List blood group systems classified as other blood group systems.
- Identify antigens contained within each of the blood group systems.
- State the frequency of phenotypes and specify ethnic group differences.
- Diagram and explain the biochemistry for each antigen system.
- Relate the Lewis system to secretor status and H genotype.
- Describe the genetic mechanism for each antigen system.
- Discuss the serological characteristics of antibodies that correspond to each of the antigens.
- Relate the methods of antibody stimulation for each of the antigen-antibody systems.
- List and discuss unique characteristics of each antigen-antibody system.

GLOSSARY

Chronic Granulomatous Disease (CGD)   an inherited disorder of phagocytic cells in which the cells do not properly capture and destroy foreign invaders; this leads to recurrent life-threatening bacterial and fungal infections

cold hemagglutinin disease   autoimmune disease with high concentrations of antibodies to red blood cells. The antibodies react at temperatures below body temperature

Donath-Landsteiner antibody   an IgG autoantibody that binds to red cells in the cold and fixes complement; lysis occurs when cells are warmed to 37°C

glycophorin   a glycoprotein that projects through a red cell membrane; may carry blood group antigens

hydatid cyst fluid   fluid from a cyst of the liver (hydatid cyst) caused by a tapeworm; the fluid is used to inhibit anti-P_1

paroxysmal cold hemoglobinuria (PCH)   a cryopathic hemolytic syndrome; is an autoimmune hemolytic anemia due to cold-reacting autoantibodies

123

sialoglycoproteins   glycoproteins that carry sialic acid; the sialic acid lends a negative charge to the red blood cell membrane

universal antigen   an antigen found on the red cells of a large percentage of the population approaching 100%

INTRODUCTION

In previous chapters, the antigens and antibodies of the ABO and Rh blood group systems have been discussed. These two systems play a major role in pre-transfusion testing and are the most critical for successful transfusion outcomes. More than 200 unique antigens, belonging to additional blood group systems, have been identified on the surface of red blood cells. The International Society for Blood Transfusion (ISBT) has identified and classified antigens in 23 blood group systems. Each individual does not possess all possible antigens but rather a genetically derived set of alleles inherited from each parent.

A complementary antibody specific for each of these antigens have been documented. With rare exceptions, the antibodies are not "naturally" found in the individual's plasma. Unlike ABO antibodies, these are red cell stimulated and formed following exposure to an antigen that is not present on the surface of the stimulating red cells. Most often, this antigenic exposure occurs during either pregnancy or blood transfusion.

WEB 🖧 ACTIVITIES

1. Type http://ibgrl.blood.co.uk/ into your browser.
2. Choose "ISBT Terminology and Workshops."
3. Click on the location that states: "*Click Here* for the **ISBT Committee on Terminology for Red Cell Surface Antigens** pages."
4. Choose "Table of blood group antigens within systems."
5. Scan the antigens listed and note the corresponding ISBT numbers for each.

WEB 🖧 ACTIVITIES

1. Type www.ncbi.nlm.nih.gov into your browser.
2. Choose "Books" from the toolbar at the top of the web page.
3. Choose the book: *Blood Groups and Red Cell Antigens.*
4. As each blood group system is discussed in this chapter, refer to the information on that system in the on-line book.
5. Continue to use this site as a reference, as needed.

Antigens and the corresponding antibodies of the major blood group systems play a role in the blood bank and in transfusion therapy. Molecular techniques have provided additional information related to the structure of the specific antigens as well as additional roles the antigens play, including the structure and physiology of the red blood membrane.

The antigen-antibody systems are broadly categorized by optimal temperature of reactivity. The individual systems are discussed, in this chapter, temperatures of reactivity are not exclusive. This classification is used for the purpose of organization, but should only be employed as a performance guideline blood group antibodies. Processes for screening and identification of antibodies will be outlined in Chapter 8.

SYSTEMS WITH COLD-REACTING ANTIBODIES

Antigen systems with antibodies that characteristically react at room temperature (25°C) or colder are included in this section. These systems are listed in Table 7-1.

TABLE 7-1 Antigen Systems with Cold-Reacting Antibodies	
SYSTEM	**MAJOR ANTIGENS**
Lewis	Le^a, Le^b
P	P$_1$
I	I, i
MNSs	M, N, S, s

TABLE 7-2 Frequencies of Antigens in the Lewis Blood Group System		
PHENOTYPE	**% FREQUENCY ADULTS IN THE UNITED STATES**	
	Caucasian	*Black*
Le (a+b−)	22	23
Le (a−b+)	72	55
Le (a−b−)	6	22

While these antibodies are typically IgM cold reactive antibodis, examples of IgG warm reactive antibodies may be encountered.

Antibodies that react best at temperatures less than body temperature (37°C) are not considered clinically significant. The antibodies are identified in the test tube at colder temperatures. Comparable reactions, however, will not be seen at 37°C or in the anti-human globulin (AHG) phase of testing. While the cold-reacting antibodies may be encountered and identified in testing, they are not likely to cause a transfusion-related reaction.

Lewis Blood Group System

The Lewis system contains two major antigens, Le^a and Le^b. These antigens are unique. In contrast to most blood group systems, such as ABO and Rh, the Lewis antigens are not an integral part of the red cell membrane. They are formed in secretions and adsorbed onto the surface of the red blood cells. Newborns have no Lewis antigens. They type as Le (a−b−). The antigens begin to develop as early as a week after birth, and this development continues for up to six years. As antigen development occurs, the laboratory technologist will visualize a progression of antigen typing results. These antigen typing results progress from Lewis (a−b−) → Lewis (a+b−) → Lewis (a+b+) → Lewis (a−b+). This final antigen typing will not be apparent until, approximately, the age of six. Frequencies of Lewis antigens are summarized in Table 7-2.

The development of Lewis antigens involves the interaction of three sets of genes. These genes are H, Secretor (Se), and Lewis (Le). Products of the Le, Se, and H genes are glycotransferases. The amorphic variants of these genes (le, se, and h) produce no detectable product. This three-way gene interaction occurs as follows:

1. The Le gene codes for the glycotransferase that produces Le^a antigen. The Le^a antigen is formed by the addition of a fucose to a type 1 precursor (see Figure 7-1). Le^a is initially present in the secretions and becomes adsorbed onto the surface of the red cells. This occurs regardless of secretor status.

2. The Se gene encodes for the H transferase to be present in secretions.

3. When a combination of Le, H, and Se exist together, the Le glycotransferase will covert the available H antigen to Le^b. The Le^b will be adsorbed onto the red blood cell instead of the Le^a. See Figure 7-1 for a summary of the biochemistry of the Lewis blood group system.

4. See Table 7-3 for a summary of gene combinations and the resulting phenotypes.

If any of the three genes, Le, Se, H, is present in the amorphic form (le, se, h), the production of Le^b cannot occur. See Table 7-3 for a summary of gene combinations and the phenotypes that accompany them.

Lewis Blood Group Antibodies

Lewis antibodies are encountered in individuals with no Le^a or Le^b antigens, Le (a−b−). Individuals who are Le (a−b+) do not produce antibodies to the Le^a antigen. It is also very rare to find an anti-Le^b in a phenotypically Le (a+b−) individual. Characteristics of the antibodies are summarized in Table 7-4. These antibodies are characteristically IgM antibodies. However, IgG anti-human globulin reacting varieties may be seen. They may be formed naturally, without direct stimulation. Lewis antibodies are unique—they may appear during pregnancy and then disappear.

Lewis antibodies are not typically clinically significant. They are rarely seen at 37°C or AHG phases

H Antigen

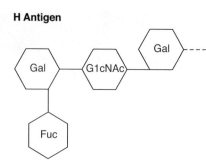

Le^a

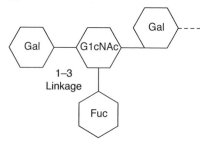

Le^b

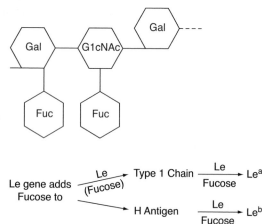

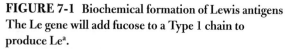

FIGURE 7-1 Biochemical formation of Lewis antigens
The Le gene will add fucose to a Type 1 chain to produce Le^a.
In the presence of the Se and H genes the Le gene will add fucose to the H antigen structure to produce Le^b.
Adapted from Brecher, Mark, editor. American Association of Blood Banks Technical Manual *15th edition. AABB, 2005.*

of testing. These antibodies are not threatening to a transfusion recipient's welfare unless they react at AHG phase or cause *in vitro* hemolysis. If a unit of blood with Lewis antigens is transfused to an individual with Lewis antibodies, the soluble antigens in the donor's plasma will neutralize the antibodies in the recipient's plasma.

Lewis antibodies do not cause Hemolytic Disease of the Fetus and Newborn (HDFN). As previously discussed, the Lewis antigens are not developed on the surface of the baby's red cells. In addition, most Lewis antibodies are IgM and do not cross the placenta.

MNSs Blood Group System

The MNSs system is composed of more than 40 antigens. The most frequently discussed are M, N, S, s, and U. Frequencies of these antigens are summarized in Table 7-5. The two genes that code for the gene pairs, M/N and S/s, are located on chromosome 4. The genes, GYPA and GYPB, code for glycophorin A (GPA) and glycophorin B (GPB), respectively. GPA codes for the M and N antigens and GPB codes for the S and s antigens. The genes are located in close proximity and are inherited as a haplotype rather than independently. Possible haplotypes are Ms, MS, Ns, and NS. The most frequently inherited haplotype is Ns. Inheriting M or N in the homozygous state enhances the strength of the antigenic expression, known as the dosage effect. For example, M+N− cells will react more strongly with anti-M than M+N+ cells.

Biochemically, MNSs antigens are attached to glycoproteins (glycophorins) that are an integral part of the red cell membrane. These glycoproteins are sialic acid-rich and are called **sialoglycoproteins**. The immune epitope is composed of protein and carbohydrate. M and N are at the extreme terminus of GPA. There are 200,000 to 1,000,000 copies of GPA per red blood cell. S and s antigens are substitutions on GPB. There are 50,000 to 250,000 copies of GPB per red cell (see Figure 7-2). The U antigen is a universal antigen found in the majority of individuals. This antigen is found on GPB and near the surface of the red cell. It is present whenever S and/or s antigens are present.

MNSs Blood Group System Antibodies

Antibodies to the MN antigens are most often cold reacting antibodies of the IgM classification. These antibodies are non-red cell stimulated or stimulated by exposure. Anti-M is most often a clinically insignificant antibody and rarely implicated in HDFN. Anti-N has identical characteristics to anti-M. It is found less

TABLE 7-3 Summary of Lewis, Secretor, and H Genes and Their Detectable Products

GENE COMBINATION	PHENOTYPE	SECRETION ANTIGENS
lele sese hh	Le (a−b−)	None
Le sese hh	Le (a+b−)	None
lele sese H	Le (a−b−)	None
lele Se hh	Le (a−b−)	None
Le sese H	Le (a+b−)	Le^a
lele Se H	Le (a−b−)	H
Le Se hh	Le (a+b−)	Le^a
Le Se H	Le (a−b+)	Le^a Le^b H

TABLE 7-4 Summary of Lewis Antibodies

SYMBOL	ISBT NUMBER	WHO CLASS	TEMPERATURE OF REACTIVITY	CLINICAL SIGNIFICANCE	PHASES OF REACTIVITY
Le	007	IgM	Room Temp or Colder	No HDFN or HTR	IS*, 4°C, RT**, Enhanced by Enzymes

*IS = Immediate Spin
**RT = Room Temperature

TABLE 7-5 MNSsU Frequencies in Adults

ANTIGEN	% FREQUENCY	
	White	*Black*
M	78	74
N	72	75
S	55	31
s	89	94
U	99.9	99

frequently than anti-M. The antibodies anti-M and anti-N are non-reactive in enzymes.

In contrast, antibodies to the Ss and U antigens most often react at 37°C and in the AHG phase of testing. They are IgG antibodies that are clinically significant and may cause HDFN and decreased red cell survival. Anti-U is rarely found. Obtaining compatible blood for recipients with this antibody is difficult and a rare donor file may need to be utilized. The temperature of reactivity removes these antibodies from the cold-reacting category. They are considered in this section since they

are related to the M and N antigens. All of these antibodies are summarized in Tables 7-6 and 7-7.

P Blood Group System

The P blood group system is composed of four antigens. These antigens are defined by the ISBT classification as part of two systems: P$_1$ antigen is in the P1 system (ISBT 003) while P, Pk, and Luke are in the GLOB (Globside) collection (ISBT 209). Collectively, these antigens comprise the P blood group system. The predominant antigen is P$_1$. A characteristic of the P$_1$ antigen is that it varies in strength on the cells of those that possess it. When this antigen is not present, the cells are labeled P$_2$. P P^k antigens are high frequency antigens present on greater than 99% of red cells. The antigens, phenotypes, and frequencies are summarized in Table 7-8.

The interactions of genes from two independently inherited loci create the antigens of the system. The alleles found at one locus are P^{1k}, P^k, and p. The alleles at the second locus are P^2 and P$^{2.0}$. These two genes code for transferases that attach carbohydrates to an oligosaccharide chain. The P$_1$ antigen is formed from the

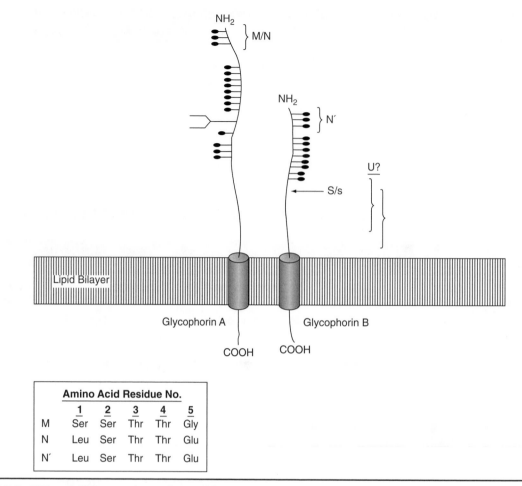

	Amino Acid Residue No.				
	1	**2**	**3**	**4**	**5**
M	Ser	Ser	Thr	Thr	Gly
N	Leu	Ser	Thr	Thr	Glu
N′	Leu	Ser	Thr	Thr	Glu

FIGURE 7-2 GPA and GPB are an integral part of the bilayer of the red cell membrane. M/N antigens are the end terminus of GPA. S/s antigens are at amino acid 29 of GPB. U antigen is located in close proximity to the S/s antigens on GPB. *This article was published in* Clinical Diagnosis and Management. Henry, John Bernard, *p. 679. Copyright Elsevier (2001).*

TABLE 7-6 Summary of MN Antibodies

SYMBOL	ISBT NUMBER	WHO CLASS	TEMPERATURE OF REACTIVITY	CLINICAL SIGNIFICANCE	PHASES OF REACTIVITY
MNS1 (Anti-M)	002	IgM, IgG (rare)	Room temp or colder	No HDFN or HTR	IS* (most), RT**, destroyed by enzymes, may be pH dependent
MNS2 (Anti-N)	002	IgM, IgG (rare)	Room temp or colder; 37°C (rare-IgG)	No HDFN or HTR	IS* (most), RT**, destroyed by enzymes, may be pH dependent

*IS = Immediate Spin
**RT = Room Temperature

TABLE 7-7 Summary of Ss Antibodies

SYMBOL	ISBT NUMBER	WHO CLASS	TEMPERATURE OF REACTIVITY	CLINICAL SIGNIFICANCE	PHASES OF REACTIVITY
MNS3 (Anti-S)	002	IgG, IgM (few)	37°C, some room temp	Yes, HDN or HTR	37°C, IAT***, destroyed by enzymes
MNS4 (Anti-s)	002	IgG	37°C	37°C, some room temp	37°C, IAT

*** IAT—Indirect Antiglobulin Test; AHG phase of testing

TABLE 7-8 P Antigens and Frequencies

PHENOTYPE	ANTIGENS	PERCENT FREQUENCY	
		Caucasian	*Black*
P_1	$P_1P\ P^k$	79	94
P_2	$P\ P^k$	21	6
P_1^k	P_1P^k	Very Rare	
P_2^k	P_2P^k	Very Rare	
p	None	Very Rare	

same precursor as the H antigen. The P_1 antigen exists in soluble form. It can be detected in serum and plasma. It can also be detected in **hydatid cyst fluid**. This fluid can be used to confirm the presence of anti-P_1. The soluble antigen in the fluid will bind to the antibody and neutralize antibody present in the serum or plasma. Following neutralization, the antibody will no longer appear in the serum or plasma. This confirms the presence of the antibody.

P Antigen Biochemistry

The antigenic determinants of this blood group system are carbohydrates. The genes at the two P loci code for transferases. These transferases attach carbohydrates to glycosphingolipids on the surface of the red blood cells. See Figure 7-3 for a summary of the biochemistry of the P antigen system.

P System Antibodies

The anti-P_1 antibody is a cold reacting antibody. It is a naturally occurring antibody found in the serum of P_2 individuals. The antibody is a cold-reacting IgM

agglutinin enhanced by enzymes. If anti-P_1 is suspected, the serum is tested at 17°C. These antibodies are not clinically significant unless they react at 37°C or the AHG phase. Generalized summary of P system antibody characteristics is provided in Table 7-9.

Autoanti-P

An autoanti-P can be produced. It is an IgG antibody and has been called the **Donath-Landsteiner antibody**. It is associated with **paroxysmal cold hemoglobinuria (PCH)** that is an immune hemolytic anemia. In PCH, the autoanti-P binds to the P-positive red blood cells when the extremities are exposed to low temperatures. The antigen-antibody complex then binds complement. When the complex warms, hemolysis occurs. This condition is usually transient and is difficult to diagnose. There is a test for the Donath-Landsteiner antibody. The procedure for this test is summarized in Figure 7-4.

Patients displaying the Donath Landsteiner antibody often have a weakly positive direct antiglobulin test caused by the bound complement. If a transfusion is required, it is not necessary to provide antigen-negative

Type 2 H Chain

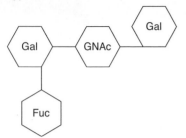

Type 2 Precursor Chain (Paraglobside)

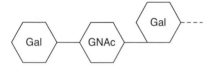

P₁ Antigen

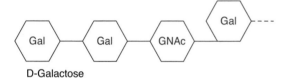

D-Galactose

Pᵏ (Ceramide Trihexoside)

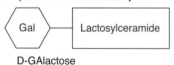

D-GAlactose

P (Globoside)

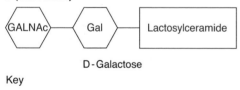

D - Galactose

Key

GAL = Galactose
GNAc = N-AcetylGlucosamine

FIGURE 7-3 The P₁ antigen is produced with the attachment of D-galactose to the Type 2 precursor chain. The P and Pᵏ antigens are exclusive of the P₁ antigen. The structure of these globoside antigens uses lactosylceramide as a precursor substance.

Source: Delmar, Cengage Learning

blood. Prewarmed crossmatch techniques and transfusion of warmed blood may be required to provide test results without agglutination. Complications of PCH may be avoided with temperature control of the patient.

Ii Antigen Collection

Antigens I and i are not considered an antigen system, but rather a collection of antigens. They are formed by the action of genes that code for glycosyltransferases. These antigens are not antithetical antigens. The i antigen is present on umbilical cord cells and the red blood cells of newborns. All adult red blood cells are positive for I antigen and the i antigen is absent. The i antigen has a linear chain structure and the I antigen has a branched structure. As the straight chains develop into branched chains, the I antigen develops and the i disappears.

Biochemically, the I/i antigens exist on the same oligosaccharide chains as A, B, and H antigens. However, the location of the I/i antigens is at a position closer to the red blood cell membrane than the position of the ABH antigens. I and i antigens are type 2 chain oligosaccharides (see Figure 7-5). The I and i antigens are present on both glycolipid and glycoprotein structures of the red blood cell membrane. Both I and i antigens are also found as soluble glycoproteins in body secretions such as human milk and amniotic fluid.

I and i Antibodies

Antibodies to either antigen react best at temperatures colder than room temperature and are not frequently seen in routine testing. They are IgM and clinically

TABLE 7-9 Basic Characteristics of P Antibodies

SYMBOL	ISBT NUMBER	WHO CLASS	TEMPERATURE OF REACTIVITY	CLINICAL SIGNIFICANCE	PHASES OF REACTIVITY
P1	003	IgM	Room Temp or Colder	No HDFN or HTR	IS*, RT**, Enhanced by Enzymes

*IS = Immediate Spin
**RT = Room Temperature

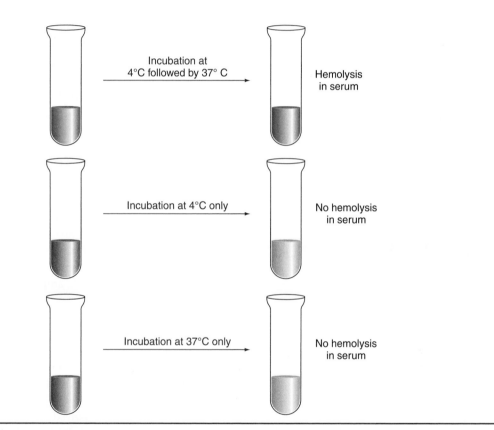

FIGURE 7-4 A patient's freshly drawn serum and red blood cells are incubated at 4°C followed by 37°C. If the Donath Landsteiner antibody is present, it will bind at 4°C and hemolysis will occur on warming to 37°C. If incubation takes place at either 4°C or 37°C alone, the hemolysis will not occur.
Source: Delmar, Cengage Learning

insignificant. Since these antibodies are often complement binding antibodies, polyspecific antiglobulin reagents may detect the bound complement. Pre-warming of all reagents and samples and the use of monospecific AHG sera (without anti-complement components) will prevent the interference of these antibodies in routine testing. Autoanti-I is a cold autoagglutinin that may be observed frequently if the test conditions permit. A strong autoanti-I is seen in persons with *Mycoplasma pneumoniae* infections and cold hemagglutinin disease. Anti-i is seen in the plasma of persons who have recently had infectious mononucleosis. Characteristics of I/i antibodies are summarized in Table 7-10.

I Antigens
Branched Type 2 Chains

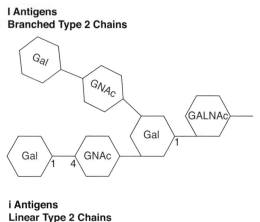

i Antigens
Linear Type 2 Chains

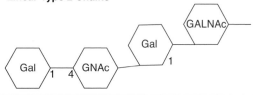

FIGURE 7-5 I antigens are constructed using Branched Type 2 Chains.
i antigens are constructed using Linear Type 2 Chains.
Source: Delmar, Cengage Learning

SYSTEMS WITH WARM-REACTING ANTIBODIES

In contrast to the cold-reacting antibodies discussed in previous sections, warm-reacting antibodies are clinically significant and may create life-threatening consequences when antigen-antibody reactions occur *in vivo*. The warm-reacting antibodies react at 37°C and in the AHG phase of testing. Antibody screen and identification cells should provide sufficient antigen diversity and test procedures must include reagents and methodologies with sufficient sensitivity to detect clinically significant antibodies.

Kell Blood Group System

The Kell blood group system was discovered by Coombs and his associates. The original antibody was associated with hemolytic disease of the newborn. The specific antibody was labeled anti-Kell and the corresponding antigen was labeled "Kell." The Kell system has been assigned the ISBT number 006. The original Kell antigen has been assigned K1. The Kell system is one of the most significant blood group systems. The antigens are strong immunogens, and the corresponding antibodies may be causative agents of transfusion reactions when antigen positive cells are transfused to recipients with Kell-specific antibodies. The antibodies are also implicated in severe neonatal anemia when antigen-positive infants are born to mothers with antigen-specific antibodies. Since the time that Coombs discovered the original Kell antigen, more than 20 additional Kell-system antigens have been discovered.

Genetics of the Kell System

The Kell blood group system genes are located on chromosome 7. The locus for the generation of the Kell system antigens is composed of five sets of genes. The antigens that summarily compose this system are genetically coded by these five sets of genes. The sets of antithetical antigens are summarized in Table 7-11.

The two principle antigens in this blood group system are the K (KEL1) and k (KEL2) antigens. The possible genotypes for an individual are *KK*, *Kk*, and *kk*. The k (Cellano) antigen is a high incidence antigen present in approximately 98% of the Caucasian population. Therefore, the *KK* genotype is rare. Each of the five sets of alleles is inherited in the Mendelian fashion with three possible sets of genotypes. Kell antigens and their frequencies are summarized in Table 7-12.

Genetically, each of these antigens arises from a single nucleotide substitution in KEL. Each nucleotide

TABLE 7-10 Basic Characteristics of I Antibodies					
SYMBOL	**ISBT NUMBER**	**WHO CLASS**	**TEMPERATURE OF REACTIVITY**	**CLINICAL SIGNIFICANCE**	**PHASES OF REACTIVITY**
I	207	IgM	4°C; RT	No HDFN or HTR	IS*, Enhanced by Enzymes

*IS = Immediate Spin

TABLE 7-11 Antithetical Antigens of the Kell Blood Group

K (KEL1)/k (KEL2)
Kp^a (KEL3)/Kp^b (KEL4)/Kp^c (KEL21)
Js^a (KEL6)/Js^b (KEL7)
KEL11/KEL17
KEL14/KEL24

TABLE 7-12 Phenotype Frequencies of Kell Antigens

	PHENOTYPE FREQUENCY (%)	
Phenotype	Caucasian	Black
K−k+	91	98
K+k−	0.2	<0.1
K+k+	8.8	2
Kp(a+b−)	<0.1	0
Kp(a−b+)	97.7	100
Kp(a+b+)	2.3	<0.1
Js(a+b−)	0	1
Js(a+b−)	100	80
Js(a+b−)	<0.1	19

substitution results in an amino-acid substitution. These single substitutions determine the specificity of each antigen.

Biochemistry of the Kell Antigens

The Kell blood-group antigens are located on a glycoprotein integral to the red blood cell membrane. The structure of the glycoprotein is a complex tertiary structure with an extensively folded disulfide bond region. It is this highly folded structure that protects the molecule from degradation by proteolytic enzymes and creates sensitivity to sulfhydryl reducing agents such as dithiothreitol (DTT), 2-mercapto-ethanol (2-ME) and ZZAP, which is a combination of DTT and cysteine-activated papain (see Figure 7-6).

Kx Antigen

A gene, XK1, is located on the X chromosome codes for a protein that produces the Kx antigen. Kx is assigned to the Xk blood group system and has been assigned the ISBT number 019. The Kx antigen is inherited independently of the Kell antigens. The Kx antigen is carried on the Xk protein. Studies of red blood cells that lack the Kx antigen, McLeod phenotype, show a very weak expression of the Kell antigens. Kell$_{null}$ cells that have no Kell antigens exhibit an increased amount of Xk protein. Structurally, it appears that the Kell glycoprotein partially covers the Kx epitope. When the Kell antigens are absent, the Kx epitope is fully exposed.

McLeod and Kell$_{null}$ Phenotypes

Kell$_{null}$ or K_0 is a phenotype completely lacking Kell antigens. Chown and associates originally identified this phenotype in 1957. The inheritance of two K_0 genes ($K_0 K_0$) produces the Kell$_{null}$ phenotype. These individuals do express the Kx antigen. Kell$_{null}$ individuals may produce an anti-Ku or an anti-K5 antibody. The K_u antigen is present on all Kell cells except for Kell$_{null}$. Transfusion of individuals with anti-K5 must be performed using K_0 red cells. These may be obtained by using the services of a rare donor file.

The McLeod phenotype is created when the XK1 gene is not inherited. This inheritance is an X-linked recessive phenotype. Since the XK1 gene is inherited on the X chromosome, the McLeod phenotype is exhibited almost exclusively in males. In this case, the Kx antigen is not found on the red cell surface and consequently the Kell blood-group antigens are produced in markedly reduced amounts. The red cells have morphologic and functional abnormalities. They display decreased permeability to water and a decreased survival rate. A peripheral smear will reveal acathocytosis and polychromasia. The polychromasia results from an increased number of reticulocytes. **Chronic Granulomatous Disease**, an x-linked condition, is at times associated with the McLeod phenotype. This condition presents with white blood cells that have a decreased ability to phagocytize. The inheritance of both the McLeod phenotype and chronic granulomatous disease results from mutation of genetic material on the X chromosome.

Kell Blood-Group Antibodies

Antibodies to the Kell blood group antigens are summarized in Table 7-13. They are primarily IgG antibodies reactive at 37°C and optimally react in the AHG phase of testing. All Kell-system antibodies are capable of causing Hemolytic Disease of the Fetus and Newborn as well as hemolytic transfusion reaction.

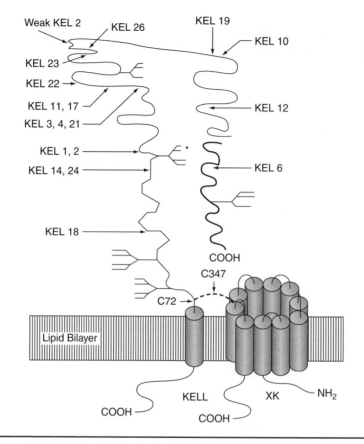

FIGURE 7-6 A diagram of the KELL and XK protein. KELL is covalently linked to the XK protein by a disulfide bond. The arrows indicate Kell-antigen sites. *Reprinted with permission by Elsevier, Inc. from Henry, John Bernard. This article was published in* Clinical Diagnosis and Management, Henry, Jon Bernard. p. 682. Copyright Elsevier (2001).

TABLE 7-13 Basic Characteristics of Kell Antibodies					
SYMBOL	**ISBT NUMBER**	**WHO CLASS**	**TEMPERATURE OF REACTIVITY**	**CLINICAL SIGNIFICANCE**	**PHASES OF REACTIVITY**
KEL	006	IgG	37°C	HDFN and HTR	IAT*, not affected by enzymes, inactivated by DTT

*IAT = indirect antiglobulin test

Kidd Blood-Group Antigens

The Kidd blood-group system is a simple blood-group system compared to other systems that consist of multiple antigens and variable antibody characteristics. The outstanding feature of this system is that the antibodies tend to be weak and short-lived. This characteristic has earned these antibodies the label "treacherous Kidds" and contributes to the notoriety of the system.

The Kidd blood group system has been assigned ISBT number 009. It is composed of three antigens: Jk^a, Jk^b, and Jk3. The Kidd locus is on chromosome 18.

TABLE 7-14 Phenotype Frequencies of Kidd Antigens

| Phenotype | PHENOTYPE FREQUENCY (%) | |
	Caucasian	Black
Jk(a+b−)	26.3	51.1
Jk(a−b+)	23.4	8.1
Jk(a+b+)	50.3	40.8
Jk(a−b−)	Rare	Rare

Within the Kidd blood group, there are two primary antithetical alleles. These alleles are Jk^a and Jk^b. Three possible genotypes exist. These are Jk^{a}Jk^a, Jk^{a}Jk^b, and Jk^{b}Jk^b. The frequencies of these antigens are summarized in Table 7-14. JK3 is present whenever either Jk^a or Jk^b is present.

Biochemically, these antigens are glycoprotein. The glycoprotein is a transmembrane protein that has 10 RBC membrane spanning domains. The Jk^a and Jk^b polymorphism is found on the fourth extracellular loop (see Figure 7-7). These antigens are involved in urea transport and, hence, Kidd antigens are also found on the cells of the kidney.

Kidd Blood Group Antibodies

Kidd antibodies were originally discovered in the 1950s. These antibodies are stimulated by direct exposure via either pregnancy or transfusion. They are typically IgG, AHG reactive antibodies. Characteristics of these antibodies are summarized in Table 7-15.

These antibodies have several characteristics that define them as the "treacherous Kidds." The antigens are not very antigenic, and do not stimulate a strong antibody response, resulting in a low antibody titer. The titer decreases to an undetectable level in the patient's plasma with the passage of time. If, inadvertently, the patient receives the corresponding antigen via transfusion, the antibody will be restimulated in a secondary immune response. This may cause a delayed transfusion reaction. Transfusion reactions will be discussed further in Chapter 12.

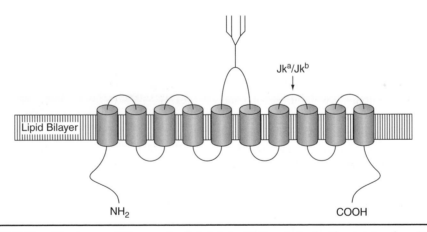

FIGURE 7-7 The Kidd/Urea Transporter Glycoprotein. *Reprinted with permission by Elsevier, Inc. from Henry, John Bernard. This article was published in* Clinical Diagnosis and Management, Henry, John Bernard, p. 687. Copyright Elsevier (2001).

TABLE 7-15 Basic Characteristics of Kidd Antibodies

SYMBOL	ISBT NUMBER	WHO CLASS	TEMPERATURE OF REACTIVITY	CLINICAL SIGNIFICANCE	PHASES OF REACTIVITY
JK	009	IgG	37°C	HDFN and HTR	IAT, Enhanced by Enzymes

*IAT = indirect antiglobulin test

The fact that Kidd antibodies decrease in strength is important for the laboratory worker. These antibodies also display dosage. The weakened antibody will react more strongly with cells that are homozygous and consequently possess a stronger antigen. These test results may be confusing at first, but should be carefully evaluated if there is potential for the existence of a Kidd antibody.

Duffy Blood Group Antigens

The Duffy blood group system was discovered in 1950 when an antibody was detected in a multi-transfused hemophiliac, Mr. Duffy. The corresponding antigen was labeled Fy^a. The antithetical antigen, Fy^b, was discovered the following year. These two antithetical antigens are the major components of this blood group.

The Duffy antigens are glycoprotein and an integral part of the red blood cell membrane. This glycoprotein is also expressed on nonerythroid cells including the endothelium, brain, colon, lung, spleen, kidney, thyroid, and thymus. The glycoprotein is related to the family of IL-8 receptors and serves as an erythrocyte receptor for proinflammatory chemokines. Chemokines play a major role in inflammation as well as malarial infection. Duffy antigens serve as a member of the superfamily of chemokine receptors as well as the receptor for the human malarial parasite, *Plasmodium vivax*.

The Duffy glycoprotein is made up of seven transmembrane spanning domains with intracellular and extracellular loops. The glycoprotein has an exocellular N terminal domain and an endocellular C terminal domain (see Figure 7-8). The two major antigens, Fy^a and Fy^b, are inherited in a Mendelian fashion and differ by a single codon. There are three genotypes possible: Fy^aFy^a, Fy^a-Fy^b, and Fy^bFy^b. The phenotype frequencies are summarized in Table 7-16. The phenotype frequencies differ considerably between Caucasian and Black populations. Note the differences in frequencies as summarized in Table 7-16. Most remarkable is the wide difference in the Fy(a-b-) frequencies.

Antibodies to Duffy Blood Group

These antibodies are characteristically IgG, AHG reactive antibodies that have been actively stimulated through direct antigen exposure. The antibodies are capable of causing Hemolytic Disease of the Fetus and Newborn and hemolytic transfusion reaction. Characteristics of these antibodies are summarized in Table 7-17.

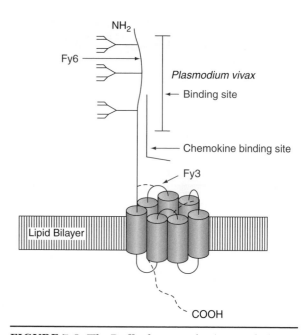

FIGURE 7-8 The Duffy glycoprotein. Arrows designate binding sites for chemokines and Plasmodium vivax. *Reprinted with permission by Elsevier, Inc. from Henry, John Bernard. This article was published in* Clinical Diagnosis and Management, Henry, John Bernard. *p. 685. Copyright Elsevier (2001).*

TABLE 7-16 Phenotype Frequencies of Duffy Antigens

	PHENOTYPE FREQUENCY (%)	
Phenotype	*Caucasian*	*Black*
Fy(a+b−)	17	9
Fy(a−b+)	34	22
Fy(a+b+)	49	1
Fy(a−b−)	Rare	>68

Lutheran Antigens and Antibodies

The Lutheran system consists of 19 antigens. It has been assigned ISBT number 005. The LU locus is on chromosome 19 along with H and Le. The LU locus is also linked to the secretor locus. Most of the Lutheran antigens are high incidence. The primary antigens are the antithetical pair Lu^a (LU1) and Lu^b (LU2). The frequencies of Lu^a and Lu^b antigens are summarized in Table 7-18.

TABLE 7-17 Basic Characteristics of Duffy Antibodies

SYMBOL	ISBT NUMBER	WHO CLASS	TEMPERATURE OF REACTIVITY	CLINICAL SIGNIFICANCE	PHASES OF REACTIVITY
FY	008	IgG	37°C	HDFN and HTR	IAT*, Destroyed by Enzymes

*IAT = Indirect Antiglobulin Test

CRITICAL THINKING ACTIVITY

Creating a Genotype
This exercise may be performed by each student or in small groups. The instructor will provide antigrams from cell identification panels to each student or group (or the antigram in Figure 2-8 may be used). Using this antigram, each student or group should:

1. Examine one cell on the antigram and determine whether that cell is positive or negative for each of the antigens discussed in the above sections on warm reactive antibodies.

2. Explain your determination to either the instructor or a partner.

3. Create a genotype for the antigram cell considering Kell, Kidd, and Duffy blood group systems.

As with other blood group systems, Lutheran null phenotypes occur rarely and result from varying genetic mechanisms. Recessive mechanisms include the inheritance of a rare Lu amorph at this locus and an X-linked suppressor gene. A dominant mechanism is an inhibitor gene In(Lu) located at a separate locus from Lu^a and Lu^b. Therefore, antibodies to these antigens are very rarely.

Antibodies to the Lutheran antigens are found occasionally in the plasma of antigen-negative individuals. Lutheran antigens are found on the glycoprotein portion of the red cell membrane.

TABLE 7-18 Phenotype Frequencies of Lutheran Antigens

PHENOTYPE	FREQUENCY
Lu(a+b−)	0.2
Lu(a−b+)	92.4
Lu(a+b+)	7.4
Lu(a−b−)	Rare

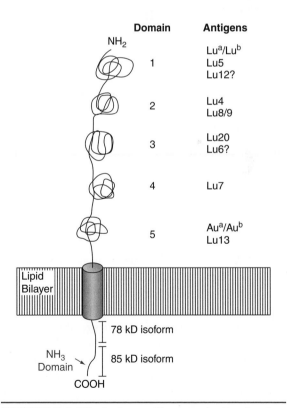

FIGURE 7-9 The Lutheran Glycoprotein. *Reprinted with permission by Elsevier, Inc. from Henry, John Bernard. This article was published in* Clinical Diagnosis and Management, Henry, John Bernard. *p. 681. Copyright Elsevier (2001).*

TABLE 7-19 Basic Characteristics of Lutheran Antibodies					
SYMBOL	**ISBT NUMBER**	**WHO CLASS**	**TEMPERATURE OF REACTIVITY**	**CLINICAL SIGNIFICANCE**	**PHASES OF REACTIVITY**
LU	005	IgG/IgM	Room Temperature/ 37°C	HDFN and HTR (Anti-Lu^b)	RT* (Anti-Lu^a), IAT** (Anti-Lu^b)

*RT = Room Temperature
**IAT = Indirect Antiglobulin Technique

Lutheran antibodies, when present, vary in characteristics. The characteristics of these antibodies are summarized in Table 7-19. Anti-Lu^a is rarely clinically significant. Anti-Lu^b is encountered more rarely, but is more often clinically significant. These antibodies are summarized in Table 7-19.

Molecular Techniques

The continued development of molecular testing methods holds a bright future for expansion of phenotyping red cells of both donors and recipients. Accessible and affordable testing continues to challenge widespread applications of molecular techniques. Some future applications include:

- Applications to counteract the dwindling supply of reagent antisera and the unavailability of antisera to rare antigens.

- The ability to create a quick, comprehensive phenotype for a patient's red blood cells, white blood cells, and platelets.

- Potential to solve typing discrepancies in recently or chronically transfused patients. These patients present unique challenges to the blood bank, since typing through traditional methods frequently produces discrepant or erroneous results. PCR methods are likely more reliable then traditional serological methods for resolving discrepancies in patients who have been transfused within the last 30 days.

- Obtaining donor blood for patients with multiple antibodies is difficult and time-consuming with traditional serological methods. Advances in microarray technology allow for patients to be genotyped for many of the most common blood-group antigens.

- Molecular genotyping of blood donors will allow for antigen-specific blood to be provided for recipients. This method is predicted to have the potential to prevent 80% to 90% of alloimmunization.

A few pitfalls to the use of molecular biology in the blood bank include:

- Molecular techniques determine a patient's genotype. The genotype does not necessarily equate to a phenotype. Genotyping a patient demonstrates antigens on red blood cells, not the true antigenic composition of the cells.

- All of a blood group's alleles may not be known. This can lead to possible problems when attempting to genotype with a rare phenotype that may not have been mapped. Point mutations with no effect on the actual phenotype may have significant effects on single nucleotide polymorphism (SNP) detection if the mutation interferes with primer binding.

- The excessive cost of molecular equipment presents a current challenge. This technology remains limited to large reference labs.

SUMMARY

■ Red blood cells have a variety of genetically determined surface antigens. These antigens are present in different combinations in each individual. With rare exceptions, the antigens are inherited in a Mendelian fashion with the antigens being codominant to each other.

■ These antigens, when not present in a recipient, may serve as immunogens and stimulate antibody production.

■ Red cell stimulated antibodies are significant if they react at warm (body) temperatures and particularly in the AHG phase.

■ Cold-reacting antibodies present interference in testing, but are most often not clinically significant nor will they be incriminated in transfusion reactions.

■ Antibody characteristics are summarized in the table below.

SYMBOL	ISBT NUMBER	WHO CLASS	TEMPERATURE OF REACTIVITY	CLINICAL SIGNIFICANCE	PHASES OF REACTIVITY
Le	007	IgM	Room Temp or Colder	No HDFN or HTR	IS*, 4°C, RT**, Enhanced by Enzymes
MNS1 (Anti-M)	002	IgM, IgG (rare)	Room Temp or Colder	No HDFN or HTR	IS* (most), RT**, Destroyed by Enzymes, may be pH Dependent
MNS2 (Anti-N)	002	IgM, IgG (rare)	Room Temp or Colder; 37°C (Rare-IgG)	No HDFN or HTR	IS* (most), RT**, Destroyed by Enzymes, may be pH Dependent
MNS3 (Anti-S)	002	IgG, IgM (few)	37°C, Some Room Temp	Yes, HDN or HTR	37°C, IAT***, Destroyed by Enzymes
MNS4 (Anti-s)	002	IgG	37°C	37°C, Some Room Temp	37°C, IAT
P1	003	IgM	Room Temp or Colder	No HDFN or HTR	IS*, RT**, Enhanced by Enzymes
I	207	IgM	4°C; RT	No HDFN or HTR	IS*, Enhanced by Enzymes
KEL	006	IgG	37°C	HDFN and HTR	IAT*, not Affected by Enzymes, Inactivated by DTT
JK	009	IgG	37°C	HDFN and HTR	IAT, Enhanced by Enzymes
LU	005	IgG/IgM	Room Temperature/ 37°C	HDFN and HTR (Anti-Lu^b)	RT* (Anti-Lu^a), IAT** (Anti-Lu^b)
FY	008	IgG	37°C	HDFN and HTR	IAT*, Destroyed by Enzymes

- Specific facts to summarize the major blood groups are:
  - Lewis antigens are not developed on the surface of newborns.
  - Lewis antigens develop by the interaction of Le, H, and Se genes.
  - Lewis antibodies are infrequent. Most often they develop during pregnancy and disappear after the pregnancy.
  - The GYPA and GYPB genes code for glycophorin A and B code for MNSs antigens.
  - M and N antigens are at the end terminus of GPA.
  - S and s antigens are at the end terminus of GPB.
  - U is a universal antigen found on GPB.
  - P antigens are formed by the interaction of two separate systems as defined by ISBT (ISBT 003 and ISBT 209).
  - P_1 is the primary antigen in this system.
  - P_1 antigen is found in soluble form in hydatid-cyst fluid.
  - Autoanti-P is an IgG antibody called Donath-Landsteiner antibody and is associated with paroxysmal cold hemoglobinuria.
  - I and i are not considered an antigen system. They are a collection of antigens.
  - i is found on cord blood cells and I is present on adult cells.
  - Anti-i is often detected after infectious mononucleosis.
  - The Kell system is significant since potent antibodies can cause HDFN and decrease red cell survival following incompatible transfusion.
  - k is a high incidence antigen found in 98% of the population.
  - A gene on the X chromosome produces Kx antigen. It is inherited independently from the Kell antigens and codes for the Xk protein. Disulfide bonds bind the Kell glycoprotein and the Xk protein.
  - The McLeod phenotype exists when the Kx gene is not inherited. This phenotype is often associated with CGD.
  - Kidd blood group is historically known for its labile antibodies known as the "treacherous Kidds."
  - Kidd antigens are involved with urea transport and hence are also found on the surface of the kidney.
  - The Kidd antibodies display dosage and disappear over time. The antigens are also known to decrease in strength with storage.
  - Duffy antigen frequency is very different in Caucasian and African-American populations.
  - Duffy antigens are found on nonerythroid cells such as kidney, lung, liver, spleen, and endothelium.
  - The Duffy antigens also serve as receptors for malarial parasites.
  - Lutheran antigens are mostly high frequency antigens. Antibodies to them are encountered rarely.
  - Molecular techniques continue to present promise and challenges to antigen typing and the ability to provide antigen-matched donor blood and prevent alloimmunization.

REVIEW QUESTIONS

1. The antibody that is enhanced by enzymes is:
   a. Anti-Fy^a
   b. Anti-Jk^a
   c. Anti-K
   d. Anti-M

2. The antigen that is associated with urea transport is:
   a. Le^a
   b. Lu^a
   c. Jk^a
   d. S

3. The phenotype of any newborn will include which of the following:
   1. Le (a−b−)
   2. Le (a+b−)
   3. Le (a−b+)
   4. I −, i +
   5. I +, i −
   a. 1 and 4 are correct
   b. 1 and 5 are correct
   c. 2 and 4 are correct
   d. 2 and 5 are correct
   e. 3 and 4 are correct
   f. 3 and 5 are correct

4. An individual with a Bombay phenotype, who is Le+ and Se+ will have a Lewis phenotype of:
   a. Le (a−b−)
   b. Le (a+b−)
   c. Le (a−b+)
   d. Le (a+b+)

5. The antibody that is not ever a cold-reacting antibody is:
   a. Anti-Lu^a
   b. Anti-Kell
   c. Anti-M
   d. Anti-P

6. An antibody identification is performed using ficin. Which of the following antibodies will not be detected?
   a. Anti-Le^a
   b. Anti-Kell
   c. Anti-M
   d. Anti-P

7. The antigen system that binds chemokines is:
   a. Lewis
   b. Lutheran
   c. Kell
   d. Duffy

8. The antigen systems that are carbohydrate do not include:
   a. P
   b. I
   c. Lewis
   d. Duffy

9, 10, and 11 Looking at the antigram below, answer the following questions:

9. The cell(s) that represents homozygous for K is
   a. cell 1
   b. cell 2
   c. cells 1 and 2

10. An anti-Jk^a will react more strongly with:
    a. cell 1
    b. cell 2
    c. cells 1 and 2

11. The Js^b antigen is present on:
    a. cell 1
    b. cell 2
    c. cells 1 and 2

12. The Globside group is associated with which antigen system:
    a. Lewis
    b. Kell
    c. I
    d. P

13. Antigen systems that are associated with HDFN include:
    1. Lewis
    2. Kell
    3. P
    4. Kidd
    5. Duffy
    a. 1, 2, and 5 are correct
    b. 1, 3, and 4 are correct
    c. 2, 4, and 5 are correct
    d. 2, 3, and 5 are correct

Cell #			Rh-hr						KELL						DUFFY		KIDD		Sex Linked	LEWIS		MNS				P	LUTHERAN	
	D	C	E	c	e	f*	C^w	V	K	k	Kp^a	Kp^b	Js^a	Js^b	Fy^a	Fy^b	Jk^a	Jk^b	Xg^a	Le^a	Le^b	S	s	M	N	P$_1$	Lu^a	Lu^b
1	+	+	0	0	+	0	0	0	0	+	0	+	0	+	0	+	+	+	+	0	+	+	0	+	+	+s	0	+
2	+	0	+	+	0	0	0	0	+	0	0	+	0	+	+	+	0	+	0	+	0	+	+	+	0	+	0	+

Source: Delmar, Cengage Learning

14. Glycophorin A is associated with the antigen:
    a. I
    b. P
    c. N
    d. S

15. The folded nature of the _____ antigen prevents enzymatic degradation.
    a. Duffy
    b. Lewis
    c. Kell
    d. Kidd

16. A 16-year-old female was recently diagnosed with *Mycoplasma pneumonia*. She is now having a type and antibody screen for an upcoming surgery. The immediate spin antibody screen was positive in both cells. The antibody that one would expect to identify is
    a. Anti-Le^a
    b. Anti-Lu^a
    c. Anti-k
    d. Anti-I

17. An anti-P$_1$ is suspected when an immediate spin antibody screen is positive in one cell. The ideal temperature for identification is:
    a. 17°C
    b. 25°C
    c. 37°C
    d. 42°C

18. Which of the following combinations will not allow Le^b antigen to be produced:
    a. Lele, Sese, HH
    b. LeLe, sese, HH
    c. LeLe, SeSe, HH
    d. Lele, Sese, Hh

19. Which of the following antibodies would you have to go to a rare donor file to find compatible blood?
    a. Anti-K
    b. Anti-s
    c. Anti-p
    d. Anti-U

20. Antigens that are integral to the red cell membrane belong to the _____ blood group.
    a. Kell
    b. Lewis
    c. I, i
    d. Secretor

CASE STUDY

1. You are working in a regional Blood Bank that performs paternity testing. The following request comes to you. These children have been typed for MNSs. The phenotypes are listed below. Your job is to determine which child cannot have the same father. The mother's phenotype is MNs and the alleged father is NSs
   Child 1: Ns
   Child 2: MNSs
   Child 3: Ms
   Child 4: MNs

2. An individual presents with a positive antibody screen. The antibody reacts with one antibody screen cell in the anti-human globulin phase. Answer the following questions.
   a. List 5 possible antibodies.
   b. State the temperature of reactivity for this antibody.
   c. This patient needs to be transfused. What special steps should be taken to assure compatible blood for this recipient.

REFERENCES

Akane, A, et al. "Classification of Standard Alleles of the MN Blood Group System." *Vox sanguinis*. Vol. 79, Issue 3. pp. 183–187.

Blaney, Kathy and Howard, Paula. *Basic and Applied Concepts of Immunohematology*. Mosby, Philadelphia, 2000.

Brecher, Mark, editor. *American Association of Blood Banks Technical Manual 15th edition*. AABB, 2005.

Castillo, Lilian. "The value of DNA Analysis for Antigens in the Duffy Blood Group System." *Transfusion*. Vol. 47; Issue 1 supplement; 2007, pp. 28S–31S.

Harmening, Denise. *Modern Blood Banking and Transfusion Practices*. F. A. Davis, Philadelphia, 2005.

Hakomore, Sen-itiroh. "Blood Group ABH and Ii Antigens of Human Erythrocytes: Chemistry, Polymorphism, and Their Developmental Change." *Seminars in Hematology*. Vol 18, No. 1, pp. 39–58.

Henry, John Bernard, *Clinical Diagnosis and Management by Laboratory Methods*. W. B. Saunders Co. 2001.

Issitt PD, Anstee DJ (1998). *Applied Blood Group Serology. 4th edition*, Durham, NC, USA: Montgomery Scientific Publications.

Lee, Soohee. "The Value of DNA Analysis for Antigens of the Kell and Kx Blood Group Systems." *Transfusion*. Vol. 47, Issue, 1 supplement, 2007, pp. 32–39S.

Lomas-Francis, Christine. "The Value of DNA Analysis for Antigens of the Kidd Blood Group System." *Transfusion*. Vol. 47, Issue 1 supplement, 2007, pp. 23–27S.

Marcus, Donald M. Kundu, Samar K. and Suzuki, Akemi. "The P Blood Group System: Recent Progress in Immunochemistry and Genetics." *Seminars in Hematology*. Vol. 18, No. 1, 1982.

McCullough, Jeffrey. *Transfusion Medicine 2nd edition*. Elsevier. 2005.

Mizukame, Hajime, Akane, A., Nakayashiki, N., Yasuhiro, A., and Shiono, Hiroshi. "Systematic Classification of Alleles of the Glycophorin A (MN Blood Group) Gene." *Journal of Human Genetics*. October 2005.

Montalvo, Lani, Walker, Phyllis, et al. "Clinical Investigation of Posttransfusion Kidd Blood Group Typing Using a Rapid Normalized Quantitative Polymerase Chain Reaction." *Transfusion*. Vol. 44, May 2004, pp. 694–702.

Palacajornsuk, P. "Review: Molecular Basis of MNS Blood Group Variants." *Immunohematology*. Vol. 22, Issue 4, 2006, pp. 171–182.

Parsons, S. F. et al. "The Lutheran Blood Group Glycoprotein, Another Member of the Immunoglobulin Superfamily, is Widely Expressed in Human Tissues and is Developmentally Regulated in Human Liver." *Proceedings of the National Academy of Sciences of the United States of America*. Vol. 92, No. 12, 1995, pp. 5496–5500.

Poole, Joyce and Daniels, Geoff. "Blood Group Antibodies and Their Significance in Transfusion Medicine." *Transfusion Medicine Reviews*. Vol. 21, Issue 1, January 2007, pp. 58–71.

Prager, Martina. "Molecular Genetic Blood Group Typing by the use of PCR-SSP Technique." *Transfusion*. Vol. 47, Issue 1 supplement, 2007, pp. 54–59S.

Pu, Jeffrey J. "Onset of Expression of the Components of the Kell Blood Group Complex." *Transfusion*. Vol. 45, Issue 6, 2005, pp. 969–974.

Quill, Elizabeth. "Blood-Matching Goes Genetic." *Science*. Vol. 319, Issue 5869, 2008, pp. 1478–1479.

Reid, Marion E. and Lomas-Francis, Christine. *The Blood Group Antigen: Facts Book*. Elsevier, 2004.

Reid, M. "Contribution of MNS to the study of Glycophorin A and Glycophorin B. *Immunohematology*." Vol. 15, Issue 1, 1999, pp. 5–9.

Reid, Marion and Lomas-Francis, Christine. *The Blood Group Antigen Facts Book*. Elsevier, 2004.

Reid, Marion E, McManus and Zelinski, Teresa. "Chromosome Location of Genes Encoding Human Blood Groups." *Transfusion Medicine Reviews*. Vol. 12, Issue 3. July 1998, pp. 151–161.

Ridgwell, K. "Production of Soluble Recombinant Proteins with Kell, Duffy and Lutheran Antibodies." *Transfusion Medicine*. Vol. 17, Issue 5, 2007, pp. 384–94.

Schenkel-Brunner, Helmut. *Human Blood Groups: Chemical and Biochemical Basis of Antigen Specificity*. Springer Wien, 2000.

Storry, Jill R. "New Technologies to replace current blood typing reagents." *Current Opinion in Hematology*. Vol. 14, Issue 6, 2007, pp. 677–681.

Sheffield, William P. "Detection of Antibodies with the Antithetical Duffy Blood Group Antigens Fy(a) and Fy(b) Using Recombinant Fusion Proteins Containing the Duffy Extracellular Domain." *Transfusion and Apheresis Science*. Vol. 35: No. 3, 2006, pp. 207–216.

Turgeon, Mary Louise. *Fundamentals of Immunohematology*. Williams and Wilkins, Media, PA, 1995.

Patient
Pre-Transfusion
Testing

Antibody Screening and Antibody Identification

LEARNING OUTCOMES

At the completion of this chapter, the reader should be able to:

- Define atypical antibody and outline its formation.
- Describe antibody screening methods and explain positive and negative outcomes.
- Diagram a step-by-step procedure for antibody screen tests continuing to the identification process.
- Describe the antibody identification panel procedure and interpret the results.
- Define phase of reactions and list phases used for antibody identification.
- List three specific ways that reaction strength can be used for resolution of antibody identification.
- Describe select cell panel and the choice of select cells that compose a panel.
- Incorporate previous knowledge of antigen systems with methodology to identify antibodies.
- Discuss the effects of high titer low avidity (HLTA) antibodies on antibody screening and identification testing.
- Outline and discuss antigen typing methods to include the use of quality control.
- Define the rule of three and selection of cells for confirmation of each antibody.
- Define and relate the necessity for absorption and elution studies in antibody identification procedures.
- Discuss enzyme tests and list antibodies that are enhanced and destroyed by these enzymes.
- Outline prewarming techniques and list antibodies that would be eliminated with prewarming.
- Resolve discrepancies in the interpretation of antibody studies.

GLOSSARY

alloantibody   antibody directed at antigens not present on an individual's red cells

allogeneic adsorption   adsorption of antibody from serum with selective cells that are not autologous cells

autocontrol   mixture of serum and cells from the same individual; used to determine the presence of antibody coating the patient's red cells

eluate   liquid harvested after an elution is performed

elution   method used to remove antibodies from the surface of red cells for testing purposes

idiopathic   without a detectable cause

parallel testing   series of tests performed using conditions identical to the patient or control tests; used to rule out contamination or other interferences

warm autoimmune hemolytic anemia (WAIHA)   anemia caused by hemolysis of red cells caused by an antibody directed against autologous cells; the etiology of the antibody is a warm-reacting antibody

INTRODUCTION

Detection and identification of an antibody in the plasma, or coating the red blood cells, often presents a challenge for the testing personnel. These antibodies are labeled "atypical" and are often unexpected. They are in contrast to ABO antibodies that are "expected" and present a problem when they are *not* detected. This chapter will present methods for detection and identification of specific antibodies outlined in Chapters 6 and 7. Many of these antibodies are clinically significant, while others may present interference in test methods, but are not significant to the well-being of the patient. The atypical antibodies are the result of direct antigen exposure either through transfusion of red cells or maternal exposure to fetal red blood cells during pregnancy. The division of antibody screening and identification falls into two broad categories: antibodies found on red cells and those present in plasma. A logical progression begins with an antibody screen to detect "atypical" antibodies in the plasma or a direct antiglobulin test (DAT) to detect antibody on the surface of the red blood cells. The step-wise progression follows with the identification of the detected antibody(ies). The interpretation of antibody screen and antibody identification tests uses a systematic approach. Specific procedures for identification are outlined in this chapter. Each sample is unique and requires a series of test procedures to obtain an accurate final result. The application of principles in this chapter will require extended practice and experience to obtain proficiency and confidence in the problem-solving process. For a summary of antibody detection techniques and the methods of testing that lead to the identification of these antibodies, refer to the flow chart in Figure 8-1.

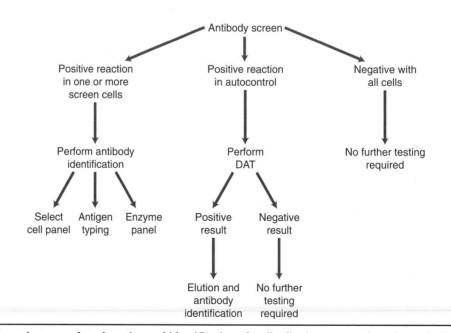

FIGURE 8-1 **A systematic approach to detection and identification of antibodies in serum and coating red cells**
Source: Delmar, Cengage Learning

ANTIBODY DETECTION

Antibody Screen Test

When exposed to foreign antigens, via transfusion or pregnancy, an individual may produce an antibody directed against foreign antigens. This antibody is an **alloantibody** and is found in the plasma. A test performed for detection of antibody in the plasma is the antibody screen test. A list of individuals screened for atypical antibodies is summarized in Table 8-1.

Antigens discussed in Chapters 6 and 7 are the most common immunogens for atypical or red cell stimulated antibodies. Recall Landsteiner's law, which states that antibodies are developed only if the antigens are not present on the individual's red cells. If the antibody screen is positive and antibodies are present in the plasma, a more definitive test known as the antibody identification panel is performed. For both antibody screen and identification tests, serum or plasma are acceptable specimens.

Test Method for Detection of Antibodies in Serum

Patient and donor plasma is screened for atypical antibodies using commercially prepared cells. They are group O cells that have been tested for the presence of the most commonly encountered antigens. The cells are provided from the manufacturer in sets of either two or three vials. Each vial contains cells from a single, unique donor. The vials are provided with a description of the antigen content of each of the cells. This description is provided in a chart known as an antigram. Sample antigrams were provided for use in activities in Chapter 2. See Figure 8-2 for a sample antigram.

Testing the plasma of the patient or donor with the commercially prepared cells is the basic antibody screen procedure. Testing incorporates varying conditions of reactivity including temperature and use of potentiating media. The media of reactivity includes immediate spin saline, potentiating media such as low ionic strength substance (LISS), and anti-human globulin (AHG) sera. Testing protocols are established at the discretion of the institution.

Results of each phase are recorded and evaluated. This is a screening test and test results indicate the presence of an antibody, but not the identity of the antibody. The use of antigrams and incorporation of knowledge of optimal temperature and media of reactivity for the potential antibodies allows the possibilities to be narrowed. For specific identification an antibody identification panel must be utilized and results evaluated.

Autocontrol

Antibody screen testing may include the use of an **autocontrol**. The autocontrol is an additional test that contains the individual's red cell suspension and plasma and is tested in parallel with the antibody screen cells. The results of the autocontrol are recorded along with the screen results. A positive result in the autocontrol at the AHG phase indicates an antibody coating the red cells. This antibody may be removed from the cells and identified

---

TABLE 8-1 Individuals Who May be Screened for Atypical Antibodies

Indications for Antibody Screen
Blood and Pheresis Donors
Prenatal Patients
Surgical Patients
Blood Component Transfusion Candidates
Transfusion Reaction Work-Up Testing

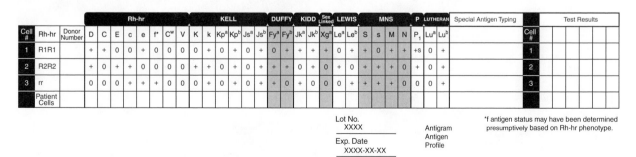

Cell #	Rh-hr	Donor Number	D	C	E	c	e	f*	Cʷ	V	K	k	Kpᵃ	Kpᵇ	Jsᵃ	Jsᵇ	Fyᵃ	Fyᵇ	Jkᵃ	Jkᵇ	Xgᵃ	Leᵃ	Leᵇ	S	s	M	N	P₁	Luᵃ	Luᵇ	Special Antigen Typing	Cell #	Test Results
1	R1R1		+	+	0	0	+	0	0	0	0	+	0	+	0	+	0	+	+	+	+	0	+	0	+	0	+	+s	0	+		1	
2	R2R2		+	0	+	+	0	0	0	0	+	+	0	+	0	+	+	+	0	+	0	+	0	+	+	+	0	+	0	+		2	
3	rr		0	0	0	+	+	+	0	0	0	+	0	+	0	+	+	0	+	0	0	0	+	+	+	+	0	0	0	+		3	
Patient Cells																																	

Lot No.
XXXX

Exp. Date
XXXX-XX-XX

Antigram Antigen Profile

*f antigen status may have been determined presumptively based on Rh-hr phenotype.

FIGURE 8-2 Sample antigram for a set of antibody screen cells
Source: Delmar, Cengage Learning

in the same manner as antibody in plasma. The use of an autocontrol is optional. Alternately, a direct antiglobulin test may be performed if the antibody screen is positive.

Alloantibody vs. Autoantibody

One must first evaluate whether the antibody is an alloantibody or an autoantibody. This assessment starts with one major factor, the autocontrol. If the autocontrol is negative, the antibody is an alloantibody. The process of identification of an alloantibody will no longer consider the results of the autocontrol.

If the autocontrol is positive, the technician must determine if this is a true autoantibody or if the positive

result is interference from the potentiating agent. When a positive autocontrol exists, a direct antiglobulin (DAT) should be performed. If the DAT is negative, then the positive reactions may be the result of interference from the potentiating agent. In this case, the panel and autocontrol should be repeated using a different potentiating agent *or* no potentiator.

If the DAT is positive, an autoantibody exists. An alloantibody may also exist. These two types of antibodies must be differentiated. The process for removing the autoantibody from the cell surface (elution) and identification of the resulting antibody will be discussed later in this chapter. See Box 8-1 for sample evaluations of antibody screen results.

Box 8-1

A.
Antibody Screen Results

Screen Cell	Immediate Spin	37°C	AHG	CC
1	0	0	0	√
2	0	1+	3+	NT
Autocontrol	0	0	0	√

Direct Antiglobulin Tests

Polyspecific		IgG	C3
0	√	NT	NT

Interpretation: Alloantibody; IgG Antibody; Most likely Single Antibody Specificity

B.
Antibody Screen Results

Screen Cell	Immediate Spin	37°C	AHG	CC
1	0	0	2+	NT
2	0	1+	3+	NT

Direct Antiglobulin Tests

Polyspecific		IgG	C3
0	√	NT	NT

Interpretation: Alloantibody; IgG; Most likely Multiple Antibodies

C.
Antibody Screen Results

Screen Cell	Immediate Spin	37°C	AHG	CC
1	1+	0	0	√
2	1+	0	0	√

Direct Antiglobulin Tests

Polyspecific		IgG		C3	
0	√	0	√	0	√

Interpretation: Alloantibody; IgM; Most likely single antibody

D.
Antibody Screen Results

Screen Cell	Immediate Spin	37°C	AHG	CC
1	0	0	0	√
2	0	0	0	√

Direct Antiglobulin Tests

Polyspecific		IgG		C3	
2+	NT	2+	NT	0	√

Interpretation: Autoantibody; IgG specificity

Key: AHG = Anti-Human Globulin G Phase
37°C = Incubation at 37°C
CC = Check Cells (Coombs Control Cells)
IgG = Monospecific IgG Antiglobulin Sera
C3 = Anti-Complement Antiglobulin Sera
0 = Negative Test Result
NT = Not tested
√ = Check cells reactive

Direct Anti-globulin Test

A second screening test for antibodies is the direct antiglobulin test or DAT. It is a test that detects antibodies coating the surface of the red blood cells *in vivo*. Individuals with a positive DAT will also have a positive autocontrol in the antibody screen. Using a combination of different AHG sera can provide additional information related to the specificity of the substance(s) coating the red cells. Polyspecific AHG contains a mixture of anti-IgG and anti-C3. Monospecific AHG is either anti-IgG OR anti-C3. Reactivity in one or more AHG sera provides specificity of the substance(s) coating the red cells. See Figure 8-3 for examples of interpretations.

The antibodies detected on the red cell surface may be removed using elution. The elution process

Polyspecific 2+	Polyspecific 1+	Polyspecific 2+
Anti-IgG 2+	Anti-IgG 0	Anti-IgG 1+
Anti-C_3 0	Anti-C_3 1+	Anti-C_3 1+

Interpretation: IgG Substances Immunoglobulins Coating Red blood Cells.	C_3 Complement	IgG Immunoglobulins C_3 Complement

FIGURE 8-3 **A positive DAT may be caused by immunoglobulins, complement, or a combination of the two. A break down of the specific coating substance can be determined by using multiple AHG sera and comparison of the results.**
Source: Delmar, Cengage Learning

removes antibodies from the cell surface and releases them into the eluting fluid. The antibody removal may be accomplished with a chemical or physical destruction

CRITICAL THINKING ACTIVITY

In small groups, students will use a sample antigram provided by the instructor (or the antigram represented in Figure 8-2). Each group should answer the questions 1 and 2 for each of these antibodies:

a. Anti-C
b. Anti-Fy^a
c. Anti-K
d. Anti-Jk^b

1. With which screening cell(s) does the antibody react?
2. List three additional antibodies that would react with the same cell(s).

CRITICAL THINKING ACTIVITY

Examination of Antibody Identification Panel Sheets
    Examine the panel sheets provided by the instructor or use the sample in Figure 2-8.
    Find the following items:

1. The lot number of the panel

    Note: It is imperative that the antigram sheet being used corresponds to the lot number on the panel. Otherwise the results obtained will not provide a pattern useful for identifying the antibody or antibodies present.

2. The patient identification section. Pertinent patient information is recorded here.
3. The results section. The interpretation of antibody or antibodies identified is recorded here.
4. The blank spaces for patient typing results. Patient cell typings are recorded in the blank space at the bottom of each antigen column.
5. The ABO testing results. These test results should be recorded for use with the identification process.
6. The DAT results. These results should be recorded for use in the identification process.

Share all of your findings with fellow students or the instructor.

of the antigen-antibody bond. The antibody is released into the eluting fluid. This fluid is tested for the presence of the eluted antibody.

Clinical Indications of a Positive Direct Antiglobulin Test

When the DAT is positive, it indicates that the red blood cells are coated with an autoantibody or complement components. An autoantibody is directed against an antigen present on the surface of the patient's red cells and defies Landsteiner's Law. Autoantibodies occur in clinical conditions such as warm or cold autoimmune hemolytic anemia (AIHA), drug-induced AIHA, hemolytic disease of the fetus and newborn (HDFN) and hemolytic transfusion reaction (HTR).

Antibody Identification

The presence of a positive antibody screen or DAT requires identification of the antibody. If one or more antibody screen cells present with a positive result, then an antibody identification panel is performed. If only the autocontrol is positive, a DAT is necessary. A positive DAT will require removal of the antibody by elution and testing of the eluate.

    As described in Chapter 2, an antibody identification panel is a series of 8 to 16 red cells from unique Group O donors that have been antigen typed for the common red cell antigens. The panel is tested using the same test parameters as an antibody screen. The patient's plasma is the unknown component of the test with the potential for having an unknown antibody. The reagent red cells contribute the known antigens. Varying temperatures and potentiators are used to enhance the antigen-antibody reaction. Results are interpreted and either provide a definitive identification or indicate that further testing is necessary. A summary of guidelines for interpretation of an antibody identification panel is presented in Table 8-2.

TABLE 8-2 Guidelines for the Interpretation of an Antibody Panel

LOOK AT	RESULT	INTERPRETATION
Autocontrol	Negative	Alloantibody
	Positive	1. Autoantibody or 2. Delayed transfusion reaction; transfused cells are sensitized with antibody
Phases	Reaction Temperature or Immediate Spin	Cold or IgM antibody
	37°C Reactions	1. May be cold (IgM) if reactions started at room temperature or 2. May be warm (IgG) if reactions are not seen at room temperature but noticed at AHG
	AHG	Warm or IgG antibody; clinically significant
Reaction Strength	Single Strength	Probably one antibody specificity
	Varying Strength	More than one antibody or one antibody showing dosage
Ruling Out	Negative Reactions	1. If no reaction was observed, the antibody to the antigen on the panel was probably not present 2. If the antigen on the panel is heterozygous, the antibody may be showing dosage; rule out carefully
	Positive Reactions	Never rule out with positive reactions
Matching the Pattern	Single antibody	If the specificity is a single antibody, the pattern matches one of the antigen columns
	Multiple antibodies	When more than one antibody is present, it is difficult to match a pattern unless the phases or reaction strengths are unique
Rule of Three	Three positives	Is the suspected antibody reactive with at least three panel cells that are antigen positive?
	Three negatives	Is the suspected antibody negative with at least three panel cells that do not possess the antigen?
Phenotype the Patient	Negative	If the patient does not possess the antigen, it is possible to make the antibody
	Positive	1. Transfused red blood cells are present if patient received a unit of red blood cells within 120 days 2. Suspected antibody is incorrect

Reprinted with permission by Elsevier, Inc. from Henry, John Bernard. This article was published in Basic and Applied Concepts of Immunohematology. Blaney, Kathy D. and Howard, Paula R. Mosby, St. Louis, MO, 2000. Copyright Elsevier (2000).

Single Antibody Identification Panel Interpretation

Once testing is completed and all results are recorded on the panel sheet, these results are interpreted using a methodical approach. The assessment of the antibody or antibodies may be simple and involve few steps *or* may be more complex and involve multiple steps dependent on the number of antibodies and reaction patterns of the antibodies.

Elimination Method

Elimination is a systematic process for interpretation of antibody identification panels. Elimination is performed using cells with no reactivity (0) at any phase

CRITICAL THINKING ACTIVITY

For this exercise, students may use results from completed antigrams provided by the instructor.

Equipment
Completed antigrams
Ruler
Pencil

1. Examine the antigram(s) provided by the instructor.
2. Following the steps in Sample Procedure 8-1 and referring to Figures 8-4 and 8-5, identify the antibody(ies) present on the antigram.
3. Share results with classmates or instructor.

to eliminate potential antibodies to antigens present on that cell. The method is useful but not foolproof. Antibodies to antigens that display dosage or combinations of antibodies will present a challenge, and the elimination method may not provide a definitive resolution. Sample Procedure 8-1 outlines the elimination procedure.

Phases of Reactivity

Elimination will narrow the possible antibodies. After the elimination process, it may be necessary to consider the temperature of reactivity for the antibody or combination of antibodies (referring to Chapters 6 and 7 and the detailed discussion of antibodies, temperatures, and phases of reactivity). Table 8-3 summarizes the antibodies and temperatures of reactivity for key antibodies.

Rule of Three

When identifying antibodies, the antibody assigned must be statistically justified. There is a "rule of three" that provides this statistical confirmation. It is necessary to identify each antibody with sufficient data to establish that the probability value (p value) is <0.05. This establishes that the event is not random with 95% confidence. This is accomplished by testing a minimum of three antigen positive cells and three antigen negative cells against the test plasma. If the original panel does not meet these criteria, then additional cells from a different panel must be tested to satisfy the statistical criteria.

Antigen Typing

Phenotyping or typing patient's autologous cells for the presence of antigen is used as confirmation of the antibody present in the serum. If the antigen is not present,

SAMPLE PROCEDURE 8-1

Elimination Method to Interpret Antibody Identification Panels

1. Place the panel sheet on a flat surface and examine the results columns. Do not consider the check cell results.
2. Determine the first cell that displayed completely negative reactions (0) when reacted with the plasma.
3. Place a straightedge under the cell typings and find results for that cell (see Figure 8-4).
4. Examine the typing results for that cell. For each antigen that typed positive on that cell, place a line through that antigen designation on the top of the page (see Figure 8-4).
5. Repeat this step with each cell that produced no reaction (0) until all of the non-reactive cells have been considered.
6. Antigens not crossed with a line are those for which the corresponding antibody has not been eliminated.
7. The vertical pattern of reactivity of the plasma is examined and compared to the vertical pattern of reactivity for each antigen. If an exact match is found, this is most likely the antibody present. It is ideal to rule out all possible antibodies since a combination of more than one antibody may be encountered (see Figure 8-5).

SAMPLE PROCEDURE 8-1

8. If an exact pattern of reactivity is not seen, additional test methods are necessary to determine the antibody or antibodies present. These techniques will be discussed in the following sections.

9. Note that some antigens are not found on any of the cells in the panel. It is impossible to rule them out with a panel that does not have the antigen present. The elimination system cannot eliminate antibodies directed against these antigens. A select cell panel may be useful in this situation.

10. Examine the pattern of reactivity on the antigram and determine if there is an exact match of patterns. For example, positive reactions were seen in cells 2 and 7 at AHG. Cells 2 and 7 are positive for the E antigen. Therefore, anti-E is an exact match. If a match is not achieved, list all possible antibodies.

11. List the possible antibodies in the area of the antigram that is designated for this purpose. The proper way to list them is as "anti-C" or using the Greek letter alpha followed by the antibody e.g. "α - C." This is an example of a potential antibody identification result.

TABLE 8-3 Temperatures and Media of Reactivity for Major Antibodies

ANTIGEN-ANTIBODY SYSTEMS	ROOM TEMPERATURE AND IMMEDIATE SPIN REACTIVE	37°C AND AHG REACTIVE	IMMUNOGLOBULIN CLASS
MN, Lewis, I, P	Yes	No	IgM
Rh, Kell, Kidd, Duffy, Ss	No	Yes	IgG

then the antibody may be present as an alloantibody. According to Landsteiner's Law, individuals develop antibodies to antigens that are not present on their red cells. Therefore, phenotyping may help to confirm the presence of the suspected antibody.

If one or more antibodies cannot be eliminated with the original panel, phenotype information may be helpful. The autocontrol must be negative at all phases of testing. For each antibody not excluded, the patient's cells may be typed for specific antigens. If the antigen is present, then the antibody is not present in the plasma. If the antigen is absent, then the antibody cannot be excluded. The results of the antigen typings are recorded on the bottom of the panel sheet where patient cell results are indicated. See Figure 8-5 for an example of antigen typing.

Additional Antibody Identification Tests

When results of the initial antibody identification are not definitive, phases and temperatures of reactivity and red cell phenotyping results are considered. When all of these factors have been assessed and a definitive result has not been obtained, further testing may be performed to narrow the possibilities. Further testing may include enzyme testing, select cell panels, cold panels, elution, and absorption.

Enzyme Testing

Enzymes are used in blood bank testing to aid in identification of antibodies. Proteolytic enzymes, such as ficin and papain, affect antigen-antibody reactions

Cell No.	D	C	E	c	e	f	K	k	Fy^a	Fy^b	Jk^a	Jk^b	Xg^a	Le^a	Le^b	S	s	M	N	P_1	IS	37°	AHG	C.C.
1	+	+	0	0	+	0	0	+	+	+							+	+	0	0	0	1+	2+	
2	+	+	0	0	+	0	+	+	+	+^w								+	0	0	0	1+	2+	
3	+	0	+	+	0	0	0	+	+	0	0					+	0	+	+^s	0	0	0		+
8	0	0	0	+	+	+	+	+	+	0	+	0	+	0	0	+	+	+	+	0	0	0	0	+
9	0	0	0	+	+	+	0	+	+	0	+	0	+	+	0	+	0	+	0	+^w	0	0	0	+
10	0	0	0	+	+	+	0	+	0	+	0	+	+	+	0	0	+	0	+	+	0	0	0	+
11													0	0							0	0	0	+

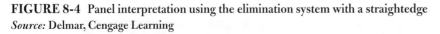

FIGURE 8-4 Panel interpretation using the elimination system with a straightedge
Source: Delmar, Cengage Learning

Cell No.	D	C	E	c	e	f	K	k	Fy^a	Fy^b	Jk^a	Jk^b	Xg^a	Le^a	Le^b	S	s	M	N	P_1	IS	37°	AHG	C.C.
1	+	+	0	0	+	0	0	+	+	+	+	0	+	0	+	+	+	+	0	0	0	1+	2+	
2	+	+	0	0	+	0	+	+	+	+^w	+	+	+	0	+	+	+	+	0	0	0	1+	2+	
3	+	0	+	+	0	0	0	+	+	0	0	+	+	0	+	0	+	0	+	+^s	0	0	0	+
4	+	0	0	+	+	+	0	+	0	0	+	+	+	0	0	0	+	+	+	+^s	0	0	0	+
5	0	+	0	+	+	+	0	+	0	+	+	+	0	0	+	0	+	0	+	+	0	1+	2+	
6	0	0	+	+	+	+	0	+	0	+	+	+	+	0	+	0	+	+	0	+	0	0	0	+
7	0	0	0	+	+	+	+	+	0	+	0	+	+	0	+	0	+	+	+	0	0	0	0	+
8	0	0	0	+	+	+	+	+	+	0	+	0	+	0	0	+	+	+	+	0	0	0	0	+
9	0	0	0	+	+	+	0	+	+	0	+	0	+	+	0	+	0	+	0	+^w	0	0	0	+
10	0	0	0	+	+	+	0	+	0	+	0	+	+	+	0	0	+	0	+	+	0	0	0	+
11	0	0	0	+	+						0	0									0	0	0	+

Interpretation: Anti-C.

FIGURE 8-5 Antigen typing of the patient's cells is performed and the results are recorded on the panel sheet.
The specific antigen typing result is recorded in the blank space directly below the column of antigen typing results for the panel cells.
Source: Delmar, Cengage Learning

TABLE 8-4 Effects of Enzymes on Antigens

ANTIGENS ENHANCED BY ENZYMES	ANTIGENS DESTROYED BY ENZYMES
Rh	Duffy
Kidd	MN
I	
Lewis	
P_1	

by either enhancing (strengthening) or inhibiting (eliminating) the reactivity. Enhancement makes antigens more accessible. Destruction of antigens on the surface of the cells by the enzyme creates inhibition of some reactions. See Table 8-4 for a summary of the effects of enzymes. Because enzymes inhibit the reactions of some antibodies, inclusion in the identification process may rule out additional antibodies in the plasma. Enzymes use two mechanisms of antibody exclusion. First, an antibody's existence may be proven with destruction of its reactivity. Alternately, removing an enzyme susceptible antibody may reveal additional masked antibodies. Exclusive use of enzyme panels is a dangerous practice since enzymes may result in destruction of clinically significant antibodies. Figures 8-6 and 8-7 show examples of antibody identification panels where reactions have been enhanced and destroyed by enzymes.

Two methods of enzyme treatment are used in blood bank testing: indirect and direct. In the indirect method, cells are treated with enzymes and the excess enzyme is washed away. These pretreated cells are used to test the plasma. In the direct method, enzyme is added to the plasma/cell test mixture as an enhancement media. The indirect method is more sensitive and provides a stronger effect but is more time-consuming. See Sample Procedure 8-2 for a sample set of instructions for pretreating red cells with enzyme.

Multiple Antibody Resolution

While resolution of single antibodies may present challenges, multiple antibodies present a larger challenge. After the initial elimination process, multiple options for the exhibited antibodies may still exist. As previously

PATIENT NAME: ______________ Lot No. XXXX Exp. Date XXXX-XX-XX

PATIENT ID: ______________ **Panel**

DATE: ________ TECH: ________

CONCLUSION: ______________

			Rh-hr								KELL						DUFFY		KIDD		Sex Linked	LEWIS		MNS				P	LUTHERAN		Special Antigen Typing
Cell #	Rh-hr	Donor Number	D	C	E	c	e	f*	C^w	V	K	k	Kp^a	Kp^b	Js^a	Js^b	Fy^a	Fy^b	Jk^a	Jk^b	Xg^a	Le^a	Le^b	S	s	M	N	P_1	Lu^a	Lu^b	
1	R1wR1		+	+	0	0	+	0	+	0	0	+	0	+	0	+	0	+	+	+	0	0	+	0	+	0	+	0	0	+	
2	R1R1		+	+	0	0	+	0	0	0	+	+	0	+	0	+	+	+	+	0	0	0	0	0	+	0	+	+s	0	+	
3	R2R2		+	0	+	+	0	0	0	0	0	+	0	+	0	+	0	+	+	0	+	0	+	+	0	+	0	+	0	+	
4	Ror		+	0	0	+	+	+	0	0	0	+	0	+	0	+	+	+	+	+	0	0	+	+	0	0	+	+	0	+	
5	r′r		0	+	0	+	+	+	0	0	0	+	0	+	0	+	0	+	+	0	0	+	0	+	+	+	+	+	0	+	
6	r″r		0	0	+	+	+	+	0	0	0	+	0	+	0	+	+	0	0	+	+	0	+	0	+	0	+	+s	0	+	
7	rr		0	0	0	+	+	+	0	0	+	+	0	+	0	+	0	+	+	0	+	0	0	0	+	+	0	+	0	+	
8	rr		0	0	0	+	+	+	0	0	0	+	0	+	0	+	+	0	0	+	+	+	0	+	+	+	0	+s	0	+	
9	rr		0	0	0	+	+	+	0	0	0	+	0	+	0	+	0	+	0	+	+	0	+	+	0	+	0	+	0	+	
10	rr		0	0	0	+	+	+	0	0	0	+	0	+	0	+	+	0	+	+	+	0	+	0	+	0	+	0	0	+	
11	R1R1		+	+	0	0	+	0	0	0	+	+	0	+	0	+	0	+	0	+	+	0	+	0	+	+	0	+s	0	+	
	Patient Cells																														
Mode of Reactivity			37°C/Antiglobulin								Antiglobulin											Variable				Cold			Var.		

	Test Results				Enzyme		
Cell #	IS	37°	AHG	c.c.c.	IS	AHG	c.c.c.
1	0	1+	2+		0	4+	
2	0	1+	2+		0	4+	
3	0	0	0	✓	0	0	✓
4	0	0	0	✓	0	0	✓
5	0	1+	2+		0	4+	
6	0	0	0	✓	0	0	✓
7	0	0	0	✓	0	0	✓
8	0	0	0	✓	0	0	✓
9	0	0	0	✓	0	0	✓
10	0	0	0	✓	0	0	✓
11	0	1+	2+		0	4+	
	0	0	0	✓	0	0	✓

Interpretation: Anti-C; Enhanced with Enzymes.

FIGURE 8-6 An antibody enhanced by enzymes
Source: Delmar, Cengage Learning

PATIENT NAME: _____   Lot No. _____   Exp. Date _____

PATIENT ID: _____   **Panel**   CCYY-MM-DD

DATE: _____   TECH: _____

CONCLUSION: _____

Cell #	Rh-hr	Donor Number	D	C	E	c	e	f	Cw	V	K	k	Kpa	Kpb	Jsa	Jsb	Fya	Fyb	Jka	Jkb	Xga	Lea	Leb	S	s	M	N	P1	Lua	Lub	Special Antigen Typing	Cell #	IS	37°	AHG	c.c.c	IS	AHG	c.c.c
1	R1wR1		+	+	0	0	+	0	+	0	0	0	+	0	+	0	0	+	+	+	0	0	+	0	+	0	+	0	0	+		1	0	1+	3+		0	4+	
2	R1R1		+	+	0	0	+	0	0	0	+	+	0	+	0	+	+	+	+	0	0	0	0	0	+	0	+	+s	0	+		2	0	1+	3+		0	4+	
3	R2R2		+	0	+	+	0	0	0	0	0	0	+	0	+	0	0	+	+	0	+	0	+	+	0	+	0	+	0	+		3	0	0	2+		0	0	✓
4	Ror		+	0	0	+	+	+	0	0	0	0	+	0	+	0	+	+	+	+	0	0	+	0	+	0	0	+	0	+		4	0	0	2+		0	0	✓
5	r'r		0	+	0	+	+	+	0	0	0	0	+	0	+	0	0	+	+	0	0	+	0	+	+	+	+	+	0	+		5	0	1+	3+		0	4+	
6	r'r		0	0	+	+	+	+	0	0	0	0	+	0	+	0	+	0	0	+	+	0	+	0	+	0	+	+s	0	+		6	0	0	0	✓	0	0	✓
7	rr		0	0	0	+	+	+	0	0	+	+	0	+	0	+	0	+	+	0	+	0	0	0	+	+	0	+	0	+		7	0	0	2+		0	0	✓
8	rr		0	0	0	+	+	+	0	0	0	0	+	0	+	0	+	0	0	+	+	+	0	+	+	+	0	+	+s	0	+		8	0	0	0	✓	0	0	✓
9	rr		0	0	0	+	+	+	0	0	0	0	+	0	+	0	0	+	0	+	+	0	+	+	0	+	0	+	0	+		9	0	0	2+		0	0	✓
10	rr		0	0	0	+	+	+	0	0	+	+	0	+	0	+	+	0	+	+	+	0	+	+	0	+	0	0	0	+		10	0	0	0	✓	0	0	✓
11	R1R1		+	+	0	0	+	0	0	0	+	+	0	+	0	+	0	+	+	0	+	0	+	0	+	+	0	+s	0	+		11	0	1+	3+		0	4+	
Patient Cells																																	0	0	0	✓	0	0	✓
Mode of Reactivity		37°C/Antiglobulin									Antiglobulin								Variable					Cold				Var.											

Interpretation: Anti-C and Anti-Fyb.
  Anti-Fyb is not seen in Enzyme Panel.
  Anti-C is Enhanced and Maintained in the Enzyme Panel.

FIGURE 8-7 An antibody destroyed by enzymes
Source: Delmar, Cengage Learning

SAMPLE PROCEDURE 8-2

Enzyme Treatment of Red Blood Cells

1. Place one drop of cells into each tube to be tested.
2. Add one drop of the prepared enzyme solution to each tube.
3. Incubate at 37°C for 10 minutes.
Note: Do not overincubate.
4. Wash all tubes with saline three times. Blot dry on third wash.

Proceed with testing. Do not add any albumin or enhancement media. The enzyme serves as the enhancement media.

CRITICAL THINKING ACTIVITY

Each student should interpret sample panel sheets provided by the instructor. Careful attention should be paid to antibodies that are enhanced or destroyed by enzymes. Follow the protocol below when examining each antigram:

1. Examine the original panel and compare the results to the enzyme panel.
2. Determine if one or more antibodies has been enhanced or destroyed.
3. Check each antibody that was enhanced or destroyed on the list of possible antibodies and try to achieve a match.
4. Discuss the results with a fellow student.
5. Have instructor check the results.

discussed, using procedures such as phenotyping, enzyme treatment, temperature variation, and consideration of reactivity phases, as well as some additional considerations will assist in separation of multiple antibodies into single modalities. Steps to be considered in multiple antibody resolution are summarized in Table 8-5.

Select Cell Panel

A select cell panel consists of multiple cells obtained from additional panels on hand in the blood bank. These cells should be chosen specifically to eliminate antibodies

WEB 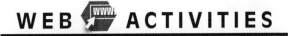 ACTIVITIES

TABLE 8-5 Steps for Resolution of Multiple Antibody Resolution

1. Consider the results of autocontrol testing to determine if the antibody is an alloantibody and/or autoantibody.
2. Perform DAT, if indicated.
3. Use elimination method for determining possible antibodies present.
4. List possible antibodies.
5. Perform phenotyping of patient's red cells to assist in ruling out possible antibodies.
6. Perform an enzyme panel, if indicated.
7. Organize and perform a select cell panel to narrow possible antibody choices. A select cell panel may also be necessary to confirm with the rule of three.
8. Consider media and temperatures of reactivity to rule out possibilities.

that could not be excluded with elimination and other appropriate methods. When choosing select cells, each cell should be positive for one antigen and negative for all remaining possibilities. For example, the possible antibodies include anti-c, anti-E, and anti-K. The anti-c may mask possible anti-E and anti-K, if they are present in the patient's serum. Select cells for this scenario are:

- Cell 1 is c negative, E negative, K positive
- Cell 2 is c negative, E positive, K negative
- Cell 3 is c positive, E negative, K negative

CRITICAL THINKING ACTIVITY

Construct a select cell panel that contains cells for ruling out anti-C, anti-Fy^b, and anti-K. Outline additional steps for eliminating possibilities. Share these results with the instructor.

After the cells are chosen, they are tested against the plasma in the same manner as the original panel. Results are recorded and antibodies eliminated or included in the final analysis, as indicated. When constructing select cell panels, be certain to include the necessary cells for completing the rule of three for each antibody. See Figure 8-8 for an example of a select cell panel, which corresponds with the antibodies displayed in Figures 8-6 and 8-7.

Dithiothreitol (DTT) Treatment

ZZAP, a reagent composed of a combination of 0.1M dithiothreitol (DTT) and 0.1% cysteine-activated papain, may be used to dissociate IgG immunoglobulins from the red cells. This reagent is used to remove antibodies from cells that have exhibited a positive autocontrol. The antibody removal allows the cells to be typed for specific antigens once the antibodies have been dissociated. DTT also destroys antigens from the Kell blood group. Therefore, it can be used to eliminate antibodies to this blood group, as well. This may be useful when an antibody to a high incidence antigen such as anti-k (cellano) is encountered.

Cold Alloantibodies

Cold alloantibodies are encountered at immediate spin, room temperature, and sometimes in a weakened state at 37°C. These antibodies are clinically insignificant, but may mask clinically significant antibodies. Since the temperature of reactivity of the antibody is below body temperature, the cold reacting antibodies will not cause hemolysis if the individual is transfused with antigen-positive blood. Specific antibodies that may react at cold temperatures include, anti-I, -H, -P$_1$, -Le^a, -Le^b, -M, and -N antibodies.

It is, however, necessary to eliminate the interference of these antibody reactions. This may be accomplished by neutralizing the antibodies or by prewarming all of the reagents and samples for testing. Alternately,

Cell #	Additional Cells			Rh-hr									KELL							DUFFY		KIDD		Sex Linked	LEWIS		MNS				P	LUTHERAN		Special Antigen Typing	Cell #	Test Results					
	Rh-hr	Donor Number	D	C	E	c	e	f*	C^w	V	K	k	Kp^a	Kp^b	Js^a	Js^b	Fy^a	Fy^b	Jk^a	Jk^b	Xg^a	Le^a	Le^b	S	s	M	N	P_1	Lu^a	Lu^b			IS	37°	AHG	c.c.c.		
			0	+													0	+																0	0	2+			
	C Neg		0	+													+	+		Fy^bPos														0	0	2+			
			0	+													0	+																0	0	2+			
			+	0													+	0																0	1+	2+			
	C⊕		+	+													+	0		Fy^bNeg														0	1+	2+			
			+	+													+	0																0	1+	2+			
		c⊕↑																																					

FIGURE 8-8 Select cell panel for resolution of anti-C and anti-Fy^b

Source: Delmar, Cengage Learning

SAMPLE PROCEDURE 8-3

Procedure for Prewarming Blood Bank Tests

1. Separately, prewarm the appropriate amount of all patient samples and reagents to be tested at 37°C for 10 minutes.

2. Concurrently, prewarm saline for washing to 37°C.

3. Following the standard operating procedure designated by the institution, add the proper amounts of patient sample and reagents and incubate at 37°C for 30 minutes. Polyethylene glycol (PEG) may be added to increase the sensitivity.

4. Wash three times with the prewarmed saline.

5. Add IgG AHG, centrifuge, and read.

6. Add Coombs control cells to the negative tubes.

Lewis antibodies may be neutralized by Lewis substance. This commercially available substance contains soluble Lewis antigen, and will neutralize a suspected Lewis antibody. Removal of these interfering antibodies is vital for obtaining compatible blood for transfusion. Sample Procedure 8-3 summarizes the procedure for prewarming tests to eliminate interference from cold antibodies. Figure 8-9 presents an example of a cold antibody in combination with a warm antibody. The prewarmed panel demonstrates the removal of the cold antibody with only the warm alloantibody remaining in the serum. Table 8-6 demonstrates an example of neutralization of an anti-Le^b.

High Titer Low Avidity (HTLA) Antibodies

Weak reacting antibodies may be produced in response to some high-incidence antigens. These antibodies are weak reacting but can be diluted to high titers in spite of the weak reactions: hence the label "high titer low avidity" (HTLA) antibodies. These antibodies provide inconsistent test results, lack of enhancement with potentiators such as PEG, and react in the AHG phase of testing. Increasing the incubation time or addition of more plasma cannot enhance reaction strength. In spite of reacting in AHG, HTLA antibodies are clinically insignificant, do not cause either hemolytic disease of the fetus and newborn or transfusion reactions, but may mask some clinically significant antibodies. A few of the antigens associated with these antibodies are: Chido (CH), Rogers (Rg), John Milton Hagen (JMH), Knops (Kn^a) and McCoy (McC^a). If HTLA antibodies are suspected, an attempt must be made to work around them in an effort to not miss a clinically significant finding.

Warm Autoantibodies

Autoantibodies present a challenge to the blood bank. They can mask the presence of clinically significant alloantibodies. Warm autoantibodies are more common and more clinically significant than cold autoantibodies. Individuals exhibiting a warm autoantibody may have a condition labeled **warm autoimmune hemolytic anemia (WAIHA)**. This condition may be associated with a specific clinical condition or **idiopathic** (without known cause). Medical history and medications may help to determine the etiology of WAIHA. Some clinical conditions and medications may produce a positive autocontrol that may or may not result in a definable antibody.

PATIENT NAME: _____   Lot No. _____ Exp. Date _____

PATIENT ID: _____   **Panel**

DATE: _____ TECH: _____

CONCLUSION: _____

Cell #	Rh-hr	Donor Number	D	C	E	c	e	f*	Cw	V	K	k	Kpa	Kpb	Jsa	Jsb	Fya	Fyb	Jka	Jkb	Xga	Lea	Leb	S	s	M	N	P1	Lua	Lub	Special Antigen Typing	Cell #	IS	37°	AHG	c.c.c.
1	R1wR1		+	+	0	0	0	+	0	+	0	0	+	0	+	0	0	+	+	+	0	0	+	0	+	0	+	0	0	+		1	0	0	0	✓
2	R1R1		+	+	0	0	0	+	0	0	+	+	0	+	0	+	+	+	+	0	0	0	0	0	+	0	+	+s	0	+		2	2+	2+	2+	
3	R2R2		+	0	+	+	0	0	0	0	0	+	0	+	0	+	0	+	+	0	+	0	+	+	0	+	0	+	0	+		3	1+	0	0	✓
4	Ror		+	0	0	+	+	+	0	0	0	+	0	+	0	+	+	+	+	+	0	0	+	0	0	+	0	+	+	0	+		4	1+	0	0	✓
5	r'r		0	+	0	+	+	+	0	0	0	+	0	+	0	+	0	+	+	0	0	+	0	+	+	+	+	+	0	+		5	1+	0	0	✓
6	r"r		0	0	+	+	+	+	0	0	0	+	0	+	0	+	+	0	0	+	+	0	+	0	+	0	+	+s	0	+		6	2+	0	0	✓
7	rr		0	0	0	+	+	0	0	0	0	+	0	+	0	+	0	+	+	0	0	0	0	0	+	+	0	+	0	+		7	1+	1+	2+	
8	rr		0	0	0	+	+	0	0	0	0	+	0	+	0	+	+	0	0	+	+	0	+	+	+	0	+	+s	0	+		8	2+	0	0	✓
9	rr		0	0	0	+	+	0	0	0	0	+	0	+	0	+	0	+	0	+	+	0	+	+	0	+	0	+	0	+		9	1+	0	0	✓
10	rr		0	0	0	+	+	0	0	0	0	+	0	+	0	+	+	0	+	+	+	0	+	0	+	0	+	0	0	+		10	0	0	0	✓
11	R1R1		+	+	0	0	0	+	0	0	+	+	0	+	0	+	0	+	0	+	+	0	+	0	+	+	0	+s	0	+		11	2+	2+	2+	
	Patient Cells																																	0	0	0	✓
	Mode of Reactivity		37°C/Antiglobulin								Antiglobulin											Variable				Cold			Var.								

Interpretation: Anti-P₁ at Immediate Spin.
 Anti-Kell at 37°C and AHG.
 Note Cells 2 and 11 are +s for P₁, so the P₁ is also still being Exhibited.
 Anti-Kell seen at 37°C.

FIGURE 8-9 Warm alloantibody in combination with a cold alloantibody
Source: Delmar, Cengage Learning

TABLE 8-6 Neutralization of Anti-Le^b

Cells Tested	ORIGINAL TEST RESULTS Serum with no pretreatment	NEUTRALIZATION Serum + Le Substance	Coombs Control Cells
1. Le(a–b+)	1+	0	+
2. Le(a–b+)	1+	0	+
3. Le(a–b+)	1+	0	+

As previously discussed, presence of a positive autocontrol in the antibody screen or antibody identification process suggests that a DAT should be performed. If the DAT is positive, an autoantibody is most likely present. It is important to identify the etiology of the positive autocontrol/DAT. Table 8-7 summarizes potential causes of a positive autocontrol and provides suggestions for identifying the etiology.

Elution

Elution is used to remove a substance coating the red cells. The fluid produced in the elution process is used for identification of the causative antibodies. All elution methods use a series of steps to remove the antibody from the cells. The type of elution technique employed is dependent on the suspected nature of the antibody or the clinical condition causing the positive DAT. Some elution procedures are simple and require no special equipment or chemicals and some methods are commercially available in kit form. A major disadvantage to elution methods is that most methods destroy the red cells rendering them no longer be available for testing. Elution techniques are summarized in Table 8-8.

Once the elution has been completed, the harvested liquid, or **eluate**, is tested in the same manner as plasma.

TABLE 8-7 Summary of Test Results following Elution

ETIOLOGY	SPECIFIC SUBSTANCE DETECTED	TEST REACTION SUMMARY
Warm Autoimmune Disease	IgG	Reacts with all test cells and autocontrol cells at the AHG phase
Cold Autoimmune Disease	IgM, C3	Reacts with all test cells and autocontrol cells at room temperature and immediate spin
Drug Interaction	IgG	Autocontrol positive at AHG, plasma may or may not be reactive
Transfusion Reaction	IgG	Specific alloantibody
Hemolytic Disease of the Fetus and Newborn; Baby's Cells Coated with Antibody	IgG	Specific alloantibody or ABO IgG antibodies

TABLE 8-8 Elution Methods

METHOD	MECHANISM OF ANTIBODY REMOVAL	ADVANTAGES	LIMITATIONS
Heat Freeze-Thaw	Physical destruction of red cells	Rapid, inexpensive; effective for ABO antibodies	Only effective for ABO antibodies
Glycine Acid	Decreased pH	Commercially available; sensitive	More expensive
Chloroform Methylene Chloride Ether	Organic solvent dissolves the red blood cell bilipid layer	Sensitive; inexpensive	Chemicals hazardous or carcinogenic

When the eluate is tested, parallel testing of the last wash is included to prove that the antibody detected in the eluate results from the elution procedure rather than contamination from insufficient washing of the real cells.

Testing of the eluate is performed using an antibody identification panel. If the test results define a specific antibody, that antibody denotes the cause of the positive DAT. At times, particularly when the positive DAT is drug related, the antibody is either non-specific, *or* no antibody is detected in the eluate. In these cases, clinical history is important for determination of the etiology. See Figure 8-10 for an example of eluate testing results.

Adsorption

Adsorption is the removal of antibodies from the plasma. Removal of antibody is achieved by creating an environment to allow the autoantibodies to attach to red cells.

Autoadsorption may be accomplished by pretreating the patient's cells with DTT and/or enzymes. This enhances the removal of plasma antibodies. The patient's red cells are incubated with autologous plasma. The adsorption step may need to be repeated if the autoantibody

PATIENT NAME: _____ Lot No. _____ Exp. Date _____

PATIENT ID: _____ **Panel**

DATE: _____ TECH: _____

CONCLUSION: _____

Cell #	Rh-hr	Donor Number	D	C	E	c	e	f*	Cʷ	V	K	k	Kpᵃ	Kpᵇ	Jsᵃ	Jsᵇ	Fyᵃ	Fyᵇ	Jkᵃ	Jkᵇ	Xgᵃ	Leᵃ	Leᵇ	S	s	M	N	P₁	Luᵃ	Luᵇ	Special Antigen Typing	Cell #	IS	37°	AHG	c.c.c.
1	R1wR1		+	+	0	0	+	0	+	0	0	+	0	+	0	+	0	+	+	+	0	0	+	0	+	0	+	0	0	+		1	0	0	2+	
2	R1R1		+	+	0	0	+	0	0	0	+	+	0	+	0	+	+	+	+	0	0	0	0	0	+	0	+	+s	0	+		2	0	0	2+	
3	R2R2		+	0	+	+	0	0	0	0	0	+	0	+	0	+	0	+	+	0	+	0	+	0	+	0	+	+	0	+		3	0	0	0	✓
4	Ror		+	0	0	+	+	+	0	0	0	+	0	+	0	+	+	+	+	+	0	0	+	0	+	0	+	+	0	+		4	0	0	2+	
5	r′r		0	+	0	+	+	+	0	0	0	+	0	+	0	+	0	+	+	0	0	+	0	+	+	+	+	+	0	+		5	0	0	2+	
6	r″r		0	0	+	+	+	0	0	0	0	+	0	+	0	+	+	0	0	+	0	0	+	0	+	0	+	+s	0	+		6	0	0	2+	
7	rr		0	0	0	+	+	+	0	0	+	+	0	+	0	+	0	+	+	0	0	0	+	0	+	+	0	+	0	+		7	0	0	2+	
8	rr		0	0	0	+	+	f*	0	0	0	+	0	+	0	+	+	0	0	+	+	0	+	+	+	+	0	+s	0	+		8	0	0	2+	
9	rr		0	0	0	+	+	+	0	0	0	+	0	+	0	+	0	+	0	+	+	0	+	+	0	+	0	+	0	+		9	0	0	2+	
10	rr		0	0	0	+	+	+	0	0	+	+	0	+	0	+	+	0	+	+	+	0	+	0	+	0	+	0	0	+		10	0	0	2+	
11	R1R1		+	+	0	0	+	0	0	0	+	+	0	+	0	+	0	+	0	+	+	0	+	0	+	+	0	+s	0	+		11	0		2+	
	Patient Cells																																			

Mode of Reactivity	37°C/Antiglobulin	Antiglobulin	Variable	Cold	Var.

Interpretation: Eluate contains anti-e as the most likely antibody. There are other choices that cannot be excluded.

FIGURE 8-10 Example of results of eluate testing results
Source: Delmar, Cengage Learning

is present in high titers. After removing autoantibodies, the plasma is tested for the presence of an underlying alloantibody. Autoadsorption is only appropriate if the patient has not been transfused within the last three months. Recently transfused patients may have transfused cells present. The transfused cells may adsorb out a clinically significant alloantibody.

Previously transfused patients must have a **differential adsorption** or **allogeneic adsorption**. This differential adsorption uses known red cells that match the patient's phenotype or those that will selectively remove specific antibodies while leaving others in the plasma. The cells are pretreated with enzyme followed by incubation with the patient's plasma. The adsorbed plasma is then used for testing. See Figure 8-11 for an illustration of these two adsorption methods.

Cold Autoantibodies

Cold autoantibodies are encountered in blood bank testing and are not usually clinically significant. They may produce positive reactions in all the cells of the antibody identification panel as well as the autocontrol. Positive reactions are typically exhibited in the immediate spin

phase and decrease or disappear completely with incubation at 37°C and in the AHG phase. See Figure 8-12 for an example of a cold-reacting autoantibody.

When a cold autoantibody is suspected, a DAT on the patient's red cells should involve the use of a monospecific C3 AHG reagent. This would demonstrate the attachment of complement to the surface of the red cells. These cold antibodies may be demonstrated in conditions such as *Mycoplasma pneumoniae*. It is useful to identify the etiology of the antibody to assist in the resolution of interference from these antibodies. Since the antibodies are not clinically significant, providing antigen negative red cells is not necessary for successful transfusion of these individuals.

Identification of Cold Antibodies

A cold reacting antibody is suspected when an antibody screen is positive at immediate spin. A cold panel is a selection of cells that will identify the suspected cold antibody. The common etiology of most cold antibodies is anti-I, -IH, or -H. Since I antigen is not developed at birth, the use of cord cells is important for the differentiation of these antibodies. These cells are available commercially. See Figure 8-12 for sample cold panels.

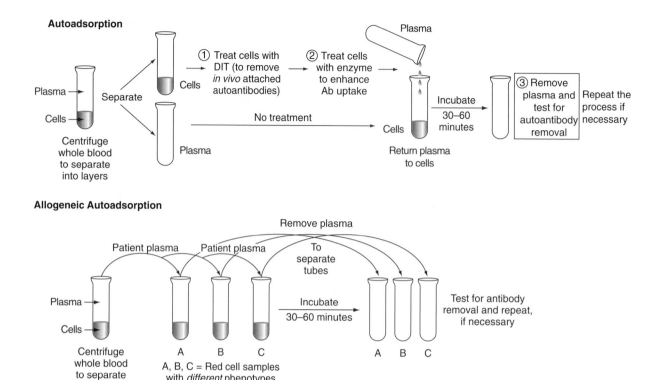

FIGURE 8-11 Illustration of autoadsorption vs. allogeneic adsorption
Source: Delmar, Cengage Learning

PATIENT NAME: _____ Lot No. _____ Exp. Date _____

PATIENT ID: _____ **Panel**

DATE: _____ TECH: _____

CONCLUSION: _____

Cell #	Rh-hr	Donor Number	D	C	E	c	e	f	C^w	V	K	k	Kp^a	Kp^b	Js^a	Js^b	Fy^a	Fy^b	Jk^a	Jk^b	Xg^a	Le^a	Le^b	S	s	M	N	P_1	Lu^a	Lu^b	Special Antigen Typing	Cell #	IS	37°	AHG	c.c.c.
			Rh-hr								**KELL**						**DUFFY**		**KIDD**		**Sex Linked**	**LEWIS**		**MNS**				**P**	**LUTHERAN**					**Test Results**			
1	rr		0	0	0	+	+	+	0	0	0	+	0	+	0	+	+	0	0	+	0	0	+	0	+	0	+	0	0	+		1	1+	0	0	✓
2	rr		0	0	0	+	+	+	0	0	0	+	0	+	0	+	0	+	0	+	+	0	+	+	0	+	0	+s	0	+		2	1+	0	0	✓
3	rr		0	0	0	+	+	+	0	0	+	+	0	+	0	+	+	0	+	0	+	0	+	+	+	+	+	+	0	+		3	1+	0	0	✓
4	R2R2		+	0	+	+	0	0	0	0	0	+	0	+	0	+	+	+	0	+	+	+	0	0	+	+	+	+	0	+		4	1+	0	0	✓
5	R2R2		+	0	+	+	0	0	0	0	0	+	0	+	0	+	+	0	+	0	0	0	+	+	+	+	+	+	0	+		5	1+	0	0	✓
6	R2R2		+	0	+	+	0	0	0	0	0	+	0	+	0	+	0	+	+	+	+	0	+	0	+	+	+	+	0	+		6	1+	0	0	✓
7	R1R1		+	+	0	0	+	0	0	0	0	+	0	+	0	+	+	0	+	0	+	0	0	+	0	+	0	0	0	+		7	1+	0	0	✓
8	R1R1		+	+	0	0	+	0	0	0	0	+	0	+	0	+	0	+	0	0	0	0	+	+	0	+	+	+	+	+		8	1+	0	0	✓
9	R2R1		+	+	+	0	+	0	0	0	0	+	0	+	0	+	+	0	+	0	+	+	0	0	+	+	0	+s	+	+		9	1+	0	0	✓
10	r'r		0	+	0	+	+	+	0	0	0	+	0	+	0	+	0	+	+	0	+	0	+	0	+	+	+	+	0	+		10	1+	0	0	✓
11	R1R1		+	+	0	0	+	0	0	0	+	0	0	+	0	+	0	+	+	+	0	+	0	+	0	+	0	+	0	+		11	1+	0	0	✓
	Patient Cells																																1+	0	0	✓
Mode of Reactivity			37°C/Antiglobulin								Antiglobulin										Variable	Cold					Var.									

Interpretation: Cold reacting autoantibody most likely anti-I.

FIGURE 8-12 An example of a cold reacting antibody that is not present in the AHG phase
Source: Delmar, Cengage Learning

Cold reacting antibodies may mask a clinically significant antibody. Once the existence of a cold antibody is established and its specificity determined, additional steps might be used to avoid the interference of cold autoantibodies. Table 8-9 summarizes the steps that can be utilized to avoid cold autoantibodies.

Adsorption Techniques

If the steps outlined in the previous section cannot avoid the cold antibody, adsorption may be necessary. If the patient has been transfused in the previous three months, the adsorption must be completed with allogeneic red blood cells or rabbit stroma. Rabbit stroma will remove antibodies to the I antigen. If the patient has not been transfused within three months, an autoadsorption may be used. After the antibodies have

TABLE 8-9 Steps for Avoiding Cold Antibody Reactivity
1. Use IgG antiglobulin reagent rather than polyspecific reagent. This will avoid the detection of complement attachment.
2. Omit the immediate spin and room temperature reaction phases. This minimizes the attachment of cold antibodies to the surface of the red cells.
3. Avoid the use of LISS. LISS is more likely to enhance the attachment of cold autoantibodies.
4. Prewarm all test procedures, if necessary.

been adsorbed from the patient's plasma, the treated serum may be tested for the presence of clinically significant alloantibodies.

SUMMARY

The detection and identification of antibodies is important for safe transfusion and diagnosis and management of hemolytic disease of the fetus and newborn. Antibodies may be detected in plasma and/or attached to red blood cells. The methods for detecting these antibodies are the antibody screen and direct antiglobulin tests. The results of the screen tests will determine the need for further testing.

- Detection of antibody in the antibody screen test with a negative autocontrol indicates the presence of an alloantibody. An antibody identification panel is then performed.

- If the antibody identification panel does not produce a specific single antibody, other test methods may be employed to aid in the identification of the

antibody mixture present. These methods include: antigen typing, select cell panels, enzyme panels, variation in temperature, and media of reactivity.

- DAT is useful in diagnosis of autoimmune disorders such as autoimmune hemolytic anemia, drug induced autoimmune hemolytic anemia, HDRN, and HTR. Physicians and technicians frequently work together to combine patient history with test results to reach a diagnosis and institute correct treatment for the patient.

- Elution and adsorption are techniques used to separate antibodies from the cells and remove them from plasma, respectively. These techniques are useful for identification of antibodies that may mask other clinically significant antibodies.

REVIEW QUESTIONS

1. The elution method that is most effective for ABO antibodies is:
   a. acid
   b. chloroform
   c. freeze-thaw
   d. ether

2. Rabbit stroma will remove:
   a. anti-D
   b. anti-P_1
   c. anti-Le^a
   d. anti-I

3. Choose the antibody that would not be present as a cold alloantibody:
   a. anti-C
   b. anti-H
   c. anti-I
   d. anti-M

4. The blood group antigens that are destroyed by DTT are:
   a. ABO
   b. Rh
   c. Kell
   d. Duffy

5. The methods that would be used for removal of antibodies from the surface of red cells include:
   1. enzyme pre-treatment
   2. freeze-thaw
   3. adsorption
   4. acid
   5. LISS enhancement
   a. 1 and 3 only
   b. 2 and 4 only
   c. 1, 2, and 5
   d. 3 and 4 only

6. From the following examples choose the condition that would not exhibit a positive DAT:
   a. HDFN
   b. HTR
   c. HTLA antibody
   d. WAIHA

7. Incubation of a patient's cells with the patients serum removes the antibody, the procedure that was used is:
   a. autoadsorption
   b. elution
   c. neutralization
   d. enzyme enhancement

8. An enzyme treated panel was used with an AHG reactive antibody. Some reactions were eliminated after this testing. The antibody that was most likely eliminated was:
   a. anti-E
   b. anti-S
   c. anti-Le^a
   d. anti-K

9. A DAT result is as follows:
   Polyspecific AHG = 1+
   Anti-IgG = negative (Check Cells = 3+)

The most etiology of this positive DAT is
   a. anti-IgG
   b. anti-C3
   c. anti-I
   d. anti-A$_1$ in an A$_1$ individual

10. In a cold panel, the cord cell is negative at all phases of testing while all panel cells are positive at immediate spin and non-reactive at all other phases. The most likely etiology of this antibody is:
    a. anti-i
    b. anti-I
    c. anti-e
    d. HTLA antibody

11. An antibody is reacting with five panel cells in the AHG phase. Two of the cells react one degree less in agglutination. Possible causes for this difference in degree of agglutination may be:
    1. multiple antibodies
    2. cold reacting antibody
    3. dosage effect
    4. enzyme sensitivity
    5. DTT effect
    a. 1, 3, and 5 are correct
    b. 2, 3, and 4 are correct
    c. 1 and 3 are correct
    d. 1 and 4 are correct
    e. 2 and 5 are correct

12. An antibody screen demonstrates a positive result *only* in the autocontrol in the AHG phase. An additional test that would most likely result in a positive result is:
    a. neutralization with Lewis substance
    b. enzyme-treated antibody screen
    c. freeze/thaw elution
    d. direct antiglobulin test

13. DTT is useful when an antibody to the _____ antigen is suspected.
    a. Duffy
    b. Lewis
    c. Kidd
    d. Kell

14. An elution procedure is performed using freeze/thaw. An advantage for using this method is that it is:
    a. requires no special equipment or reagents
    b. effective for all antibodies
    c. requires the used of a commercial kit
    d. does not destroy the red cells

15. A patient was transfused two weeks before his current testing. He is exhibiting a positive DAT and a positive antibody screen in both cells at the AHG phase. The autoantibody may be removed form the serum using:

    a. heat elution
    b. enzyme treated cells
    c. autoadsorption
    d. allogeneic adsorption

CASE STUDY

1. A 61-year-old male patient was admitted for a laparotomy. Two units of blood were ordered to be crossmatched for possible transfusion. Since no previous records were available for this patient, the technician performed an ABO, an Rh, and an antibody screen prior to performing the crossmatch. The antibody screen showed positive results. An antibody identification panel was performed. The results of this panel are summarized in Panel A.

Panel A

	D	C	E	c	e	f	K	k	Fya	Fyb	Jka	Jkb	Xga	Lea	Leb	S	s	M	N	P₁	IS	37°	AHG	C.C.
1	+	+	0	0	+	0	0	+	+	+	+	0	+	0	+	+	+	+	0	0	0	0	1+	
2	+	+	0	0	+	0	+	+	+	+ʷ	+	+	+	0	+	+	+	+	0	0	0	0	1+	
3	+	0	+	+	0	0	0	+	+	0	0	+	+	0	+	0	+	0	+	+ˢ	0	0	0	+
4	+	0	0	+	+	+	0	+	0	0	+	+	+	0	0	0	+	+	+	+ˢ	0	0	1+	
5	0	+	0	+	+	+	0	+	0	+	+	+	0	0	+	+	0	+	0	+	0	0	1+	
6	0	0	+	+	+	+	0	+	0	+	+	+	+	0	+	0	+	+	0	+	0	0	1+	
7	0	0	0	+	+	+	+	+	0	+	0	+	+	0	+	0	+	+	+	0	0	0	0	+
8	0	0	0	+	+	+	+	+	+	0	+	0	+	0	0	+	+	+	+	0	0	0	1+	
9	0	0	0	+	+	+	0	+	+	0	+	0	+	0	+	0	+	0	+	+ʷ	0	0	1+	
10	0	0	0	+	+	+	0	+	0	+	0	+	+	+	0	0	+	0	+	+	0	0	0	+
CORD														0	0						0	0	0	+

Source: Delmar, Cengage Learning

    a. Interpret Panel A. What is the antibody(ies) most likely present?
    b. If an enzyme panel were performed, what effect would the enzyme have on the reactions of this antibody?
    c. What would you expect to be the patient's results of antigen typing for the antigen specific to the antibody?

(continues)

CASE STUDY (CONTINUED)

2. A 72-year-old man admitted for possible bowel obstruction is being prepared for surgery. The surgeon has ordered ABO, Rh, and antibody screen tests as well as a crossmatch for two units of blood. The antibody screen was positive in the autocontrol but not in either of the screening cells.
   a. What test would be performed next? What specific reagent(s) would be useful? Why?
   b. If the tests performed in #1 were positive, what test would be performed next? Why?
   c. Since the antibody screen test is negative, is an identification panel on the patient's serum necessary? Why or why not?
3. A prenatal specimen demonstrated a positive antibody screen. The antibody identification results are summarized in Panel B.

Panel B

	D	C	E	c	e	f	K	k	Fyᵃ	Fyᵇ	Jkᵃ	Jkᵇ	Xgᵃ	Leᵃ	Leᵇ	S	s	M	N	P₁	IS	37°	AHG	C.C.
1	+	+	0	0	+	0	0	+	+	+	+	0	+	0	+	+	+	+	0	0	0	0	0	✓
2	+	+	0	0	+	0	+	+	+	+ʷ	+	+	+	0	+	+	+	+	0	0	0	0	0	✓
3	+	0	+	+	0	0	0	+	+	0	0	+	+	0	+	0	+	0	+	+ˢ	0	1+	3+	
4	+	0	0	+	+	+	0	+	0	0	+	+	+	0	0	0	+	+	+	+ˢ	0	0	2+	
5	0	+	0	+	+	+	0	+	0	+	+	+	0	0	+	+	0	+	0	+	0	0	2+	
6	0	0	+	+	+	+	0	+	+	+	+	+	0	+	0	+	+	0	+	0	1+	3+	
7	0	0	0	+	+	+	+	+	0	+	0	+	+	0	+	0	+	+	+	0	0	0	2+	
8	0	0	0	+	+	+	+	+	+	0	+	0	+	0	0	+	+	+	+	0	0	0	2+	
9	0	0	0	+	+	+	0	+	+	0	+	0	+	+	0	+	0	+	0	+ʷ	0	0	2+	
10	0	0	0	+	+	+	0	+	0	+	0	+	+	+	0	0	+	0	+	+	0	0	2+	
CORD													0	0							0	0	0	✓

Source: Delmar, Cengage Learning

   a. Interpret Panel B. What is the antibody(ies) most likely present?
   b. What additional test procedures would be performed on this specimen to confirm and expand the initial antibody identification?
   c. What would you expect to be the patient's results of antigen typing for the antigen specific to the antibody?
4. A presurgical antibody screen is performed on a 17-year-old female who was also exhibiting a mild viral illness with low-grade fever and sore throat with exudates for the previous 10 days. The antibody screen results are weakly positive on both cells on immediate spin. These results disappeared with 37°C incubation. The blood bank supervisor recommends a cold panel.

CASE STUDY

a. What cells should be included in the panel?
b. What results are expected when testing the cold panel?
c. Is this antibody clinically significant?
d. If the patient requires a transfusion, will antigen-negative blood be required?

5. A patient is being screened for pre-transfusion. The patient was previously identified with an auto-anti-I. At that time, the patient was recovering from *Mycoplasma* pneumonia. On this admission, the patient's sample is negative at all temperatures and in all phases of antibody screening. All crossmatches are compatible at all temperatures and phases of testing.

a. What steps should be taken to assure safe transfusion of the red cells for this patient?
b. Why is the antibody screen negative at this time?

6. A patient with idiopathic anemia returned to the hospital for an outpatient transfusion. The patient had been transfused 4 months previously. Test results for previous and current antibody screens are displayed below:

Previous Testing:

Anti-A	Anti-B	Anti-D	A₁ Cells	B Cells	Interpretation
4+	0	3+	0	4+	A positive

	IS	37° C	AHG	Interpretation
		LISS		
Screen Cell I	0	0	0	Negative
Screen Cell II	0	0	0	Negative

Current Testing:

Anti-A	Anti-B	Anti-D	A₁ Cells	B Cells	Interpretation
4+	0	3+	0	4+	A positive

	IS	37° C	AHG	Interpretation
		LISS		
Screen Cell I	0	0	0	Negative
Screen Cell II	0	0	2+	Positive

a. What are the interpretations of the two antibody screens?
b. Explain any differences in the antibody screen results. What might be the explanation for any discrepancies.
c. What additional testing and considerations should be made for this patient in light of the current test results?

REFERENCES

Blaney, Kathy and Howard, Paula. *Basic and Applied Concepts of Immunohematology*. Mosby, Philadelphia, 2000.

Branch, Donald R. and Petz, Lawrence D. "A New Reagent (ZZAP) Having Multiple Applications in Immunohematology." *American Journal of Clinical Pathologists*. Vol. 78, No. 2, 1982, pp. 162–167.

Brecher, Mark, editor. *American Association of Blood Banks Technical Manual 15th edition*. AABB, 2005.

Brown, Michelle and Crim, Peggy. "Organizing the Antibody Identification Process." *Clinical Laboratory Science*. Vol. 20, No. 2, 2007, pp. 122–126.

Chiaroni, Jacques, et al. "Adsorption of autoantibodies in the presence of LISS to detect alloantibodies underlying warm autoantibodies." *Transfusion*. Vol. 43, 2003, pp. 651–655.

Cid, Joan, et al. "Use of Polyethylene Glycol for Performing Autologous Adsorptions." *Immunohematology*. Vol. 45, 2005, pp. 694–697.

Diedrich, B, et al. "K, Fy(a) and Jk(a) Phenotyping of Donor RBC's on Microplates." *Transfusion*. Vol. 41, 2001, pp. 1263–1267.

Lee, Edmond "Do Patients with Autoantibodies or Clinically Insignificant Alloantibodies Require an Indirect Antiglobulin Test Crossmatch?" *Transfusion*. Vol. 47, No 7, 2007, pp. 1290–1295.

Package Insert. *Gamma Lewis Blood Group Substances*. Immucor, Georgia, 2007.

Package Insert. *Gamma PeG™*. Immucor, Georgia, 2007.

Package Insert. *MTS Buffered Gel Card*. Micro Typing Systems. Pompano Beach, Fl. 1999.

Poole, J. "Problem-Solving in Antibody Identification." *Vox Sanguinis*. Vol. 87, Supplement 1, 2004, pp. 567–569.

Poole, Joyce and Daniels, Geoff. "Blood Group Antibodies and Their Significance in Transfusion Medicine." *Transfusion Medicine Reviews*. Vol. 21, No 1, 2007, pp. 58–71.

Standards for Blood Banks and Transfusion Services, 25th Edition. AABB, Bethesda, MD. 2008.

Stroebel, Erwin. "Use of the Enzyme Method for Antibody Identification." *Clinical Laboratory*. Vol. 50, 2004, pp. 575–580.

Turgeon, Mary Louise. *Fundamentals of Immunohematology*. Williams and Wilkins, Media, PA, 1995.

CHAPTER

9

Compatibility Testing

LEARNING OUTCOMES

At the completion of this chapter, the reader should be able to:

- Identify components of compatibility testing.
- Discuss clerical components of compatibility testing.
- Describe procedure and applications of immediate spin crossmatch.
- Outline and discuss the criteria for electronic crossmatching.
- Describe appropriate specimen labeling for compatibility testing.
- Discuss release of blood under a variety of circumstances.
- Define massive transfusion.
- Outline possible procedures for compatibility testing following massive transfusion.

GLOSSARY

compatible   no evidence of agglutination or hemolysis in a crossmatch when recipient's serum and donor's cells are combined

crossmatch   the mixing of donor red cells and recipient serum to determine if *in vitro* reactions may indicate potential for an *in vivo* reaction between the donor's cells and the recipient's plasma

immediate spin crossmatch   mixing donor and recipient blood and reading for agglutination after the first spin without incubation or enhancement media

incompatible   presence of agglutination or hemolysis in a compatibility test where recipient's plasma and donor's red cells are tested in combination; these units should not be transfused

major crossmatch   compatibility test combining recipient's plasma with donor's cells

massive transfusion   a total blood volume exchange by transfusion within a 24-hour period

minor crossmatch   compatibility test combining recipient's cells with donor's plasma

recipient   individual who receives a transfusion of blood or its components

INTRODUCTION

Compatibility testing is a vital part of the blood bank laboratory. The determination of compatibility of a unit of blood for transfusion is performed each time a unit of red blood cells is to be transfused. Testing for compatibility is not exclusively the physical mixing of donor and recipient, but includes pre-analytical steps leading up to laboratory testing and post-analytical steps after the testing is complete. Compatibility testing is required by all accrediting agencies. A list of considerations for pre-transfusion testing includes:

- Accurate patient identification at time of collection.

- Collection of the correct sample type and volume.

- Review of transfusion history of recipient.

- Accurate testing of the donor blood at the time of collection and repeat testing upon arrival at the administering institution.

- Accurate testing of the recipient's blood samples as well as accurate checking of records of previous typing and antibody results.

- Correct selection of ABO and Rh compatible donor units that are negative for antigen corresponding to atypical antibodies detected in the recipient's plasma.

- Correct patient identification and observation at the time of transfusion and post-transfusion.

All of these factors will be considered in this chapter. The crossmatch or compatibility test procedure will be the main focus of the chapter with other topics covered in less detail.

OVERVIEW OF COMPATIBILITY TESTING

Compatibility testing has a long history within the medical community. As early as the 1600s, blood transfusion was attempted with animal blood and then with human blood. The results were often unsuccessful, with the recipient dying from severe reactions. Historically, the progression of transfusion and compatibility testing has proceeded from virtually no testing through performing both major and minor crossmatches to the current state of limited compatibility testing in some recipients. See Figure 9-1 for a historical timeline of blood transfusion and compatibility testing.

Timeline for History of Blood Transfusion

19th Century
1st Transfusion of Human Blood

1906 Landsteiner: ABO discovery

1908: Ottenberg Initiated Pre-Transfusion Testing (Hemolysin Test)

1911: George Minot Suggested Major and Minor Crossmatch

1917: Bernheim suggested Major and Minor Crossmatch in all circumstances

1918: Moss suggested Direct Microscopic Cross Match: Observe up to 15 minutes Microscopically

Up through 1940's all testing Was done on slides versus tubes

1945 Diamond and Denton Suggested Enhancement with Bovine Albumin and Anti-Human Globulin Technique

1947 Morton and Pickles Described the Augmenting Effective of Enzymes

1950 Carl Walter and W. P. Murphy, Jr. introduced plastic bag for blood collection

Latter 1950's Advent of antibody screening cells

1958 AABB publishes its first Edition of Standards for Blood Transfusion Service

1960's Minor Crossmatch abandoned

1965 Stratton thought inclusion of complement important for testing Standards of AABB required the Presence of complement

1967 Rh Immune Globulin commercially introduced

1972 Hepatitis B Surface antigen testing started for donor blood

1979 CPDA-1 extends the shelf-life of blood to 35 days

1983 Additive solutions extend shelf-life of blood to 42 days

1985 First screening test to Detect HIV

1990 Heptitis C test introduced

1992 Testing of Donor Blood for HIV 1 and HIV 2 antibodies

1999 Implementation of Nucleic Acid Amplification Testing (NAT) For detection of HCV and HIV

2005 FDA clears apheresis platelets collected with certain storage systems for up to 7 days when microbial detection is employed; West Nile Virus blood test for screening donors is introduced

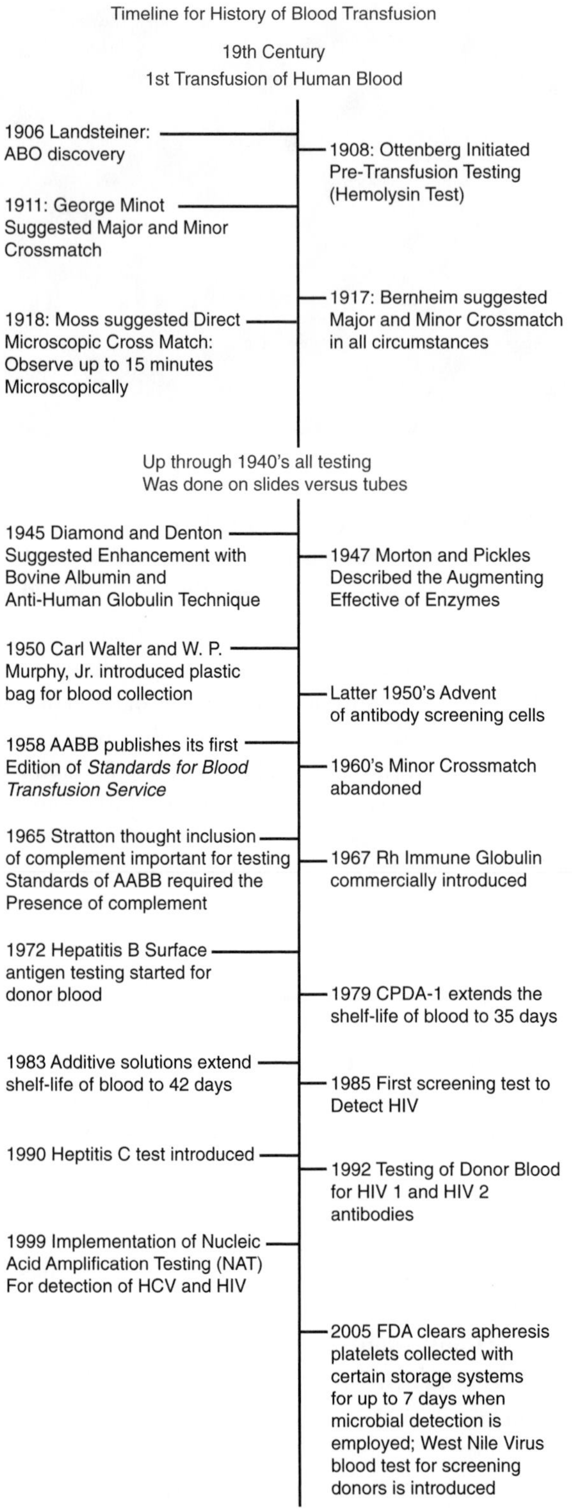

FIGURE 9-1 A historical timeline of the history of blood transfusion
Source: Delmar, Cengage Learning

Compatibility testing is a series of procedures designed to ensure the safety of blood for transfusion. Included in the compatibility test is a **crossmatch**. The crossmatch is an actual mixing of the recipient and donor's blood to insure *in vitro* compatibility. The **major crossmatch** combines plasma from the **recipient** or patient with cells from the donor. This crossmatch procedure is performed prior to transfusion of any blood product containing red blood cells. Any reaction in the major crossmatch is considered significant and the cause must be determined before transfusion of the unit should proceed. Transfusion reactions will be discussed in Chapter 12.

Recipient Blood Sample Collection and Labeling

Achieving successful results for any laboratory test begins with the pre-analytical components including the collection of the correct blood sample. Compatibility testing is no exception. Not only the type of sample collected, but also the assurance that the sample collected has been properly identified and related to the recipient is imperative. This requires appropriate labeling at the bedside. These items will be outlined in the following sections.

Sample Criteria

Serum and plasma from selective anticoagulants are acceptable for pre-transfusion testing. Acceptable collection tubes for pre-transfusion testing are summarized in Table 9-1. Historically, the use of anticoagulant for crossmatching was discouraged, since the binding of calcium inhibited the activation of complement in the compatibility test. The clinical significance of these complement-binding

antibodies has been determined insignificant. Hence, the use of anticoagulated samples has become acceptable. Anticoagulated samples are readily available for crossmatching in an emergency situation since the time required for a sample to clot prior to processing may delay testing and treatment. In addition, the formation of fibrin that may interfere with testing is less likely when using an anticoagulated specimen.

The integrity of the compatibility testing sample should be confirmed. The sample should not be contaminated with IV solutions. A sample may be collected from an infusion line only if the line is flushed with saline and a volume of blood equal to twice the test volume is withdrawn and discarded prior to obtaining the sample.

The collection process should employ a needle of sufficient size to avoid hemolyzing the red cells in the sample. The presence of hemolysis in plasma of the original sample may mask hemolysis resulting from an antigen-antibody interaction in the testing process. Lipemic serum may also provide an environment that is difficult for evaluation of serological reactions. At times it may be necessary to accept test samples with some amount of hemolysis or lipemia. Each institution should establish criteria and procedures for acceptable samples.

Sample Age

Individual institutions should establish the maximum age for pre-transfusion testing samples. However, the *AABB Standards for Blood Bank and Transfusion Services, 25th Edition,* states that a recipient sample must be collected within three (3) days of the scheduled transfusion if the patient has been transfused or pregnant in the preceding three (3) months or if the history is uncertain or unavailable. The day of collection is labeled as day zero (0). These patient samples, as well as a segment from any red cell containing component, are all refrigerated and retained for at least seven (7) days after transfusion.

Patient and Sample Identification

The AABB designates that the request for blood and blood products contain sufficient information to uniquely identify the patient. This includes a minimum of two independent identifiers. These two independent identifiers should be confirmed at the time of collection and the blood sample labeled with this unique information, the date of collection, and the phlebotomist's signature. This labeling must take place at the bedside.

TABLE 9-1 Sample Collection Tubes Acceptable for Compatibility Testing

Plain Red Tube	(No Anticoagulant; No Serum Separator)
Yellow Top Tube	(Acid Citrate Dextrose or ACD, Formula B)
Pink or Purple Top	(EDTA)
Blue Top	(Sodium Citrate)

Most institutions use hospital identification bands to identify patients. Phlebotomists should use these ID bands, and compare their information to the requisition and any other labels used to identify the blood sample. All identifying information must match. In situations where an identity cannot be determined, an established emergency identification procedure should be used. This method must continue to be used after the patient's true identity has been determined. A system of cross checking the emergency identification with the established identity should be part of the emergency identification procedure.

Commercial banding systems are available for identification of transfusion recipients. Each system has unique methods for labeling and identification. The blood bank should establish a procedure for utilization of these commercial systems. The procedure must be available to all blood bank staff and staff responsible for collection of pre-transfusion specimens. Figure 9-2 shows an example of a commercial banding system.

Review of Previous Records

As stated in the *AABB Standards for Blood Bank and Transfusion Services, 25th Edition*, compatibility testing must include a review of historical records. Past records should be compared to current test results. The requirement further states that the current ABO and Rh type must be compared to results obtained within the past 12 months. Discrepancies are investigated and resolved before any units are issued for transfusion.

Repeat Testing of Donor Blood

The AABB Standards require that all donor blood have the ABO and Rh confirmed from an attached segment

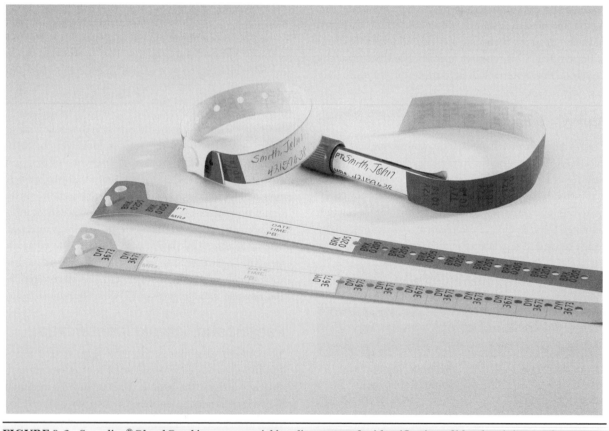

FIGURE 9-2 Securline® Blood Band is a commercial banding system for identification of blood recipients. The system includes an ID wristband with insert card, a sheet of 16 pre-numbered labels, and a specimen tube label. *Reprinted with permission of Precision Dynamics Corporation, San Fernando, CA.*

prior to transfusion of any whole blood or red blood cell component. The standards do not require that the institution issuing the blood for transfusion perform a test for the confirmation of the weak D antigen.

Required Pre-Transfusion Testing

The AABB and the FDA provide governance of all blood bank testing procedures. The AABB provides the most comprehensive guidelines. According to the AABB, patient samples must be tested for ABO, Rh, and unexpected antibodies to red cell antigens prior to transfusion of red cells. The weak D test is not required, but the antibody screen must include "incubation at 37°C preceding an antiglobulin test using reagent red cells that are not pooled."

The AABB Standards designate a serologic crossmatch be performed prior to the issue of blood components containing red cells. The recipient's serum or plasma must be tested against a sample of donor cells from the segment attached to the unit of whole blood or red cells designated for transfusion. The Standards require that test methods demonstrate "ABO incompatibility and clinically significant antibodies to red cell antigens and shall include an antiglobulin test."

The increasing use of molecular techniques may provide more accurate methods for the laboratory. These very specific methods will phenotype both donors and recipients to provide exact matches. These molecular techniques may eliminate standard serological crossmatch procedures.

The compatibility test procedure is only applicable for red cell products that are to be transfused. Plasma-based products such as cryoprecipitate, platelet concentrates, and frozen plasma contain virtually no red cells and require no compatibility testing. These components have been screened for antibodies and infectious diseases. Hence, they are transfused as ABO-compatible. Platelet-pheresis products and granulocyte concentrates may contain some red cells, but require crossmatching only if more than 2 ml of red cells are present.

Crossmatch Procedures

The major crossmatch is an *in vitro* determination that combines recipient's plasma with a 5% cell suspension of the donor's cells. This test is performed at different phases in the same manner as the antibody screen and

antibody identification. The final phase is the anti-human globulin (AHG) test. Antibodies present in the recipient that are reactive at the AHG phase are most likely to cause an *in vivo* reaction.

The **minor crossmatch** is performed by mixing donor plasma with cells from the recipient. The minor crossmatch is no longer performed. The majority of cellular products transfused are red blood cells rather than whole blood. The volume of donor plasma transfused with red cell products is very small and not significant enough to induce a reaction with recipient cells (see Figure 9-3).

Compatibility test procedures are performed and the results assessed. **Compatible** units of red cells will have no agglutination or hemolysis at any phase of testing. Tests that have either hemagglutination or hemolysis noted are **incompatible** and should not be transfused without further evaluation. The cause of the incompatibility should be determined and documented.

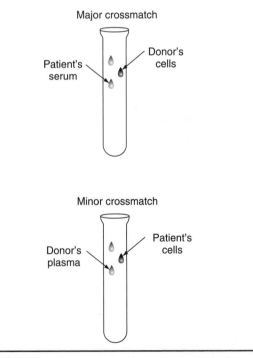

FIGURE 9-3 Major and minor crossmatch procedures. The major crossmatch is a combination of donor cells and recipients serum. The minor crossmatch is the reverse of the major crossmatch, with donor plasma and recipients cells being combined.
Source: Delmar, Cengage Learning

Immediate Spin Crossmatch

The **immediate spin crossmatch** is the first phase of the major crossmatch procedure. This crossmatch mixes recipient's plasma with donor's cells and the immediate spin phase is performed and recorded. This procedure provides a determination of compatibility that encompasses ABO incompatibility. Historically, ABO incompatibility has produced the majority of fatal transfusion reactions. The AABB Standards designate that if all pre-transfusion tests are performed as outlined, no clinically significant antibodies are detected, and there is no record of previously detected antibodies, "at a minimum, detection of ABO incompatibility shall be performed."

Electronic Crossmatch

As computer technology has developed and the sensitivity of antibody detection has increased, a process for computer or electronic crossmatch has been developed. The electronic crossmatch is a viable option when there is no current or previous history of clinically significant antibodies. A summary of electronic crossmatch guidelines outlined in the AABB Standards is provided in Sample Procedure 9-1.

Advantages of the electronic crossmatch are summarized in Table 9-2. One of the primary advantages is

maximum utilization of blood supply. When the electronic crossmatch is used with appropriate patients, wastage of units by holding units for specific patients is significantly reduced. When blood is required for a patient on whom an electronic crossmatch has been performed, a list of all available units is provided. A unit for transfusion is selection from these available units. A flow chart to outline decision-making protocol for immediate spin and electronic crossmatch as compared to traditional testing is provided in Figure 9-4.

CRITICAL THINKING ACTIVITY

Considering the information in Sample Procedure 9-1, work in small groups to answer the following:

1. List five sources of error for the electronic crossmatch.
2. Write a procedure for ABO confirmation of the recipient by two technicians.
3. List five advantages of the electronic crossmatch.

Share this information with other groups and the instructor.

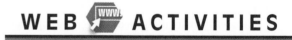

WEB ACTIVITIES

The Code of Federal Regulations (CFR) provides the guidelines for blood bank and transfusion service testing. In small groups, do the following:

1. Using this link, www.gpoaccess.gov, find the CFR. Go to that Web site.
2. Find the section that provides guidelines for Compatibility Testing (Title 21, Part 606, Section 1510).
3. Compare these guidelines to the current issue of the *AABB Standards for Blood Bank and Transfusion Services*.
4. Either write a short paragraph comparing the two sets of guidelines or discuss the differences in a small student group or with the instructor.

WEB ACTIVITIES

1. Type www.ortho-wire.com into your browser.
2. Register to be a user and choose a password.
3. When you have registered, sign on.
4. From the left hand column, choose laboratory management.
5. Choose "Electronic Crossmatching: A Step-By-Step Visual Guide of Procedures."
6. Read the information included and view all slide.
7. Log off.

SAMPLE PROCEDURE 9-1

Summary of AABB Guidelines for Electronic Crossmatch

1. The computer system being utilized has been validated on site to ensure that only ABO-compatible whole blood or red blood cell components have been selected for transfusion. This validation must also be submitted to the FDA.

2. Two determinations of the recipient's ABO group must be made as follows:
   a. One determination must be made on the current sample.
   b. A second determination must be made by
   A different technologist retesting the same sample

   or

   Testing a second current sample

   or

   Comparison of previous records

3. The computer system contains information on the donor including:
   a. Donation identification number
   b. Component name
   c. ABO group and Rh type
   d. Confirmed unit ABO group

4. The computer system contains recipient information including:
   a. The two unique recipient identifiers
   b. Recipient ABO group
   c. Rh type
   d. Antibody screen results
   e. Interpretation of compatibility

5. A method must be in place to verify all data prior to release of blood components.

6. The computer system contains a method to alert the user to discrepancies between:
   a. ABO and Rh type on the donor label and those determined by blood group confirmatory tests
   b. ABO compatibility between the recipient and donor unit

TABLE 9-2 Advantages of the Electronic Crossmatch

1. More efficient management of blood inventory
2. Less wastage of blood components due to outdate
3. More efficient use of technician time
4. Increase in staffing flexibility
5. Smaller recipient sample required
6. Potential for a centralized transfusion service data bank accessible by all interested parties

Problem Solving Incompatible Crossmatches

Incompatible results in the crossmatch must be resolved. Resolution of issues refers back to the original testing of the recipient or donor. Some possible resolutions are listed in Table 9-3.

Compatibility Testing for Autologous Transfusion

Autologous donation is the process of collecting units of blood and storing them for transfusion to the original donor. This procedure is most often used for

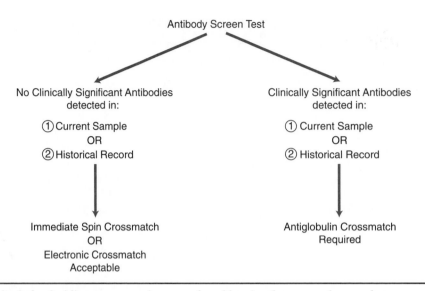

FIGURE 9-4 Criteria for deciding on appropriateness of an abbreviated crossmatch procedure
Source: Delmar, Cengage Learning

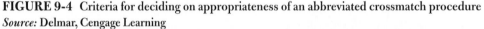

TABLE 9-3 Resolution of Incompatible Crossmatches

PROBLEM ENCOUNTERED	POSSIBLE CAUSE	RESOLUTION
ABO typing	Patient identification error; Sample identification error; Choice of unit of incompatible ABO group	Repeat the ABO group of the recipient; Recheck the label of the selected unit; Recollect a sample from the recipient
Unexpected antibodies when antibody screen is negative at AHG	Cold alloantibody; Cold autoantibody; anti-A_1 in an A_2 individual	Test with panel cells and determine clinical significance of antibody; Prewarm compatibility testing; Test plasma of recipient with A_2 cells
Positive AHG phase of compatibility test	Positive DAT in donor; Antibody to low incidence antigen in recipient with antigen positive cells in donor	Perform DAT test on donor; Choose alternate unit for compatibility test

patients anticipating elective surgery. Each institution specifies pre-transfusion testing required for autologous units. Procedures to ensure that the collected units are transfused to the intended recipient are established by the transfusing institution. This procedure may be computerized with all records retained electronically. The procedure must include a system to ascertain that the autologous units are administered before any allogeneic units are issued. The administration of allogeneic units before the stored autologous units presents a liability risk for the administering institution.

Compatibility Testing of Neonates under Four Months of Age

Neonates require special consideration. Antibodies present have originated from the mother since the neonate is unable to produce their own antibodies. Initial pre-transfusion testing uses the neonate's red cells for ABO and Rh typing. Reverse grouping is not performed on neonates due to the lack of antibody production. Antibody screen may be performed using either the infant or maternal plasma. If the initial antibody screen is negative, there is no need to perform additional antibody screens or crossmatches on the neonate during this admission, so long as ABO-compatible and Rh identical red cell products are administered.

If the antibody screen is positive, the antibody must be identified and antigen negative units administered for assured compatibility. Additionally, an antiglobulin crossmatch should be performed and only compatible units released. Crossmatching of all units needs to be continued until the maternal antibody is no longer detectable in the infant's plasma.

Units of blood are crossmatched and divided since only small quantities are administered to neonates. Blood bags with multiple satellite bags or "pedi-packs" are commercially available for this purpose. This further reduces the possibility of incompatibility or disease transmission. CMV negative units for use specifically in neonates may be obtained from the component source.

ISSUING BLOOD PRODUCTS

The choice of blood products is the responsibility of the technician performing the testing. These products are usually stored on site in the blood bank. The products may be collected on-site or in a commercial blood collection facility. Commercial blood banks that collect and provide large quantities of blood products to multiple hospitals and clinics are the norm in some areas, while on-site facilities may also be available. The collection facility, whether on-site or remote, is responsible for collecting, testing, and labeling the unit. The blood bank issuing the unit(s) for transfusion is responsible only for verifying the ABO and Rh type and completion of compatibility testing prior to transfusion.

Inspecting and Issuing Blood Products

After the compatibility testing has been completed, the appropriate units are tagged and prepared for issue. The attached tag must be labeled with appropriate information as outlined in Table 9-4. The unit is then refrigerated in a monitored refrigerator until released for transfusion.

The most commonly used method for issuing a blood component for transfusion includes direct contact between blood bank personnel and an individual from the transfusing location. Incorporating information technology into the release procedure has created a system that is less labor intensive and time-sparing. An electronic release system must include all of the manual release steps in order for the system to be in compliance with the AABB and FDA.

Procurement of blood components from the blood bank requires the involvement of two individuals. The individuals concurrently check all the paperwork and inspect the unit prior to its release. The verified items are documented and the names of both individuals recorded. An individual from the transfusing facility presents an order for release of the blood component to the blood bank. The patient identity on the order is checked against the tag on the unit. Specific information related to the unit is verified on the tag and compared to the information on the bag. The expiration date is checked to verify that the unit is not expired. Visual inspection of the unit takes

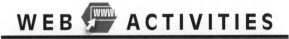

WEB ACTIVITIES

1. Go to the American Red Cross web site: www.redcross.org
2. Choose "Give Blood."
3. Choose "Local Red Cross."
4. Find a Red Cross location near you and click on the link.
5. Review the web site.
6. Discuss your findings with classmates.

TABLE 9-4 Required Information for Blood Tags
Patient's Full Name and Identification Number
Identifying number from Commercial Band System, if Appropriate
Name of the Product
Donor Number
Expiration Date of the Unit
ABO and Rh type of the Unit
Interpretation of the Crossmatch Test, if Indicated
Incompatibility or Incomplete Test Results Documented
Identity of the Individual Performing the Testing or Selecting the Unit

place by both individuals, who check for any abnormalities in appearance including discoloration, hemolysis, or clots. The date and time of issue, along with the final destination, are documented.

When the unit reaches its final destination, the information is re-verified by two individuals prior to initiation of transfusion. Identification of the patient is imperative. The hospital-issued wristband with patient name and identification number must be attached and match the information on the unit of blood exactly. At this juncture, the commercial band system numbers will also be verified. Bar coding has become more popular in hospital settings and provides further reassurance of correct patient identification.

Once the units have been issued from the blood bank, return of these units is only permitted if the units have not been entered; the temperature has not exceeded the upper or lower limits for transportation (1 to 10°C); or the unit is returned to the blood bank within 30 minutes of issue. The time limit for return of issued units is not significant if the units are stored in a monitored refrigerator while out of the blood bank. If any of the above criteria has not been met, the units may not be re-issued and must be discarded.

Miscellaneous Topics

Emergency Issue of Blood for Transfusion

At times, emergent circumstances require that blood be released for transfusion before the pre-transfusion testing is completed. At times, blood release occurs before any pre-transfusion testing has been initiated. The institution must have a protocol for emergency release of blood. In addition, these protocols should be activated only when a delay in transfusion could be detrimental to the patient.

In the case of a life-threatening emergency, the first priority for medical personnel is obtaining a sample for pre-transfusion testing. This is achieved, ideally, before any transfusions have been initiated. In addition, it is imperative that attention be given to the details of specimen labeling. This is challenging for the collecting personnel who may be treating the patient in a very chaotic environment.

Once the sample is received by the blood bank, the testing priority is to perform an ABO and Rh type on the patient in an attempt to provide ABO and Rh specific blood. If the nature of the emergency does not allow the ABO and Rh to be completed, only O negative cells and AB plasma should be administered. If O negative blood is in short supply, then it should be reserved for women of childbearing age and O positive cells should be administered to males and women over childbearing age. If ABO and Rh testing has been completed, type-specific blood should be issued. If past history indicates the presence of an antibody, blood should be screened for the corresponding antigen, if time permits.

Antibody screening should be completed as soon as possible using the original sample. Compatibility testing may be performed at the same time. If evidence of an atypical antibody or an incompatibility is detected at any time during testing, the physician of record should be notified. Ideally, further transfusion should be delayed until the discrepancy is resolved. The physician must make this determination based on the present condition of the patient.

Emergency release of blood requires the signing of a release form by the physician requesting the unit. This is a requirement stated in both the AABB Standards and CFR (Title 21 CFR 606.151). It is also required that these records be maintained. Units released must be tagged with information described in the previous section, but must also stipulate that no crossmatch has been performed. Segments from each unit must be maintained and appropriately labeled for compatibility testing. All testing must be completed even if the units have been successfully transfused. If, in the course of performing necessary testing, an antibody, discrepancy, or incompatibility is encountered, the appropriate medical personnel should be notified, immediately.

CRITICAL THINKING ACTIVITY

Students should work in pairs or small groups. Each pair or group should:

1. List at least five emergency situations that would require rapid treatment and may be encountered in the blood bank. Discuss each of these situations.
2. Have the instructor review situations.
3. Interact with other pairs or groups and compile a list of situations.

Massive Transfusion

Massive transfusion is defined as a total blood volume exchange by transfusion within a 24-hour period. The same criteria apply to adults and infants. At this point, the recipient's own blood volume has been entirely replaced by donor blood. There is no autologous blood remaining in the recipient's circulation. The blood bank should have a protocol for massive transfusion, with particular attention to the recipient sample. At the point where a complete blood exchange has occurred, the "recipient" sample is no longer autologous blood. The institution's protocol will dictate the course of action under these circumstances. The options depend on the presence or absence of atypical antibodies in the original sample. If no antibodies were present and electronic crossmatch is in place, transfusion of type specific units would be appropriate. In this situation, the immediate spin crossmatch may be omitted for a period of time. If red cell stimulated antibodies are present at the outset, type specific antigen negative units should be administered and immediate spin crossmatch performed.

Choice of blood for massive transfusion may depend on the availability of O negative and type specific, as well as the age and sex of the patient. The choice will also reflect the time available for typing at the beginning of the transfusion session. Typically, O negative is given at the outset followed by type specific. If the inventory of type specific wanes, a type switch may be made to an ABO compatible type. (ABO substitution was outlined in Chapter 5.) The future decisions to switch back to the recipient's own ABO type may impact the patient's course of care. It is necessary to determine that the level of passively administered antibody will not create a reaction with any newly transfused ABO specific cells. A new "recipient" sample should be collected and tested against the cells intended for transfusion.

SUMMARY

Compatibility testing represents a large portion of the testing within the transfusion service. With the development of the immediate spin crossmatch and electronic crossmatching, the number of serological crossmatches has declined without a decrease in safety for the recipient. Important points of compatibility testing include:

- Major crossmatch is the testing of recipient's plasma and donor's cells; minor crossmatch is the testing of recipient's cells and donor's plasma. Minor crossmatch is no longer performed.

- Collection of the recipient's sample is a vital part of the testing process. Correct labeling of the sample will prevent delay in the testing and transfusion process.

- Pre-transfusion testing may involve ABO and Rh typing, antibody screening, and a major crossmatch. When atypical antibodies do not exist, immediate spin crossmatch or electronic crossmatching may be used instead of the serological crossmatch.

- Units of blood should be properly tagged with the recipient's information, as the unit's type, and the technologist who completed the testing. If the units are released without compatibility testing the tag must clearly indicate this fact. Commercial banding systems may be in place and units should be labeled with the ID number corresponding to the band.

- The issue of the units requires a system for two individuals to check the identification information. Administration of the units requires the same crosschecking mechanism, with two individuals present at the bedside when the unit is administered.

- Emergency conditions may warrant the administration of blood components without compatibility testing. A release must be signed by the ordering physician and retained in the blood bank. All testing should then be completed even if the units have been completely administered.

- The need for massive transfusion does exist in both adults and infants. Massive transfusion is the complete replacement of a recipient's blood volume within 24 hours. O negative is most often administered at the outset with type specific substituted as soon as possible. Protocol for massive transfusion will vary by institution.

REVIEW QUESTIONS

1. Immediate spin crossmatch detects incompatibility with:
   a. ABO group
   b. Rh type
   c. AHG reactive atypical antibodies
   d. IgM atypical antibodies

2. Labeling of recipient's blood sample for pre-transfusion testing does *not* need to include the following:
   a. patient's name
   b. identification number
   c. ABO group
   d. collection date

3. An electronic crossmatch includes all of the following *except*:
   a. ABO grouping
   b. ABO grouping confirmation by second source
   c. antibody screen
   d. historical review for atypical antibodies

4. Major crossmatch consists of:
   a. recipient's serum with donor's cells
   b. recipient's cells with donor's plasma
   c. donor's serum with donor's cells
   d. recipient's serum with recipient's cells

5. Individuals with no history of atypical antibodies require which of the following compatibility tests:
   a. no additional testing required
   b. major crossmatch in AHG
   c. minor crossmatch in saline only
   d. immediate spin crossmatch

6. The recipient has a positive compatibility test at the AHG phase with a negative antibody screen. The most likely cause for this incompatibility is:
   a. ABO incompatibility
   b. antibody to a high frequency antigen
   c. donor with a positive DAT
   d. positive DAT in recipient

7. A unit of blood has been removed from the blood bank. It may be returned and reissued if it:
   a. is entered, but no blood has been removed
   b. has been stored in a monitored refrigerator at 4°C

   c. was left at the patient's bedside for 40 minutes
   d. was not entered but the original label was damaged

8. The administration of a blood to a 25 year-old woman who is hemorrhaging is necessary on an emergency basis. The best choice for initial transfusion is:
   a. type specific
   b. O positive
   c. O negative
   d. no blood should be transfused without pretransfusion testing

9. A neonate needs to be transfused. The pretransfusion testing that should take place should consist of:
   a. type specific without any serologic tests
   b. serologic tests on neonate's serum
   c. serologic tests on mother's serum
   d. electronic crossmatch after ABO grouping of neonate

10. A compatible crossmatch is:
    a. mixed field reaction at AHG phase with positive reaction with Coombs control cells
    b. negative at immediate spin; 1+ at AHG
    c. negative at the AHG phase; negative with Coombs control cells
    d. negative at AHG phase; positive with Coombs control cells

11. A recipient is AB negative, the supply of type specific blood has been exhausted. The best choice for substitution is:
    a. O negative
    b. A negative
    c. A positive
    d. AB positive

12. An electronic crossmatch was performed. The check of the patient's history indicates that an anti-Jka was found in the serum three years previously. The technologist who initiated the testing should:
    a. administer type specific units if the ABO confirmation matches
    b. collect another sample and retype the patient

c. proceed with antibody screen and crossmatch

d. perform an immediate spin crossmatch and administer compatible units

13. Donor blood is received from a source outside of the hospital. Testing that must be performed on this donor blood is:

a. antibody screen

b. infectious disease testing

c. direct antiglobulin test

d. ABO and Rh

14. When performing the visual check of a unit of blood for transfusion, the technician should look for:

1. hemolysis in the plasma
2. clots in the bag
3. separation of cells and serum in layers
4. discoloration of the contents

a. 1, 2, and 3 are correct

b. 1, 2, and 4 are correct

c. 1, 3, and 4 are correct

d. 2, 3, and 4 are correct

e. all are correct

15. If a potential recipient was transfused two months ago, the sample should be collected within _____ day(s) of the intended upcoming transfusion.

a. 1

b. 3

c. 7

d. 14

For items 16 to 20, use the following choices:

a. immediate spin or electronic crossmatch

b. AHG crossmatch

_____ 16. An 8 year-old child was injured in a car accident and requires a splenectomy. The type and screen shows no atypical antibodies in the AHG phase and there are no historical records for this patient.

_____ 17. A 22 year-old sickle cell patient requires transfusion for anemia. Historical records indicate that one year ago the patient had an anti-c.

_____ 18. A 40 year-old patient is having a type and screen for elective surgery. The type and screen shows no evidence of atypical antibodies at the AHG phase. Five years ago the patient was typed and screened and a cold autoantibody was detected then. It is not being demonstrated at this time.

_____ 19. An 89 year-old male patient is experiencing a G.I. bleed. He has had a complete replacement of his blood volume in the past 20 hours. His initial antibody screen demonstrated no atypical antibodies at the AHG phase.

_____ 20. A leukemic patient has received 20 units of leukocyte-reduced cells over the past three months. Two weeks previously the antibody screen demonstrated and anti-K.

CASE STUDY

1. A trauma center received several casualties from a multi-car automobile accident. One casualty was an 18-year old female with internal injuries. In preparation for surgery, the surgeon requested ten units of blood to be crossmatched for transfusion. The surgeon wanted two units to be started immediately. The technician collected a sample, but time was insufficient to perform an ABO and Rh type before releasing the first two units. Respond to the following questions related to this case.

   a. What ABO and Rh type should be chosen for the two units to be transfused immediately?

   b. As soon as the sample is received in the blood bank and can be used for testing, what tests will be performed on this sample?

   c. After the two emergency units have been released, will any tests need to be performed with these units? If so, what are they?

   (continues)

C A S E   S T U D Y   (C O N T I N U E D)

2. A phlebotomist is sent to collect a sample for pre-transfusion testing. The hospital uses a commercial system to identify patients and units for transfusion. The patient has no hospital ID band and no transfusion ID band. The patient is heavily medicated and is not coherent to identify herself. The phlebotomist collects the blood and labels it with the name that is on the placard on the end of the bed. She forwards this blood to the Blood Bank.

   a. What do you expect the Blood Bank to do with this sample?

   b. What errors, if any, did the phlebotomist make?

   c. What is the correct procedure for a phlebotomist to follow when expected identification methods is/are not present?

3. You have released a unit of blood for transfusion at 8 a.m. The phlebotomist calls the Blood Bank to report a unit of blood in the patient food refrigerator at noon. The phlebotomist was unsure about protocol, but felt uneasy about this scenario.

   a. What should you do about this situation?

   b. What is the disposition of the blood?

4. A teenage patient is scheduled for an orthopedic procedure that may require transfusion. The patient donated two units of autologous red cells that are being held for transfusion. The surgery is postponed due to a family emergency and cannot be rescheduled for three weeks. At this point, the units of blood will have expired.

   a. What alternatives exist for this patient?

5. A GI bleeder arrives at the Emergency Room with active bleeding. Initial testing results were a 7.0 g/dl hemoglobin and a 22% hematocrit. The ER physician ordered 3 units of packed red cells for transfusion. Pre-transfusion testing began in the Blood Bank. Previous records showed that an anti-C was found previously. Current antibody screen results are demonstrated below:

	LISS			
	IS	37°C	AHG	Interpretation
Screen Cell I	0	0	0	Negative
Screen Cell II	0	0	0	Negative

The patient is A positive.

All units of blood are compatible.

The doctor is expressing an urgency for transfusion of blood. What should you do regarding the compatible blood?

   a. What steps should be taken to assure compatible blood for this patient?

   b. Should the compatible units be transfused with no further testing?

   c. What blood types may present alternatives if the correct number of A positive units may not be found?

(continues)

CASE STUDY (CONTINUED)

6. A patient was transfused in the emergency room with 14 units of O negative red cells over a period of 6 hours. The acute bleeding was stopped and the patient transferred to the ICU for continued care. Type and screen on the original sample, revealed O positive with an antibody screen negative at all phases of testing. An H and H was performed and the results were:

Hemoglobin: 8 g/dl
Hematocrit: 24.7%

The physician ordered a crossmatch for 4 additional units.
a. What sample should be used for testing?
b. What blood type should be transfused? What made this determination?

REFERENCES

Blaney, Kathy and Howard, Paula. *Basic and Applied Concepts of Immunohematology*. Mosby, Philadelphia, 2000.

Boulton, F. "A Hundred Years of Cascading—Started by Paul Morawitz (1879–1936), a Pioneer of Haemostasis and of Transfusion." *Transfusion Medicine*. Vol. 16, 2006, pp. 1–10.

Brecher, Mark, editor. *American Association of Blood Banks Technical Manual 15th edition*. AABB, 2005.

Chapman, J. F., Milkins, C., Voak, D. "The Computer Crossmatch: A Safe Alternative to the Serological Crossmatch." *Transfusion Medicine*. Vol. 10, 2000, pp. 251–256.

Code of Federal Regulations, 21 CFR § 606.151. Food and Drug Administration.

Herman, Jay and Manno, Catherine. *Pediatric Transfusion Therapy*. AABB Press, 2002.

"Highlights of Transfusion Medicine History." *AABB Web Site*. 2006.

Hillyer, Christopher D., et al. "Integrating Molecular Technologies for Red Blood Cell Typing and Compatibility Testing into Blood Centers and Transfusion Services." *Transfusion Medicine Reviews*. Vol. 22, No. 2, 2008, pp. 117–132.

Kuriyan, Mercy and Fox, Ellen. "Pretransfusion Testing without Serologic Crossmatch: Approaches to Ensure Patient Safety." *Vox Sanguinis*. Vol. 78, 2000, pp. 113–118.

McCullough, Jeffrey. *Transfusion Medicine 2nd edition*. Elsevier. 2005.

Oberman, H. A. "The Crossmatch, A Brief Historical Perspective." *Transfusion*. Vol. 21, No. 6, 1981, pp. 645–651.

Standards for Blood Banks and Transfusion Services, 25th Edition. AABB, Bethesda, MD. 2008.

Staves, Julie, et al. "Electronic Remote Blood Issue: A Combination of Remote Blood Issue with a System for End-to-End Electronic Control of Transfusion to Provide a 'Total Solution' for a Safe and Timely Hospital Blood Transfusion Service." *Transfusion*. Vol. 48, March 2008, pp. 415–424.

Blood Components and Their Administration

10

Donor Criteria and Blood Collection

LEARNING OUTCOMES

At the completion of this chapter, the reader should be able to:

- Describe the information included in a complete donor registration.
- Discuss the administration of the donor history questionnaire.
- List screening questions intended for donor protection.
- List screening questions intended for recipient protection.
- Describe, in detail, the physical exam criteria for allogeneic donors.
- Discuss informed consent of donors.
- Outline the steps for donor arm inspection and preparation.
- List adverse donor reactions and the treatment for each.
- Differentiate autologous and allogeneic donor criteria.
- Describe intraoperative red cell salvage.
- List products of apheresis.
- Describe the procedure for apheresis.
- Define directed donation.
- Discuss the philosophy and criteria of directed donation.
- Define therapeutic phlebotomy.
- List clinical conditions that may be treated with therapeutic phlebotomy.

GLOSSARY

allogeneic donation   blood or tissue from the same species that is not genetically identical

antecubital   the area of the arm in front of the elbow

apheresis   removal of a specific component of the blood; the remaining components are returned to the donor

autologous donation   a donor's donation reserved for the same donor's use at a later time

deferral   non-acceptance of a potential donor

diastolic pressure   the second sound heard while taking a blood pressure; it represents the filling of the heart chamber

189

hemapheresis whole blood removed from a donor and separated into components; one or more of the components are retained; the remainder is returned to the donor

leukapheresis the removal of whole blood from a donor; the blood is separated into components; the leukocytes are retained and the remaining components returned to the donor

plasmapheresis the removal of whole blood from a donor; the blood is separated into components; the plasma is retained and the remaining components returned to the donor

plateletpheresis the removal of whole blood from a donor; the blood is separated into components; the platelets are retained and the remaining components returned to the donor

red cell apheresis the removal of red cells from a donor via pheresis

syncope fainting

systolic pressure the first sound heard when taking a blood pressure; the contraction of the heart

INTRODUCTION

Maintaining an adequate blood supply can be a challenge for blood banks and transfusion services. Donors and prospective donors must be actively recruited with appropriate educational materials. The general population should be educated about the blood bank's need for an adequate donor pool. "A primary goal of appropriate donor recruitment and screening is to select and retain donors whose characteristics predict a low incidence and prevalence of transfusion-transmissable diseases (TTDs)." Donor screening and physical exams for donors are imperative for maintenance of a safe blood supply. Chapter 11 will cover the processing of blood and blood components.

DONOR SCREENING

Donor screening procedures have evolved in recent years. Procedures now consider a number of components including an emphasis on the donor's health, blood products free from TTD, and the donor's protection during the collection process and post-collection recovery. The screening process consists of three phases: registration, an interview of health history, and a physical exam. Criteria for acceptance or rejection of a donor are regulated by the FDA and accrediting agencies such as the AABB.

Registration

Donor registration is required with each donation. A donor registration record must include documentation that fully identifies the donor, and identification must be verified with each donation. Computerized records have eased the burden of the registrar by maintaining information that is updated each day of donation. Information to be included in the record is:

- Date and time of donation
- Name: last, first, and middle initial (if available)
- Address: home and/or business
- Telephone: home and/or business
- Gender
- Age or date of birth
- Record of previous deferrals
- Date of last donation
- Written informed consent

Additional information that may be included:

- Driver's license or social security number
- Positive identification; e.g. photo identification
- Intended use if it is specific; e.g. directed or autologous
- Race
- Unique donor characteristics: e.g. CMV negative, O negative donors

Information from first-time donors is recorded for reference at the time of future donations. Repeat donors require verification of previous information at the time of each future donation. Eligibility to donate must be confirmed and documented on each day of donation.

Age

Donors must be at least 17-years-old to be eligible for donation. Exceptions to this age restriction may be found in some states where the minimum donation age is 16 years of age as determined by state law. Parental consent may be required for donors who are under 18 years of age. State laws determine minor status. There are no upper-age restrictions. Blood banks establish age criteria and publish them in the standard operating procedures. The medical director may accept or decline donors based on their medical condition at the time of each assessment.

Previous Donations

Whole blood donors are eligible to donate every 56 days (8 weeks). It is important to determine eligibility on each day of donation. Apheresis donors (plateletpheresis, leukapheresis, and plasmapheresis) must allow at least 48 hours to elapse after pheresis before donation of whole blood.

Donor Education

Prospective donors are provided with educational materials. These materials should include:

- Information on infectious diseases transmitted by blood transfusion.
- The signs and symptoms of AIDS.

Additional pre-donation information provided to donors includes:

- The importance of providing accurate information.
- The freedom to withdraw themselves from the donation process if for any reason they believe their blood is not suitable for transfusion.

The donor acknowledges the materials have been read and signs the acknowledgement.

Donor Consent

Prior to each donation, the donor must sign a written, informed consent for collection of the blood. The donor must have the freedom to ask questions, receive answers to these questions and, finally, the option to consent or refuse to participate in donation. Each donor is educated on risks of the procedure and infectious disease

testing that will be performed on the collected unit. An explanation is provided regarding notification of positive test results. The donor is informed that he or she will be notified if the testing of the unit reveals the potential of infectious disease transmission. In addition, the donor is informed that **deferral** from future blood donation will occur if infectious disease testing yields positive results. The donor will have the opportunity to confidentially self-defer. The donor will designate the collected unit in one of two ways: either "transfuse my blood" or "do not transfuse my blood."

Health History Interview

The Donor History Questionnaire (DHQ) is administered on the day of donation. Prospective donors should review the Donor Educational Materials prior to completing the DHQ. They are provided the Medication Deferral List and a list of bovine spongiform encephalopathy (BSE) countries to be used with the DHQ. The Full-Length DHQ obtained from the AABB Web site is represented in Figure 10-1. This questionnaire is recommended for use by the AABB and approved by the FDA. Medical directors may modify the questions to accommodate the specific needs of an individual blood bank. Local vernacular may dictate these changes.

This questionnaire should be administered according to the institution's SOP. Three modalities of administration are:

- Face-to-Face Interview (FFI): A trained donor historian administers the questionnaire by asking each question and recording the response.
- Written Donor Self-Administered (WDSA): The donor completes the form privately. A trained donor historian reviews the completed form.

WEB ACTIVITIES

1. Go to www.aabb.org
2. Choose "Donate Blood."
3. Review current AABB information on blood donation and donor testing.
4. Summarize for instructor in the form of a bulleted list.

Full-Length Donor History Questionnaire

	Yes	No	
Are you			
1. Feeling healthy and well today?	☐	☐	
2. Currently taking an antibiotic?	☐	☐	
3. Currently taking any other medication for an infection?	☐	☐	
Please read the Medication Deferral List.			
4. Are you now taking or have you ever taken any medications on the Medication Deferral List?	☐	☐	
5. Have you read the educational materials?	☐	☐	
In the past 48 hours			
6. Have you taken aspirin or anything that has aspirin in it?	☐	☐	
In the past 6 weeks			
7. Female donors: Have you been pregnant or are you pregnant now? (Males: check "I am male.")	☐	☐	☐ I am male
In the past 8 weeks have you			
8. Donated blood, platelets, or plasma?	☐	☐	
9. Had any vaccinations or other shots?	☐	☐	
10. Had contact with someone who had a smallpox vaccination?	☐	☐	
In the past 16 weeks			
11. Have you donated a double unit of red cells using an apheresis machine?	☐	☐	
In the past 12 months have you			
12. Had a blood transfusion?	☐	☐	
13. Had a transplant such as organ, tissue, or bone marrow?	☐	☐	
14. Had a graft such as bone or skin?	☐	☐	
15. Come into contact with someone else's blood?	☐	☐	
16. Had an accidental needle-stick?	☐	☐	
17. Had sexual contact with anyone who has HIV/AIDS or has had a positive test for the HIV/AIDS virus?	☐	☐	
18. Had sexual contact with a prostitute or anyone else who takes money or drugs or other payment for sex?	☐	☐	
19. Had sexual contact with anyone who has ever used needles to take drugs or steroids, or anything not prescribed by their doctor?	☐	☐	
20. Had sexual contact with anyone who has hemophilia or has used clotting factor concentrates?	☐	☐	
21. Female donors: Had sexual contact with a male who has ever had sexual contact with another male? (Males: check "I am male.")	☐	☐	☐ I am male
22. Had sexual contact with a person who has hepatitis?	☐	☐	
23. Lived with a person who has hepatitis?	☐	☐	
24. Had a tattoo?	☐	☐	
25. Had ear or body piercing?			

FIGURE 10-1 Full-Length Donor History Questionnaire (DHQ) is available at www.aabb.org. *Reprinted with permission from the AABB, Arlington, VA.*

Full-Length Donor History Questionnaire

	Yes	No
26. Had or been treated for syphilis or gonorrhea?	☐	☐
27. Been in juvenile detention, lockup, jail, or prison for more than 72 hours?	☐	☐
In the past three years have you		
28. Been outside the United States or Canada?	☐	☐
From 1980 through 1996,		
29. Did you spend time that adds up to three (3) months or more in the United Kingdom? (Review list of countries in the UK)	☐	☐
30. Were you a member of the U.S. military, a civilian military employee, or a dependent of a member of the U.S. military?	☐	☐
From 1980 to the present, did you		
31. Spend time that adds up to five (5) years or more in Europe? (Review list of countries in Europe.)	☐	☐
32. Receive a blood transfusion in the United Kingdom or France? (Review list of countries in the UK.)	☐	☐
From 1977 to the present, have you		
33. Received money, drugs, or other payment for sex?	☐	☐
34. Male donors: had sexual contact with another male, even once? (Females: check "I am female.")	☐	☐
Have you EVER		
35. Had a positive test for the HIV/AIDS virus?	☐	☐
36. Used needles to take drugs, steroids, or anything <u>not</u> prescribed by your doctor?	☐	☐
37. Used clotting factor concentrates?	☐	☐
38. Had hepatitis?	☐	☐
39. Had malaria?	☐	☐
40. Had Chagas disease?	☐	☐
41. Had babesiosis?	☐	☐
42. Received a dura mater (or brain covering) graft?	☐	☐
43. Had any type of cancer, including leukemia?	☐	☐
44. Had any problems with your heart or lungs?	☐	☐
45. Had a bleeding condition or a blood disease?	☐	☐
46. Had sexual contact with anyone who was born in or lived in Africa?	☐	☐
47. Been in Africa?	☐	☐
48. Have any of your relatives had Creutzfeldt-Jakob disease?	☐	☐

(Beside question 34: ☐ I am female)

FIGURE 10-1 (Continued)

Full-Length Donor History Questionnaire

Use this area for additional questions	Yes	No

FIGURE 10-1 (Continued)

■ Computer-Assisted Donor Self-Interviewing (CASI): The donor completes the interview using a computer-assisted system. The CASI is text format possibly in combination with audio or visual prompts.

The questionnaire contains questions with two general intents: questions intended for the protection of the donor and for the protection of the recipient. The entire questionnaire is administered prior to each donation. A confidential environment should be provided, and the donor should be encouraged to answer all questions honestly.

Questions for the Protection of Donors

Questions designed for the protection of the donor focus on health status or maintenance of an appropriate health status. Examples include:

■ Are you feeling healthy and well today?
   Donors exhibiting symptoms of a cold, influenza, nausea, and symptoms that may indicate an underlying minor illness should be deferred temporarily.

■ In the past six weeks have you been pregnant or are you pregnant now?
   Women who are currently pregnant or have been pregnant within six weeks should be temporarily deferred.

■ In the past eight weeks have you donated blood, platelets, or plasma?
   Whole blood donation, or loss of a significant volume of red cells while participating as a pheresis donor, requires an eight-week deferral from the time of whole blood donation or pheresis-associated blood loss.

Additional assessments related to a donor's health and well-being may result in temporary or permanent deferral. These include:

■ Previous surgery

■ Heart and lung disease

■ History of cancer

■ History of leukemia or lymphoma warrants a permanent deferral

■ Bleeding tendencies require deferral to avoid complications during donation

■ A trained donor historian will interview the prospective donor and determine his or her donation suitability. Questionable circumstances may be referred to the medical director for a final ruling. All deferrals should be discussed confidentially with the donor using tact and compassion. An explanation of the length of deferral should be included in the counseling session.

Questions for the Protection of the Recipient

Questions for the protection of the recipient constitute the majority of the questions on the DHQ. Donors are questioned in depth about possible exposure to TTD. Extended questioning includes: vaccinations, medications, and high-risk activities. Questions are updated frequently. The AABB Web site (www.aabb.org) should be consulted for the most recent DHQ.

Affirmative responses to screening questions related to a history of jaundice, liver disease, hepatitis, or IV drug use could indicate potential for infection with a blood-borne pathogen. Individuals who provide a positive response to any of these questions will be permanently deferred. Donor blood is screened for blood-borne pathogens. Early in the disease process the individual is infectious but the level of pathogen is undetectable by test methods.

Possible exposure to infectious agents may occur through a tattoo, body piercing, or exposure to an individual with viral hepatitis. Donors with exposure through any of these modalities should be deferred for 12 months.

A series of questions on travel to or immigration from endemic areas is the primary screening method for parasitic TTDs. Parasitic TTDs include: malaria (*Plasmodium species*), Chagas disease (*Trypanosoma cruzi*), and Babesiosis (*Babesia microti*). Donors with previous malarial infection or those receiving malarial therapy are deferred for three years. History of Chagas disease or Babesiosis requires permanent deferral. Testing for Chagas disease has decreased the likelihood of transmission of this parasite to a recipient. This testing will be discussed in Chapter 11.

A list of medications is provided for each donor as part of the screening process. Medications may result in a deferral. The deferral may result from the underlying disease process not the medication itself. Examples of

TABLE 10-1 Medications Commonly Accepted for Blood Donation

- Oral contraceptives
- Replacement hormones
- Decongestants
- Blood pressure medications; donor must be free of symptoms
- Antibiotics for acne treatment; including tetracycline
  Anti-fungal agents (oral or topical) taken for vaginal, skin, or nail infection, or ringworm. Other reasons require medical evaluation.
- Tamoxifen®, if taken to prevent cancer
  Anti-viral agents taken for cold sores, genital herpes, genital warts, or shingles. Other reasons require medical evaluation.
  Any anti-platelet medications; such as, Clopidogrel®, Plavix®, Ticlid®, or Ticlopidine® (if donating for any donation type, except defer for plateletpheresis donations)
- Mild analgesics
- Vitamins

TABLE 10-2 Temporary Deferrals following Vaccine Administration

DEFERRAL TIME	VACCINE
7 Days	Hepatitis B (Not for Exposure)
2 Weeks	Measles (Rubeola)
	Mumps
	Yellow Fever
	Polio (Oral)
	Typhoid (Oral)
4 Weeks	German Measles (Rubella)
	Measles, Mumps, Rubella Combination Vaccine
	Varicella Zoster (Chicken Pox)
8 Weeks	Smallpox
12 Months	Hepatitis B Immune Globulin
	Rabies Vaccine, Unless for Prevention
	Experimental/unlicensed Vaccine if Participating in a Research Study

TABLE 10-3 12-Month Deferrals

- Tattoo
- Mucous-membrane or skin-penetration exposure to blood
- Sexual contact with an individual at high risk for human immunodeficiency virus
- Incarceration in a correctional institution for more than 72 hours
- Victims of rape
- Return from a malarial-endemic area
- Positive test for syphilis
- Completion of therapy for syphilis or gonorrhea
- Transfusion of blood, components, or derivatives
- Organ transplant

medications that are permissible for donation are summarized in Table 10-1.

Aspirin and aspirin-containing medications affect platelet function. Donors who will serve as a source of platelets, for example plateletpheresis, are deferred for at least 48 hours following aspirin consumption.

Vaccinations may require deferral. Vaccines prepared from killed organisms or toxoids do not require deferral. The donor should be free of symptoms. Hepatitis A and meningitis vaccines do not require a deferral if they were administered for prevention rather than exposure. Routine vaccines such as influenza and tetanus do not require deferral, assuming that the donor is asymptomatic and fever-free. Table 10-2 summarizes temporary deferrals for vaccine administration:

Twelve-Month Deferrals. Additional criteria requiring a twelve-month deferral are included for protection of the recipient. These deferrals are summarized in Table 10-3.

Permanent Deferrals. Conditions with serious consequences for the recipient may require permanent deferral. These are summarized in Table 10-4.

Physical Examination

A physical examination provides a general screening of health and vital signs to ensure good health on the day of donation. The donor should appear in relative good health to the trained donor historian. Appearance

TABLE 10-4 Criteria with Potential Permanent Deferral

- Potential exposure to Creutzfeldt-Jakob Disease (CJD)
- Human pituitary growth hormone
- History of familial CJD
- Dura-matter transplants from brain surgery
- Travel for a total of three months or more in the U.K. (England, Scotland, Wales, Northern Ireland, Isle of Man, Channel Islands, Gibraltar, Falkland Islands) from 1/1/1980 to 12/31/1996
- Spending a total of six months or more on or associated with a U.S. military base in Belgium, Netherlands (Holland), or Germany from 1/1/1980 to 12/31/1996
- Spending a total of six months or more on or associated with a U.S. military base in Spain, Portugal, Turkey, Italy, or Greece from 1/1/1980 to 12/31/1996
- Spending a total of five years or more in Europe
- A sexual partner born in or lived in Cameroon, Central African Republic, Chad, Congo, Equatorial Guinea, Gabon, Niger, or Nigeria for five years or more after 1977
- History of Infectious Disease
- Viral hepatitis
- Babesiosis
- Chagas disease
- HIV
- Human T Cell Lymphotropic Virus (HTLV)
- High-Risk Behavior
- Use of a needle to take drugs not prescribed by a doctor
- Taken clotting factor concentrates to correct a bleeding problem
- AIDS
- Positive Test for AIDS
- Males who have had sex with another male since 1977
- Twelve month deferral for a female with sexual contact with a male who has had sex with another male

TABLE 10-5 Criteria for Donor Physical Examination

CRITERIA	LIMITS
Hemoglobin	≥12.5 g/dl
Hematocrit	≥38%
Blood Pressure	Systolic ≤180 mm Hg
	Diastolic ≤100 mm Hg
Temperature	≤37.5°C (99.5°F)
Pulse	Between 50 and 100 Beats/minute
Weight	≥110 lb (50 kg)

parameters are set to allow donation of 525 ml of blood, including samples for testing, without a negative impact on the donor. Acceptable criteria for physical examination are summarized in Table 10-5.

Hemoglobin or Hematocrit

Hemoglobin or hematocrit determination is performed on a sample from venipuncture, finger puncture, or earlobe puncture. For whole blood donation, the minimum hemoglobin is 12.5 g/dl. Minimum hematocrit is 38%.

The hematocrit may be spun and the hemoglobin may be determined spectophotmetrically. Previously, hemoglobin determinations were performed by dropping a drop of blood in copper sulfate and timing the descent to the bottom of the vial of $CuSO_4$. This method has been eliminated from most blood banks.

Temperature

Body temperature is measured to indicate a possible infection. The temperature must not exceed 37°C (99.5°F). Donors with elevated temperatures should be deferred for that day.

Blood Pressure

Systolic pressure is the first reported number in a blood pressure reading. A donor's systolic pressure should not exceed 180 mm hg. The diastolic pressure is the second number reported in a blood pressure reading. A donor's diastolic pressure should not exceed 100 mm Hg.

Pulse

The pulse rate should be between 50 and 100 beats per minute. No irregularities in the pulse should be present.

or suspicion of drug or alcohol use would result in a deferral for that day. Specific screening assessments are performed and the results recorded in the donor record. The minimum requirements for some of these

Athletes may exhibit low pulse rates. These individuals are acceptable as donors.

Weight

Donors must weigh a minimum of 110 lb (50 kg). Donors weighing less may donate with reduced anticoagulant. See Chapter 11 for the calculation of reduced coagulant for donors. There is no maximum weight for donation. Donors weighing more than 350 pounds should contact the medical director.

PHLEBOTOMY

Following an established protocol for donor phlebotomy is imperative for collection of an acceptable unit identification of the donor must take place before phlebotomy begins. Once the identification is completed, the collection process may commence.

Arm Preparation and Venipuncture

The phlebotomist inspects the **antecubital** area of both donor arms. This inspection locates an acceptable vein for the collection of the blood product. During the inspection process, the phlebotomist checks for evidence of intravenous drug use and presence of skin lesions. The arm used for collection must be free of skin lesions on the day of donation.

The venipuncture site is scrubbed with an acceptable arm preparation solution. The *AABB Standards for Blood Banks and Transfusion Services, 25th Edition,* states "green soap shall not be used." Use of a 70% aqueous scrub solution of iodophor compound to remove the surface dirt, followed by a prep solution of 10% PVP-iodine, provides an adequate preparation for venipuncture. The 10% PVP-iodine is applied in concentric circles beginning at the intended venipuncture site (see Figure 10-2). The prepared area should be allowed to air dry for 30 seconds and may be covered with sterile gauze prior to venipuncture.

A blood pressure cuff inflated to 40 to 60 mm Hg will sufficiently distend the vein for ease of phlebotomy. A 16-gauge needle attached to a primary blood bag is used for collection (see Figure 10-3). The venipuncture is performed using an appropriate vein in the antecubital area. The venipuncture site should be free of skin lesions.

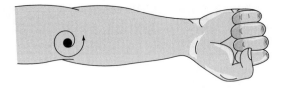

FIGURE 10-2 The 10% PVP-iodine is applied in concentric circles beginning in the center of the area designated for venipuncture.
Source: Delmar, Cengage Learning

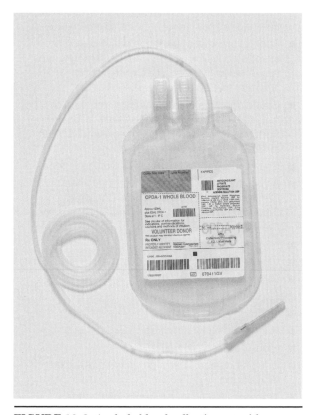

FIGURE 10-3 A whole blood collection set with integral tubing and needle. *Reprinted with permission from Terumo Medical Corporation, Somerset, NJ.*

Donation commences until the blood bag is sufficiently full. The needle is removed and pressure applied to the venipuncture site. The donor's arm is elevated. Additional tubes for testing are collected as per the institutions SOP.

Donor Reactions

Most donations are tolerated without incident, but an adverse reaction may occur at any time from donor

TABLE 10-6 Adverse Donor Reactions and Interventions

PRESENTATION	INTERVENTION
Hematoma	■ Apply pressure to site; Follow with ice
Pallor, sweating, dizziness, rapid breathing, nausea	■ Elevate feet; Lower head ■ Apply cold compresses to forehead and back of neck
Muscle spasms and twitches	■ Breathe into a paper bag
Syncope	■ Lower head and raise feet ■ Apply cold compresses to forehead and back of neck ■ Apply aromatic spirits of ammonia, if indicated in SOP
Convulsions	■ Call for emergency help ■ Maintain airway ■ Protect donor from injury until help arrives
Cardiac Symptoms	■ Call for emergency help ■ Initiate CPR or AED if indicated

screening through the post-donation period. A summary of adverse reactions is found in Table 10-6. Most reactions are minor and may be assessed and treated by blood bank staff. Serious reactions up to and including convulsions and cardiac arrest do occur, but rarely. All phlebotomists must be trained to recognize symptoms of reactions and provide treatment and first aid, when indicated.

Symptoms may include pallor, sweating, dizziness, rapid breathing, nausea, and **syncope** or fainting. At the first sign of an impending reaction, the blood pressure cuff and needle are removed. Immediate treatment is initiated. Treatment may include calling for emergency medical attention.

Post-Donation Care of Donors

Following donation, the donor should begin the rehydration process. Liquids and a light snack may be provided immediately following donation. Donors are instructed to consume extra fluids over the next 72 hours. Other specific post donation instructions should include:

■ Avoid alcohol until first consuming food.

■ Avoid smoking for 30 minutes.

■ Be aware of any pre-syncope symptoms that may indicate a possible delayed reaction.

■ Treat bleeding from phlebotomy site by elevating arm and applying pressure to the site.

ALTERNATE COLLECTIONS
Autologous Donation

Autologous donation is the collection of blood to be transfused to the donor at a later time. This is in contrast to **allogeneic donation** or the collection of blood intended for transfusion to an individual in the general population. The use of autologous blood is the safest alternative for transfusion. This procedure eliminates the possibility of disease transmission and alloimmunization to any of the cellular material in the transfused blood. These donations are often used for elective surgery. The requirements for preoperative collection of autologous donor units may differ from those previously described for allogeneic donors. The *AABB Standards for Blood Banks and Transfusion Services, 25th Edition*, states "in situations where requirements for allogeneic donor selection or collection are not applied, alternate requirements shall be defined and documented by the medical director." General guidelines are listed in Table 10-7.

This alternate system for providing blood for transfusion has advantages and disadvantages. Table 10-8 provides a summary.

Intraoperative Blood Collection

Alternately, blood may be collected from the operative field and reinfused to the patient. The collection, washing, filtering, and re-infusion of the units may be performed with an automated device designed for this purpose. See Figure 10-4 for an example of an intraoperative cell recovery instrument.

Units that are washed with 0.9% saline may be stored at room temperature for up to six hours and at 1 to 6°C for up to 24 hours provided storage at 1 to 6°C is begun within four hours of collection. This method of collection and reinfusion is not acceptable if the operative field is potentially bacterially contaminated. Written policies for use of blood collected intraoperatively must be in place and the SOP followed in all instances.

Directed Donations

Concern of the general public, related to the safety of the general blood supply, has led to the desire for potential recipients to select their own blood donors. Directed donor programs are available in most blood banks. Donor screening and testing must be the same as those for allogeneic donors. Additional policies related to pre-donation ABO testing, fees, and time for distribution of units should be institution-specific.

Therapeutic Phlebotomy

Clinical conditions may require the removal of blood from a patient as a therapeutic process. This process of "bleeding" is intended to alleviate symptoms of the medical condition. The blood is not used for transfusion purposes and must be discarded. Some clinical conditions that may warrant phlebotomy include: polycythemia vera and hemochromatosis.

Hemapheresis

Hemapheresis is a procedure that removes a unit of whole blood, separates a component by mechanical means, and returns the remainder of the blood to the donor. There are four major types of hemapheresis:

- **Leukapheresis**—the removal of white blood cells
- **Plateletpheresis**—the removal of platelets

TABLE 10-7 General Guidelines for Autologous Donations

- Donor must have a medical order from a physician.
- Hemoglobin shall be ≥11 g/dl *or* hematocrit ≥33 %—earlobe puncture must not be used for this determination.
- All autologous collections must be completed more than 72 hours before the anticipated time of surgery or transfusion.
- Autologous donor is deferred if a condition exists where bacteremia may be present.
- The unit shall be reserved for autologous transfusion.
- Testing is not required unless it is to be converted for use for allogeneic transfusion.
- Units must include standard labeling and be labeled "Autologous Donor"; untested units must be labeled "Donor Untested."
- The unit(s) must be tagged with donor identification.

TABLE 10-8 Advantages and Disadvantages of Autologous Blood Use

ADVANTAGES	DISADVANTAGES
Prevents transfusion transmitted disease	Does not affect risk of bacterial contamination
Prevents red cell alloimmunization	Does not affect risk of ABO incompatibility error
Supplements blood supply	Is more costly than allogeneic blood
Provides compatible blood for patients with alloantibodies	Results in wastage of blood not transfused
Prevents some adverse transfusion reactions	Increased evidence of adverse reactions to autologous donation
Provides reassurance to patients concerned about blood risks	Subjects patient to perioperative anemia and increased likelihood of transfusion

- **Plasmapheresis**—the removal of plasma
- **Red cell apheresis**—the removal of red cells

The removal of one component while allowing the reinfusion of the remaining components permits the collection of a greater volume of a specific component from a single donor. Apheresis is performed on a cell separator machine. The collection of each product requires a specific machine with specifications set by the manufacturer. See Figures 10-5 and 10-6 for examples of pheresis instruments for collection of platelets and red blood cells.

Pheresis instruments use centrifugal force to separate the blood into components based on specific gravity. Blood from the donor flows into the bowl. The desired component is removed and stored in a donor bag. The remaining components are returned to the donor.

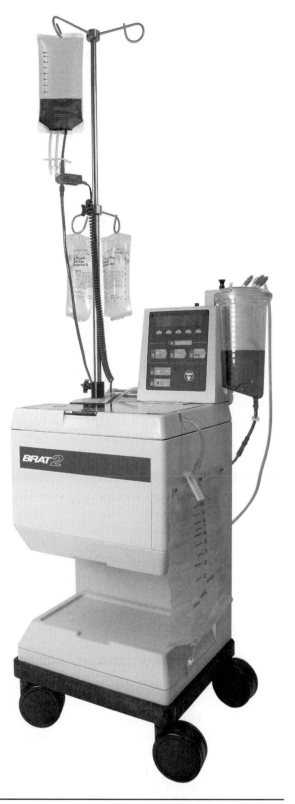

FIGURE 10-4 Brat-2 Intraoperative cell saver. *Reprinted with permission from the Sorin Group, Arvada, Co.*

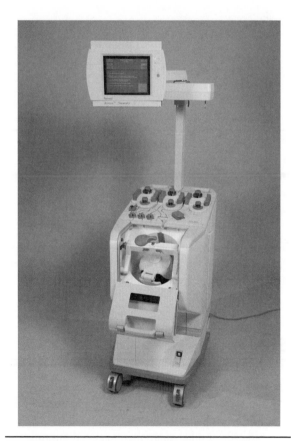

FIGURE 10-5 Amicus plateletpheresis equipment. *Amicus is a trademark and a registered trademark of Fenwal, Inc. All rights reserved. No reproduction or other use permitted without express consent of Fenwal, Inc. Reproduced with permission from Fenwal, Inc, Lake Zurich, Illinois.*

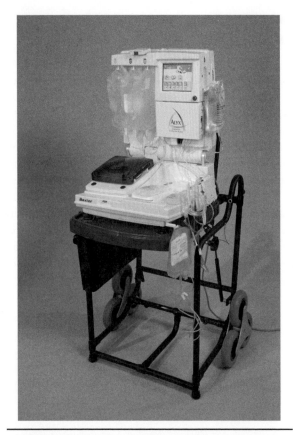

FIGURE 10-6 Alyx hemapheresis equipment. *Alyx is a trademark and a registered trademark of Fenwal, Inc. All rights reserved. No reproduction or other use permitted without express consent of Fenwal, Inc. Reproduced with permission from Fenwal, Inc, Lake Zurich, Illinois.*

This process is performed in a closed system. Multiple "passes" may be required to achieve the desired volume. The process may take from ½ TK to two hours.

Continuous flow or intermittent systems are available. In an intermittent system, a single needle is placed in one arm. The donation and reinfusion take place through this single needle. The advantage is that the donor has one venipuncture and that only one arm is incapacitated during the donation. The disadvantage is that the entire donation takes longer. Continuous flow requires a venipuncture in each arm. The donation occurs from one arm and the returned components are reinfused through the other arm. This process takes less time, but two venipunctures are required and both arms are incapacitated during the procedure.

The same standards for whole blood collection apply to pheresis donations with some exceptions:

- Two-unit red cell apheresis donors are deferred for 16 weeks following a two-unit red cell apheresis collection.

- Plateletpheresis donors must have at least 48 hours between donations.

- Plateletpheresis donors may donate a maximum of two times in a seven-day period; not to exceed 24 times in a year.

- Plateletpheresis donors who donate more frequently than every four weeks shall have a platelet count of ≥150,000 before subsequent platelet donations.

- Plasmapheresis donors who donate more frequently than every eight weeks shall have tests every four months for total plasma or serum protein determination, and a plasma or serum protein electrophoresis or quantitative immuno-diffusion test or an equivalent test to determine immunoglobulin composition of the plasma or serum (CFR 640.65).

SUMMARY

- Donor selection and screening is a vital component of health care. The provision of a safe blood supply for patients who require transfusion of red cells or other components saves thousands of lives every day. The process of donor registration, screening, and physical examination are steps to insure that collected units are as safe as possible. The protection of the donor is a major consideration. Education and informed consent of the donor continue to provide a comfortable environment for the donor and a safe blood supply for the recipients. Screening for infectious diseases, travel to areas endemic for TTDs, and high-risk behavior are important steps to insure that all areas of potential hazards are ruled out to the best of the blood banks ability.

■ The donor is positively identified and the blood collection process is carried out by a set of carefully appointed steps. Arm preparation should be performed with a two-step procedure ascertaining that bacteria are removed to prevent contamination of the unit collected. Following donation, the donor is rehydrated and observed for untoward reactions. Post donation instructions are provided.

■ Special donations include autologous donations, directed donations, therapeutic phlebotomy, and apheresis. These special donations add additional measures of safety to the blood supply, provide a measure of comfort for patients wishing to choose their own blood donors, and optimize the supply of components by fractionating whole blood. The FDA and AABB govern all donation processes.

REVIEW QUESTIONS

1. Donors for whole blood are being recruited from a local high school. Parental approval may be needed if the student:
   a. weighs 120 lb
   b. has previously experience syncope
   c. is 17 years old
   d. was immunized to rubella at age 15

2. A donor presented with the following vital signs:
   Blood pressure: 150/102
   Temperature: 37.7°C
   Pulse: 77 beats/minute
   The donor's donation status is:
   a. acceptable for donation
   b. unacceptable for donation due to blood pressure and temperature
   c. unacceptable for donation due to blood pressure and pulse
   d. unacceptable for donation due to temperature and pulse

3. A college student is donating at a blood drive on campus. The student is scheduled to study abroad in Argentina in one month. He received the following immunizations eight weeks previously:
   Yellow fever
   Hepatitis A (for prevention)
   Hepatitis B (for prevention)
   Typhoid (oral)
   The donor's donation status is:
   a. acceptable for donation
   b. unacceptable for donation due to yellow fever and typhoid
   c. unacceptable for donation due to hepatitis A and B

   d. unacceptable for donation due to hepatitis A, yellow fever, and typhoid

4. A donor is evaluated for possible exposure to CJD. A deferral could be based on which of the following characteristics:
   1. dura matter transplant
   2. lived in Europe for two years in her teens
   3. human pituitary growth hormone administration
   4. stationed on a military base in Germany 3/84 through 5/85
   5. spent eight weeks in England May and June 1999
   a. patient acceptable for donation
   b. deferred based on 1, 3, and 4
   c. deferred based on 1, 2, and 5
   d. deferred based on only 2 and 4
   e. deferred based on only 1 and 3

5. Minimum donor physical examination requirements were established to allow the collection of _____ ml of blood including samples for testing.
   a. 450 ± 45
   b. 500 ± 25
   c. 525 ml maximum
   d. 550 ml maximum

6. A donor begins to experience dizziness before the donation is complete. The phlebotomist should:
   a. continue with the donation unless the donor loses consciousness
   b. call a colleague for assistance
   c. discontinue donation
   d. finish collecting the unit regardless of the donor's condition

7. Intraoperative salvage was used to collect a unit of blood for reinfusion of a surgical patient. The unit was not reinfused during the surgery. This unit may be:
   a. used for the recipient within 24 hours when stored at 1 to 6°C
   b. used for the recipient for up to 56 days from the time of collection
   c. discarded since it was not reinfused
   d. converted to an allogeneic unit when stored at 1 to 6°C

8. Pheresis is performed to collect a specific component. The component that cannot be collected with pheresis is:
   a. granulocytes
   b. erythrocytes
   c. plasma
   d. cryoprecipitate

9. A unit of blood is collected. Upon inspection, the unit has dark purple areas. The unit should be:
   a. transfused to a recipient
   b. discarded
   c. returned to storage until quarantine period is over
   d. converted to washed red cells

10. A blood drive at a local university takes place after a mass immunization program for meningococcal vaccine. How will this affect the donor pool?
    a. no impact
    b. acceptable two weeks after immunization
    c. acceptable four weeks after immunization
    d. all recipients deferred permanently

11–20. For each of the following situations, choose:
    a. accept donor
    b. temporary deferral
    c. indefinite deferral

11. A donor documented using a needle to administer a medication for relief of migraine headaches. Her physician prescribed the medication.
_____

12. A 25-year-old female experienced a miscarriage three weeks previously.
_____

13. The principal of the local high school calls to schedule an appointment to donate. She had traveled to Africa nine months before. Antimalarial medication was taken during the trip and for one month after her return.
_____

14. A 16-year-old athlete with a pulse of 45 beats per minute.
_____

15. A 30-year-old male with a hematocrit of 49% who admits to intravenous drug us in his teenage years.
_____

16. A 75-year-old retiree with a screening and physical exam all within normal limits. He is taking no medication.
_____

17. A platelet pheresis donor who consumed aspirin one week ago for a toothache.
_____

18. A health care worker who had a needlestick and hepatitis prophylaxis seven months before.
_____

19. A new mother who gave birth 45 days ago.
_____

20. A 35-year-old male who was released from prison one month ago.
_____

CASE STUDY

1. A 25-year-old male donor's health questionnaire has the following responses:

   Vital Signs:
   Blood Pressure: 125/75
   Pulse: 78 beats/minute
   Temperature: 36.9°C
   Weight: 150 lb
   Hemoglobin: 15.8 g/dl; Hematocrit .48 L/L

   Potential significant findings in the medical history include:
   a. Received a blood transfusion nine months previously after an automobile accident.
   b. Immunized against rabies three months previously when beginning a new job at a veterinarian's office. This immunization was required for prevention in the event of accidental exposure.
   c. Received a tetanus shot following an injury with a rusty nail.
      - Can this individual donate a unit of blood at this time?
      - If not, on what criteria is the deferral based?
      - If the donor is deferred, in what time frame can he be eligible for the donor pool.

2. A donor experiences syncope while donating a unit of whole blood. How should the blood bank personnel treat the donor's condition? Is the donor eligible for future donations? Why or why not?

3. A donor comes to the blood bank to donate a unit of blood to be reinfused during a hip replacement in two weeks. This donor has a hemoglobin value of 12.0 g/dl.
   - May this donor provide this unit of blood for her upcoming surgery? Why or why not?
   - May this unit be converted to an allogeneic unit if the donor does not require a transfusion? Why or why not?
   - If she were planning to provide a directed donation for a relative, would she be acceptable as a donor? Why or why not?

4. A student anticipating study abroad has received vaccinations 30 days, previously. The vaccines he received were:
   a. Varicella
   b. Typhoid (oral)
   c. Hepatitis A and B
   d. Polio (oral)

   Discuss whether the student may donate at this time. If the donor is deferred, state which vaccine(s) caused this deferral and in what time frame he will again be eligible as a donor.

5. A donor center has recruited donors for a blood mobile visit to a local church. Fifty donors have arrived as the blood drive begins. The phlebotomist begins to process a donor who informs her that previous tests reflected a positive test for hepatitis B. The donor is a B negative. There is a shortage of B negative. The donor insists that

(continues)

CASE STUDY (CONTINUED)

her blood was accepted on her last visit and that she wants to donate. The technician collects the unit of blood and labels it.

1. What errors did the phlebotomist make with the donor?
2. Will the blood from this donor be used for transfusion? Why or why not?
3. What information will determine the future donation status of this donor? How will the donor know about his/her future donation status?

6. An O negative donor who donates on a regular schedule does NOT donate for a period of six months. Upon returning, the donor reports having had a viral illness with fatigue, low grade fevers, swollen lymph nodes and general malaise that lasted approximately three weeks. The illness occurred four months previous and the donor has been asymptomatic for three months. The donor was accepted and her blood collected without incident. Upon testing, the donor's plasma was positive for CMV antibodies. All other testing was concurrent with previous donations. She was previously a CMV-negative donor. Her blood was previously used for newborn transfusion.

1. May this donor unit be used for transfusion?
2. What additional information related to this donor's blood is significant? Why?

7. A donor presents with the following statistics:

Hemoglobin:	13.0 g/dl
Weight:	111 lb
Blood Pressure:	150/92
Pulse:	87 beats/minute
Immunization:	Hepatitis B Vaccination booster 1 year before

1. Is this donor acceptable for donation today?
2. Is there a remedial step that may be taken today?

REFERENCES

Alaishuski, Lindsay A. MD, Grim, Rodney D., Domen, Ronald E, MD. "The Informed Consent Process in Whole Blood Donation." *Archives of Pathologic Laboratory Medicine*. Vol. 132, June 2008, pp. 947–951.

Alyx Component Collection System, Operator's Manual: Revision 1.1. Baxter Healthcare, Deerfield, IL.

Blaney, Kathy and Howard, Paula. *Basic and Applied Concepts of Immunohematology*. Mosby, Philadelphia, 2000.

Blood Donor Eligibility Guide. Available from the American Red Cross, New York-Penn Region. May 2008.

Brecher, Mark, editor. *American Association of Blood Banks Technical Manual 15th Edition*. AABB, 2005.

Circular of Information: For the use of Human Blood and Blood Components. Available at www.aabb.org

"Donor History Questionnaire User Brochure." February 2007. Available at www.aabb.org

"Full-Length Donor History Questionnaire." Feb 2007. Available at www.aabb.org

"Guidance for Industry: Recommendations for Collecting Red Blood Cells by Automated Apheresis Methods Technical Correction February 2001." FDA, Available at www.fda.gov

Katz, Louis M., Cumming, Paul D., Wallace, Edward L. "Computer-Based Donor Screening: A Status Report."

Transfusion Medicine Reviews. Vol. 21, No. 1, 2007, pp. 13–25.

McCullough, Jeffrey. *Transfusion Medicine 2nd edition.* Elsevier. 2005.

Standards for Blood Banks and Transfusion Services, 25th Edition. AABB, Bethesda, MD. 2008.

Processing Blood Components

Contributions by: Kevin E. Whitlock, MT (ASCP)

LEARNING OUTCOMES

At the completion of this chapter, the reader should be able to:

- List and discuss components available for transfusion.
- Discuss the benefits of component separation.
- List the steps of collection and preparation of all blood components available in the blood bank.
- Discuss the clinical use of each blood component.
- Discuss the storage times and temperature ranges for each component.
- Outline the roles of the FDA and AABB in the regulation of blood components.
- Discuss labeling requirements for each blood component.
- Define and outline the components of ISBT 128.
- Discuss blood substitutes.
- Outline alarm and storage requirements for blood components.
- Discuss bacteria and viruses included in donor blood screening tests.
- List and describe test methods for detection of viral and bacterial agents in donor blood.
- Discuss anticipated future test methods that may be added to donor screening.

GLOSSARY

AIDS   complex of symptoms and diseases that result from damage to the immune system of the host; caused by the Human Immunodeficiency Virus (HIV)

anticoagulant-preservative solution   chemical solution that serves to prevent clotting of whole blood and provide metabolic support during storage

closed system   blood collection system that allows for fractionation of the unit without breaking the seal and exposing the blood products to the environment

components   fractions of a unit of whole blood that are used for transfusion

concatenation   reading of two bar codes as a single message

corrected count increment   anticipated increase in platelet count adjusted for the number of platelets infused and the size on the patient

cryoprecipitate   concentrated coagulation factor VIII and fibrinogen extracted from fresh frozen plasma

deglycerolized red cells   cells that have been frozen in glycerol, thawed, and washed

differential centrifugation   centrifuging at varying speeds to separate a unit of whole blood into individual parts or components; the principle of this separation is by the different specific gravities of the components

fraction   dividing a whole into parts or fractions

fresh frozen plasma   fluid portion of one unit of blood that has been centrifuged, separated, and frozen solid at $-18°C$ (or colder) within six hours of collection

frozen thawed red cells (deglycerolized cells)   a red cell product that has been frozen in glycerol, thawed, and washed prior to transfusion; a leuko-reduced component that is also used for transfusion to individuals with IgA deficiency

hepatitis   inflammation of the liver, frequently due to bacterial or viral infections

ISBT 128   a system of labeling blood components that provides an international standard

labile   not stable; will disintegrate upon storage or standing

leukocyte concentrate   white blood cells collected by pheresis from a single donor

leukocyte reduced red cells   red cell products prepared by one of several methods to create a product that has a decreased amount of white blood cells

open system   blood collection system that does not allow for fractionation of the unit without breaking the seal and exposing the blood products to the environment; red cells remaining, after plasma and platelets are removed, carry an expiration time of 24 hours

packed red cells   red cell concentrate prepared from a single unit of whole blood by removing plasma

parasite   eukaryotic organism that infects a host to its benefit, while harming the host

parenterally   route of entry of a substance into the body other than by the digestive tract; e.g. by injection

platelet concentrate   platelets removed from whole blood and stored for transfusion

platelet-rich plasma (PRP)   plasma prepared from whole blood with a "light spin; the platelets remain in the plasma after the centrifugation step; the plasma is removed to a satellite bag

preservative   chemical substance that provides metabolites to prevent deterioration of the cells

prion   presumptive infectious agent composed entirely of protein

recovered plasma   plasma that does not qualify as fresh frozen plasma

refractory   resistant to ordinary treatment

single donor plasma   plasma extracted from red cells after the time frame allowable for fresh frozen plasma or plasma with the cryoprecipitate removed; used for volume replacement

subclinical   an infection that produces no overt symptoms or only mild non-specific symptoms

virus   an infectious agent, consisting of nucleic acid, either DNA or RNA, and a protein based protective covering called a capsid

whole blood   blood that contains all components

INTRODUCTION

Whole blood, as it is collected, provides a single use product that will benefit a single patient. Whole blood may be divided into parts or components. The use of components maximizes the appropriate utilization of blood which is a limited, yet valuable resource. Fractionation of whole blood into components permits a patient to receive the most effective therapy with a product that is safer than whole blood. Division of whole blood into components provides maximum benefit to multiple recipients, as opposed to a single patient. As discussed in Chapter 10, individual components may also be collected by pheresis. Advantages of pheresis include increase in supply of available components and more frequent donation of some blood products obtained by pheresis.

The FDA regulates the collection and fractionation of whole blood. Blood banks and transfusion services that collect whole blood and prepare components must follow Good Manufacturing Practices (GMP) and strictly adhere to the FDA guidelines. Initial collection procedures, preparation of components, labeling, storage, and distribution of all components are vital processes in the blood bank. GMP was outlined in Chapter 3, while donor blood collection and pheresis procedures were discussed in Chapter 10. Components of whole blood, methods of preparation, labeling, storage, and appropriate utilization of each component will be discussed in this chapter.

BLOOD COLLECTION BAGS

Blood collection bags are commercially available in various configurations. These blood containers "shall be uncolored and transparent to permit visual inspection of the contents and any closure shall be such as will maintain a hermetic seal and prevent contamination of the contents." The container material "shall not interact with the contents under the customary conditions of storage and use."

All collection bags have a sterile interior, including the needle and all attached tubing, and contain an anticoagulant-preservative solution. Anticoagulant-preservative solution varies by manufacturer. The ideal collection system consists of a closed system. The closed system is constructed of a primary bag and one or more satellite bags. The interconnected bags allow for transfer of components from the original bag without exposing the blood product to air. This maintains sterility of the components and allows the red cells to retain the expiration date of the whole blood. An open system, as it implies, opens the airtight system of the original collection container during component preparation. This process exposes the components to an increased risk of contamination and changes the expiration date of the components. Examples of blood collection bags are featured in Figures 11-1, 11-2, and 11-3.

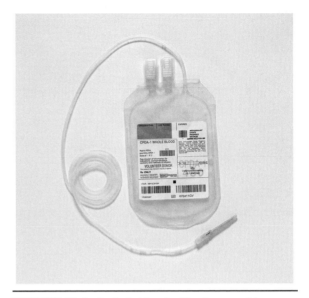

FIGURE 11-1 A whole blood collection set with integral tubing and needle. *Reprinted with permission from Terumo Medical Corporation, Somerset, NJ.*

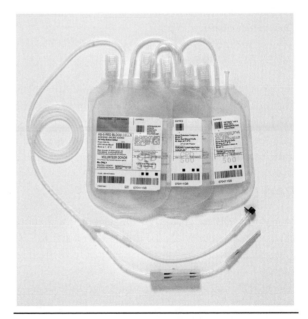

FIGURE 11-2 A whole blood three-bag collection set. The third bag contains the additive solution. *Reprinted with permission from Terumo Medical Corporation, Somerset, NJ.*

The choice of bag configuration is facility specific. The configuration of the bags is determined by the final disposition of the fractionated unit. The conditions of storage (temperature and time) are dictated by the

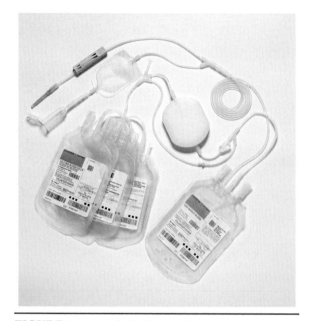

FIGURE 11-3 A whole blood collection set with three satellite bags and an in-line leukocyte reduction filter. *Reprinted with permission from Terumo Medical Corporation, Somerset, NJ.*

components prepared from the original unit. Anticipated fractionation of platelets will require room temperature storage until the platelets are removed. If platelets are not to be removed from the unit, it may be stored at 1 to 6°C until fractionated.

Red Cell Storage

Stored red cells are affected by the ongoing biochemical changes that occur while the unit is stored at 1 to 6°C. These changes are the "storage lesion" of red cells. This storage lesion contributes to reduction in the viability of the cells. During storage, there is a progressive decrease in levels of 2,3 diphosphoglycerate (2,3 DPG), adenosine triphosphate (ATP), glucose, and pH. This decrease in the level of 2,3 DPG impacts the ability of red cells to release oxygen to the tissues. As the red cells are stored in an anticoagulant, with or without additives, the 2,3 DPG levels decrease, in a linear fashion, to zero by approximately two weeks. The oxygen release of these stored cells is much less than fresh cells. The levels of ATP and 2,3 DPG are regenerated in the recipient. This regenerative process requires approximately 12 hours.

While in storage, potassium leaves the cells and sodium enters the cells. The effects of the storage lesions are negligible in most recipients. Neonates are an exception. To avoid post-transfusion complications, neonates must receive fresh cells. Fresh cells are usually designated as less than seven days old. Storage lesions are summarized in Figure 11-4.

Red cells being stored prior to transfusion must meet several criteria. These criteria include:

- Sterility
- Viability during storage
- *In vivo* survival after storage: greater than 75% 24 hours post-transfusion
- Hemolysis of ≤1%

Anticoagulant-preservative solutions are formulated to support these criteria.

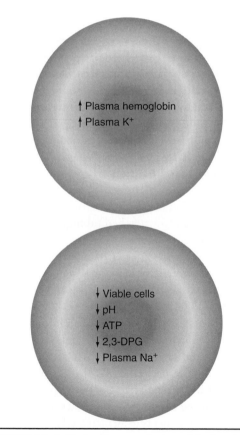

↑ Plasma hemoglobin
↑ Plasma K$^+$

↓ Viable cells
↓ pH
↓ ATP
↓ 2,3-DPG
↓ Plasma Na$^+$

FIGURE 11-4 Red cell storage lesion = biochemical changes in stored red blood cells.
Source: Delmar, Cengage Learning

Anticoagulant-Preservative Solutions

Anticoagulant-preservative solutions have two functions. The anticoagulant prevents clotting. The preservative function supports and extends the life of the cells, buffers the contents of the bag, and acts as a preservative or source of nutrients for the red cells. These functions are imperative for maintaining the integrity of the cells during storage. The volume of solution in the bag varies form 63 or 70 ml. The volume of anticoagulant-preservative solution ordains the amount of blood collected in the bag.

- A bag with 63 ml of anticoagulant will support the collection of 450 ± 45 ml of blood.

- A bag with 70 ml of anticoagulant will support the collection of 500 ± 50 ml of blood.

As discussed in Chapter 10, a donor weighing less than 110 lb may donate blood with a reduced volume of anticoagulant. Box 11-1 explains the adjustment of anticoagulant volume.

Specific anticoagulants included in blood collection bags include: citrate-phosphate-dextrose (CPD), citrate-phosphate-dextrose-adenine (CPDA-1), and citrate-phosphate-2-dextrose (CP2D). CPD and CP2D

Box 11-1

$$\frac{\text{Weight of the donor}}{110\text{ lb}} = \text{A (Factor used to reduce anticoagulant volume)}$$

$A \times 70$ ml = B (Amount of anticoagulant)
$70 - B$ = Amount of anticoagulant to remove
$A \times 500$ ml = Amount of blood that should be withdrawn

Example: A 90-lb donor wishes to donate blood

$$A = \frac{90}{110} = .82$$

$0.82 \times 70 = 57$ = Amount of anticoagulant to be used
$70 - 57 = 13$ ml of anticoagulant to be removed from bag
$0.82 \times 500 = 410$ ml amount of blood to be drawn

CRITICAL THINKING ACTIVITY

Perform the calculations for the following; A female donor weighs 100 lb. She has a rare blood type and is an antigenic match for a sickle cell patient requiring a transfusion. She may donate _____ ml of blood in _____ ml of anticoagulant.

are approved for storage for 21 days at 1 to 6°C. CPDA-1 is approved for storage for 35 days 1 to 6°C.

Additive Solutions

Additive solutions (AS-1, AS-3, and AS-5) may be used in combination with the anticoagulant/preservative solution. Additives extend the shelf-life of the units of blood. Additive solutions provide nutrients to stabilize the red cell membrane, maintain the level of 2,3 DPG, and increase the storage time for the unit of red blood cells. The solution is a mixture of glucose, adenine, and normal saline. AS-1 and AS-5 also contain mannitol as a stabilizing agent, while AS-3 uses citrate and phosphate to support red cell stability. These additives extend the shelf life of the unit to 42 days.

The additives are an integral part of the blood bag system, as demonstrated in Figure 11-5. Figure 11-5 represents a three-bag system with the additive contained in one of the satellite bags. This additive is added to the red cells after the plasma has been removed. See Figure 11-6 for a diagrammatic example of whole blood fractionation and addition of AS-1 to a unit of packed cells.

COMPONENTS OF WHOLE BLOOD

Each whole blood unit collected may be transfused without modification, or split into components that may be transfused to different recipients as the need arises. Whole blood is very rarely transfused as a single, entire unit. Dividing a unit of whole blood into components is a common practice that optimizes the use of this valuable resource. With very few exceptions, all blood is fractionated. Blood lost by bleeding can be replaced with red cells and crystalloid or colloid solutions. Components available for transfusion and some of their common uses are summarized in Table 11-1.

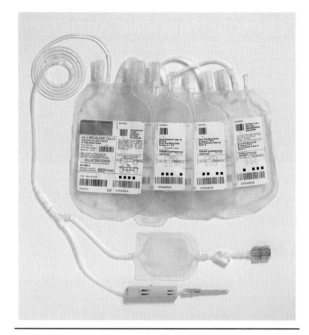

FIGURE 11-5 A whole blood collection set with additive solution in the fourth bag (far right in the photo). *Reprinted with permission from Terumo Medical Corporation, Somerset, NJ.*

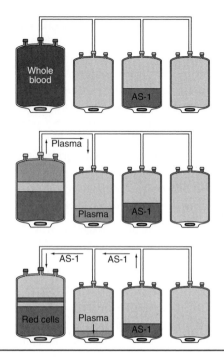

FIGURE 11-6 Component preparation with the addition of AS-1 to the packed cells. AS-1 extends the shelf life of packed cells to 42 days.
Source: Delmar, Cengage Learning

TABLE 11-1 Components Available for Transfusion

Component	Potential recipients
Whole blood	Hemorrhage
Packed red cells	Hemorrhage
	Anemia
	Surgical blood loss
Leukocyte reduced red cells	Anemia
Anemia with sensitivity to white cells	
Washed red cells	Anemia with sensitivity to white cells and/or plasma components
Deglycerolized red cells	Anemia with severe sensitivity to white cells and/or plasma components
	Transfusion to individuals with rare blood types or atypical antibodies
	Autologous storage
Fresh frozen plasma	Coagulation deficiencies
	Combined with massive red cell transfusion
	Disseminated intravascular coagulation
Stored plasma	Fluid replacement
Cryoprecipitate	Hemophiliacs
Factor VIII and fibrinogen deficiency	Disseminated intravascular coagulation
Platelet concentrate	Thrombocytopenia
	Consumption coagulopathy
Leukocyte concentrate	Severe leukopenia

Component Preparation

The preparation of components from a single unit of whole blood may be accomplished using various formats. Figure 11-7 summarizes the division of a unit to provide multiple components. Storage times and temperatures for components are summarized in Table 11-2.

Component preparation begins with centrifugation of the whole blood unit. This centrifugation provides primary separation of red cells and plasma. The centrifuge should be calibrated to provide an optimum cellular concentration. Calibration establishes optimum spin time and speed for preparation of each component. The revolutions per minute (rpm) should also be checked periodically. The *AABB Technical Manual* may be referenced for a centrifuge calibration procedure. The blood bank should institute quality control for the preparation of each component. This ensures that preparation methods are providing a maximum yield for each component.

Following primary separation, the red cells are on the bottom of the bag and the plasma and platelets are in the top of the bag. The separation of cellular components is contingent on their specific gravities. **Differential centrifugation** accomplishes this separation. The steps for differential centrifugation are summarized in Box 11-2.

Whole Blood

Whole blood is defined as the "blood collected from human donors for transfusion to human recipients." It is the component collected from a donor. As outlined in Table 11-2, storage times for whole blood are contingent on the anticoagulant-preservative solution used for collection. Additive solutions are not used for whole blood. Whole blood is fractionated into components as described in the previous section. Storage of whole blood results in decreased viability of platelets and **labile** coagulation factors. Whole blood has limited use in the treatment of clinical conditions.

Indications for Whole Blood Use.
Historically, whole blood was indicated for hemorrhaging patients with considerable blood loss, greater than 25% of the blood volume. This practice has become obsolete and replacement of blood volume is typically accomplished with red cells and crystalloids. If replacement of coagulation factors is necessary, fresh frozen plasma (FFP) provides a complete replacement of viable coagulation factors.

Red Blood Cells

Red blood cells are the component of choice for hemoglobin replacement. Hemoglobin provides oxygen to the tissues of the body. Loss of hemoglobin occurs as a result of acute or chronic blood loss, impaired production of red cells, or increased red cell destruction by physiological or mechanical means. Red blood cells are transfused to provide oxygen carrying capacity to the body.

When the hemoglobin decreases to a level that requires transfusion support, red cell transfusions are initiated. Transfusions of other appropriate components may occur concurrently. Additional components will replace coagulation factors to prevent additional bleeding or exacerbation of other clinical conditions. These components may include FFP and/or platelets. Conditions that may require transfusion of red cells include:

- Acute or chronic anemia
- Trauma
- Surgery
- Carcinoma, lymphoma, leukemia
- Thalassemia
- Sickle cell anemia
- Renal disease
- Hemolytic Disease of the Fetus and Newborn (HDFN)

The transfusion of a single unit of red cells will increase the hemoglobin approximately 1 gram. This varies by weight of the recipient, but can be used to gauge transfusion volume. Red cells may be modified for transfusion. Modifications of red cell blood cells for transfusion are summarized in the following sections.

Leukocyte-Reduced Red Blood Cells

Leukoreduction removes "99% of the allogeneic WBCs from donor blood before transfusion." **Leukocyte-reduced red cells** have several advantages:

- Reduction of the risk of non-hemolytic febrile transfusion reactions.
- Reduction of alloimmunization to HLA-A and HLA-B antigens thereby reducing the incidence

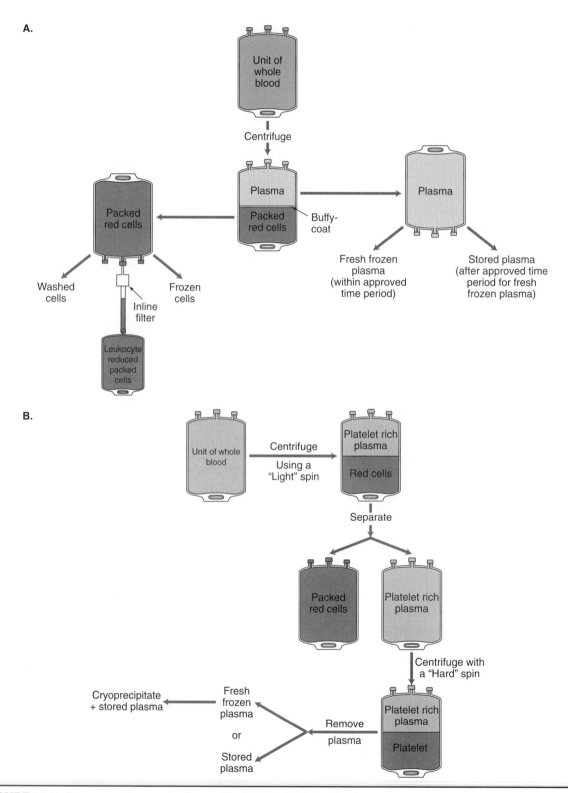

FIGURE 11-7 Component Preparation from a Single Unit of Whole Blood

A. Simple Centrifugation and Separation into Plasma and Packed Cells; Possible conversion Options for the Plasma and Packed Cells.

B. Centrifugation with a Light Spin and Conversion to Packed Cells, Plasma, and Platelet Concentrate.

Source: Delmar, Cengage Learning

Box 11-2

Whole blood is centrifuged with a "light spin." This separates the unit into red blood cells and **PRP**. The platelets are suspended in the plasma as opposed to falling into the bottom of the bag with the red blood cells. The plasma is expressed into an attached satellite bag. Expression may be accomplished with a plasma expresser that applies pressure and pushes the plasma out of the top of the bag (see Figure 11-8).

- If an additive system is used, it is added to the red cells following removal of the plasma. The red cell bag is disconnected from the collection set. A tube welder is used to maintain a closed system (see Figure 11-9). The red cell unit may be filtered to produce leukocyte-reduced cells or stored as packed red blood cells. The storage for leukocyte-reduced and packed red blood cells is 1 to 6°C. A leuko-reduction filter is seen in Figure 11-10.

- The PRP is centrifuged using a "heavy spin." The platelet concentrates will sediment to the bottom of the bag. Plasma is expressed into a satellite bag. The platelet concentrate is suspended in 50 to 70 ml of plasma. The platelet bag is sealed. The platelets are permitted to "rest" or remain unagitated for at least an hour. The platelets are placed on a rotator for gentle mixing. The storage time for platelets is 20 to 24°C for five days.

- The expressed plasma has two possible dispositions.

- Frozen as Fresh Frozen Plasma (FFP). The FFP must be frozen within the time frame designated by the anticoagulant and stored at ≤−18°C for up to one year or <−65°C for up to seven years.

- Fresh frozen plasma may be transformed into **cryoprecipitate** (CRYO). If CRYO is to be produced from FFP, the FFP is frozen with an attached satellite bag. The FFP is thawed at 1 to 6°C. A white precipitate of CRYO is present in the thawed plasma. The CRYO concentrates are in the bottom of the bag. The plasma is centrifuged with a heavy spin and removed into a satellite bag. This remaining plasma is used as **recovered plasma**. A company that manufacturers products from plasma, such as albumin, may use recovered plasma in the manufacturing process. CRYO is frozen at ≤−18°C for up to one year.

- Plasma that has been expressed more than eight hours post-collection no longer qualifies as fresh frozen plasma. It is labeled recovered plasma.

---

of platelet transfusion refractoriness, transfusion-associated acute lung injury (TRALI) and organ allograft rejection.

- Decrease in transmission of WBC-associated viruses, such as cytomegalovirus.

- Decrease in occurrence of transfusion associated graft-versus-host disease.

- Possible reduction in post-operative infection.

Transfusion reactions are discussed in detail in Chapter 12. While it is not necessary to leukocyte-reduce all units of red blood cells, the benefits of transfusion of leukocyte-reduced cells far outweigh the modest cost factor of 10 to 15%. These factors have resulted in some blood banks establishing leukocyte reduction as standard protocol. Filtration is an efficient method for removal of leukocytes. The AABB requires that leukocyte reduced red cell units have $<5 \times 10^6$ white blood cells per unit. Ideally, leukocyte reduction should take place before red blood cell storage. The methods for achieving this are:

- Using a system with an in-line filter. These systems allow for the red cell unit to be leuko-reduced before storage. See Figure 11-11 for an example of a system with a filter that is integral to the collection system.

- A leukocyte-reduction filter that is not integral, but may be attached with a sterile welding device. Once the weld has been made, the filtration may take place while a closed system is maintained.

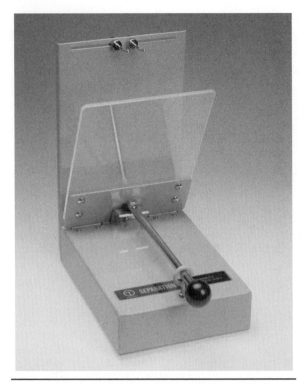

FIGURE 11-8 Plasma Expressor for removal of plasma from a unit of whole blood. *Reprinted with permission from Terumo Medical Corporation, Somerset, NJ.*

■ A filter that is used when the unit is transfused. This method creates an open system that changes the expiration date to 24 hours.

Washed Red Blood Cells

Washing a unit of red blood cells with normal saline reduces the concentration of plasma proteins in that unit. Washed red blood cells have varied uses in transfusion medicine. They may be indicated for patients with a history of febrile, allergic, or anaphylactic transfusion reactions. See Chapter 12 for a discussion of transfusion reactions. Washed red cells may also be used for intrauterine transfusions. See Chapter 13 for a discussion of intrauterine transfusions. The process of washing is performed with an automated blood processor. The cells are washed with a liter of 0.9% saline. The unit of washed cells carries an expiration date of 24 hours.

Frozen Red Blood Cells

Freezing red cells provides a method for long-term preservation and storage of the red cells. This process may be used to preserve rare units as well as extend the storage time for autologous blood. The process of freezing the red blood cells creates leukocyte-reduced units.

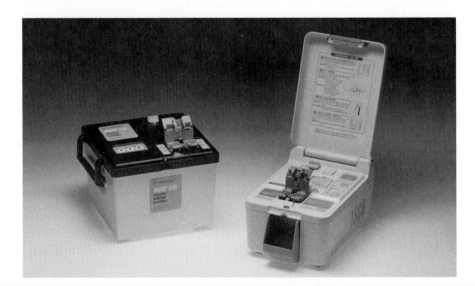

FIGURE 11-9 Tube welder used to fuse tubing and maintain a closed system when either fractionating a unit or producing a leuko-reduced unit. The sterile tube welder works on the principle of heating a copper wafer to approximately 320°C. The tubing to be welded is cut by the heated wafer and the two stubs are quickly attached to each other. The weld is completed when cool. The high temperature also serves to kill microorganisms. *Reprinted with permission from Terumo Medical Corporation, Somerset, NJ.*

Freezing red cells requires the addition of a cryopreservative to the cells. The cryopreservative prevents dehydration and the formation of ice crystals that will cause red cell lysis. Gycerol is a commonly used cryopreservative for red cells. An automated processing system slowly adds glycerol until the concentration is 40% weight per volume. The red cell/glycerol mixture is transferred to a polyvinyl chloride or polyolefin bag. The units are stored at −65°C for up to ten years. A metal canister is used to prevent breakage of the bags at low temperatures.

Deglycerolized Red Cells

Deglycerolized red cells are a product created when the frozen cells are thawed and the glycerol removed. The frozen unit is thawed at 37°C. An automated red blood cell processor is used to process the thawed cells. Multiple washes with saline solutions of decreasing osmolity are used. This process draws the glycerol out of the cells and the cells are resuspended in the saline concentration used in the final wash. The saline concentrations used are 12%, 1.6%, and 0.9%. This is an open system and the unit expires 24 hours after preparation.

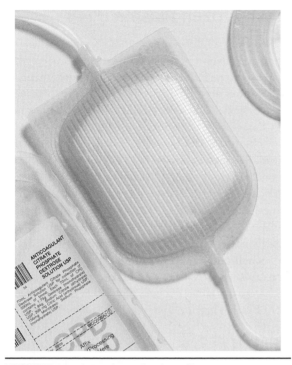

FIGURE 11-10 Leuko-reduction Filter. *Reprinted with permission from Terumo Medical Corporation, Somerset, N.J.*

TABLE 11-2 Storage Criteria for Blood Components

COMPONENT	STORAGE TEMPERATURE	STORAGE TIME LIMITS
Whole Blood	1 to 6°C	CPD, CP2D = 21 days
		CPDA-1 = 35 days
Red Blood Cells	1 to 6°C	CPD, CP2D = 21 days
		CPDA-1 = 35 days
		AS-1, AS-3, AS-5 = 42 days
Red Blood Cells, Frozen	≤−65°C	10 Years
Deglycerolized	1 to 6°C	24 Hours
Red Blood Cells, Irradiated	1 to 6°C	28 days from Irradiation *or* Original Outdate (the Shortest Outdate)
Platelet Concentrates (Single donor and pheresis)	20 to 24°C	5 Days
Pooled Platelets	20 to 24°C	4 Hours
Fresh Frozen Plasma (FFP)	≤−18°C	1 Year
	≤−65°C	7 Years
Thawed FFP	1 to 6°C	24 Hours
Cryoprecipitate	≤−18 °C	1 Year
CRYO (Pooled)	20 to 24°C	4 Hours
Granulocytes	20 to 24°C	24 Hours

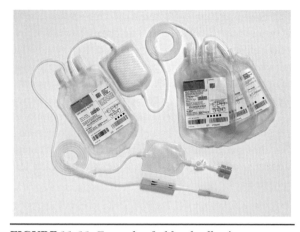

FIGURE 11-11 Example of a blood collection system with an in-line filter. *Reprinted with permission of Terumo Medical, Somerset, NJ.*

Irradiated Red Blood Cells

Gamma irradiation of red blood cells prevents the proliferation of T cells. Viable T cells that are transfused with a unit of red blood cells may cause transfusion-associated graft versus host disease (TA-GVHD). GVHD is fatal in a high percentage of cases (90%). GVHD is discussed in Chapter 12.

Irradiation of red blood cells is accomplished with a gamma irradiator. The required dose of irradiation is "a minimum of 25 Gy (2500 cGy) delivered to the central portion of the container. The minimum dose at any point in the component shall be 15 Gy (1500 cGy)." The irradiation system must be validated at inception and the dose periodically verified with the verification documented.

Irradiation for prevention of GVHD is suggested in:

- Immunoincompetent patients
- Intrauterine transfusion
- Oncology patients who are undergoing chemotherapy and irradiation
- Bone marrow recipients
- Premature newborns

Irradiated units are a closed system. The expiration date is 28 days, or the original expiration date if that is less than 28 days. The process of irradiation creates some red cell membrane damage that results in a higher potassium level and a decrease in the ATP and 2,3 DPG levels.

Fresh Frozen Plasma (FFP)

FFP contains a full complement of coagulation factors. Blood coagulation is a series of reactions or steps that terminate in the formation of a clot. The constituents of the reactions are plasma proteins, phospholipids, and calcium. Some of these factors are labile and disintegrate with storage. FFP preserves these labile factors.

The process of blood coagulation consumes the coagulation factors. It may be necessary to provide additional or supplemental coagulation factors by infusion of FFP. Congenital deficiencies of coagulation factors may also exist. FFP can replace or supplement any of the coagulation factors normally present in the plasma. Some indications for use of FFP are summarized in Table 11-3.

Single donor plasma is the second source of plasma for a transfusion. This plasma is used for fluid replacement since it is either not collected within the time frame for FFP or has had the cryoprecipitate removed.

Thawed FFP

FFP is thawed in a water bath at 30 to 37°C. This process takes 30 to 45 minutes. Waterbaths may have a mechanism for agitating the unit, and will accelerate the process of thawing. When thawed in a waterbath, the ports of the plasma bag should be protected from contact with the water to prevent bacterial contamination. The FDA has approved some microwave ovens for plasma thawing. To

---

TABLE 11-3 Indications for Use of Fresh Frozen Plasma

- Following massive transfusion where the coagulation factors have been depleted by consumption, loss through bleeding and non-replacement by transfusion of stored components.
- Management of bleeding.
- Replacement of factors II, VII, IX, X, or XI if the appropriate factors are not available.
- Patients on anticoagulation therapy who require emergency surgery or who are actively bleeding.
- Patients experiencing Disseminated Intravascular Coagulation (DIC).
- Correction of bleeding in patients with factor deficiencies.
- Exchange transfusion in conjunction with the red cells.

use microwaves for thawing, an FDA approved appliance must be used and the manufacturer's instructions followed for this specific process. Thawed FFP is stored at 1 to 6°C and expires 24 hours after thawing. ABO compatible plasma should be administered. No compatibility testing is required for thawed FFP.

Cryoprecipitated Antihemophilic Factor (CRYO)

Cryoprecipitated antihemophilic factor (CRYO) is a product prepared from plasma that is removed from red cells promptly after collection. It is a concentrate of coagulation Factors VIII, I (Fibrinogen), von Willebrand's Factor (vWF), and fibronectin. The product is prepared by removing the plasma from red cells and freezing to a slushy mixture. At that point, a "button" of concentrated material in the bottom of the plasma is cryoprecipitate. The remaining plasma is removed and the button of cryoprecipitate labeled and frozen.

Historically, CRYO was the primary treatment for hemophilia or hereditary deficiency of Factor VIII. The availability of viral inactivated Factor VIII for treatment of Factor VIII deficiency has decreased the use of cryoprecipitate for replacement therapy. Conditions treated with this viral inactivated component include: Hemophilia A, von Willebrand's disease, and Deficiency of Factor VIII:C. CRYO is still the primary treatment for Factors XIII and I deficiencies. CRYO is also used to treat congenital or acquired deficiencies of fibrinogen, including afibrinogenemia, hypofibrinogenemia, and dysfibrinogenemia.

The blood bank must perform quality control on cryoprecipitate. Each unit of CRYO must contain a minimum of 150 mg of fibrinogen and a minimum of 80 IU of coagulation factor VIII.

Dosage of factor VIII varies with weight and the desired level of replacement. Calculation of dosage if summarized in Box 11-3. Multiple units of CRYO may be administered to achieve a desired dose of the intended factor. The CRYO is thawed in a 30 to 37°C waterbath. The units may be pooled into a common bag for transfusion. The pooled CRYO must be transfused within four hours and stored at room temperature until transfusion. ABO compatible units should be chosen, when possible. If a large volume of CRYO is to be infused, ABO compatible units are indicated. Coagulation studies should be used to monitor the effectiveness of the cryoprecipitate infusion.

Box 11-3

Number of Factor VIII Units = Plasma volume × (desired level % – initial level %)
80 units/bag
e.g. Plasma volume: 40 ml/kg × body weight (kg)
Quantity of Factor VIII coagulant activity: On bottle label
Factor VIII in CRYO = 80 units/bag
Patient: 74 kg
Desired level = 60 % activity = 60 units/dl
Initial level = 4% activity = 4 units/dl
Number of Factor VIII Units = 2960 × (.60 – .04)
                            = 20.7 bags of CRYO
                            80

CRITICAL THINKING ACTIVITY

A patient requires a transfusion of cryoprecipitate. Using the following numbers, calculate the amount of CRYO that should be administered to achieve the desired effect.
   Patient: 69 kg
   Desired level = 55% activity
   Initial level = 2% activity

Platelet Concentrates

Platelet concentrate may be prepared from a single unit of whole blood, as described in the section on component preparation. These platelets are "random" donor platelets or platelet concentrates. These single donor platelets must yield a minimum of 5.5×10^{10} platelets per unit. The shelf life of stock platelets is anticoagulant dependent. The expiration date is usually five days from the date of collection. Single units may be pooled to provide a larger volume of platelet concentrate for transfusion to adult recipients. The pooling process involves combining platelets from single units in a separate transfer set using aseptic technique. This pooling process creates an open system. Pooled platelets are stored at 20 to 24°C until transfused and must be transfused within four hours.

The use of pooled platelets has decreased due to the rate of bacterial contamination of platelet concentrates. Because platelets are stored at 20 to 24°C, bacteria introduced at time of collection are more likely to multiply. The process of pooling additionally compromises the combined volume of platelets increasing the likelihood that bacteria will be introduced into the pooled environment. Pooled platelets are still administered, but platelet pheresis products are used whenever possible.

Platelets may also be collected by hemapheresis, as discussed in Chapter 10. Plateletpheresis must yield a minimum of least 3×10^{11} platelets. This is the equivalent of five to eight units of platelets prepared from whole blood. Plateletpheresis donors may donate twice per week up to a total of 24 times per year. There must be at least 48 hours between donations.

Platelets obtained by pheresis can be matched for HLA or other platelet antigens in recipients who may have antibodies to specific antigens on the platelet surface. Individuals receiving frequent platelet transfusions may develop antibodies that decrease the survival of the transfused products. These patients are said to be refractory to the transfused platelets. It is important to determine the anticipated increase in platelet count post-transfusion. This is accomplished by calculating the corrected count increment (CCI). Calculation of the corrected count increment is outlined in Box 11-4.

Leuko-reduction of platelet units may be accomplished in the pheresis process or by using a filter with prestorage or at the patient's bedside. These leuko-reduced platelets may decrease the likelihood of developing antibodies and becoming refractory to future platelet transfusions. Units of matched platelets may also be irradiated for prevention of graft vs. host disease.

Box 11-4

CCI = post-transfusion platelet count – pre-transfusion platelet count x BSA*
    Number of platelets transfused in multiples of 10^{11}
    *BSA=body surface area; calculated by using a chart for this purpose

Example: BSA= 1.6 M^2
    Pre-transfusion count = 3500/μl
    Post-transfusion count = 32,000/μl
    Platelets Transfused = 4.0 $\times$ 10^{11}
    CCI = 32,000 – 3,500 $\times$ 1.6 = 4.0
    CCI of greater than 7500 indicates adequate platelet count increment.

CRITICAL THINKING ACTIVITY

Calculate the CCI given the following data:
    BSA= 1.5 M^2
    Pre-transfusion count = 3000/μl
    Post-transfusion count = 40,000/μl
    Platelets transfused = 5.0 $\times$ 10^{11}

Granulocyte Concentrate

Granulocyte concentrate is prepared by hemapheresis. This component will contain platelets as well as some red blood cells. Granulocyte concentrates my be stored for up to 24 hours at 20 to 24°C, but deteriorate rapidly on storage. At least 75% of the units tested must contain a minimum of 1.0×10^{10} granulocytes. A crossmatch is required if greater than 2 ml of red cells present. Transfusion of granulocyte concentrate should take place through a filter that will not remove the granulocytes. The component should be irradiated since the recipients are often immunosuppressed individuals.

The use of granulocyte concentrates is rare due to potential for reactions, the use of improved antibiotics, and development of bone marrow stimulating substances such as recombinant growth factor. Indications for transfusion of granulocytes include:

■ Neutropenia: $<0.5 \times 10^9/L$

■ Infection

■ Lack of response to antibiotics

Coagulation Factors VIII and IX

The use of manufacturing processes for extraction of coagulation factors, protease inhibitors and IgG from plasma has been used to provide alternatives to blood component therapy. These processes have provided products with improved safety and purity. The use of Factors VIII and IX has increased for the treatment of Hemophilia A, von Willebrand's Disease, and Hemophilia B, consecutively. These products maybe distributed from the pharmacy or the blood bank.

Blood Substitutes

The use of blood substitutes has been controversial since their inception. Substitutes have been used with

CRITICAL THINKING ACTIVITY

A leukemia patient has been admitted to the local hospital with fatigue and a localized infection that has not been responsive to antibiotics. The hematologist on call orders a complete blood count and coagulation testing. The results reflected decreased values for the red blood cell count, white blood cell count, and platelet count. The coagulation tests reflected normal levels of coagulation factors. This patient has been previously transfused. When the records are checked, fever and chills were noted with previous red cell transfusions. The director of the blood bank had reviewed these records and indicated that the cause was probably a sensitivity to white blood cells.

1. Does this patient need transfusion therapy? If so, what components?

2. What consideration needs to be given to the sensitivity to white blood cells? Does this information alter the type of red cell component that will be chosen?

3. Is the decreased platelet count significant for transfusion therapy? Why or why not?

WEB ACTIVITIES

1. Go to www.aabb.org

2. Choose "About Blood and Cellular Therapies."

3. Choose "Circulars of Information."

4. Choose "Circular of Information for the Use of Cellular Therapy Products"

5. Review the information on the use of the blood components that were discussed in previous sections.

varying success and levels of controversy. Development and testing of substitutes continues. Examples of blood substitutes include hemoglobin-based oxygen carriers (HBOCs) and perfluorocarbons.

Advantages to blood substitutes include:

- Overcoming blood components shortages
- Extended storage times
- Room temperature storage
- No crossmatching necessary
- Decrease of risks inherent in allogeneic blood transfusions including
- Infectious disease transmission
- Transfusion reactions
- TRALI
- Delayed postoperative wound healing
- Immunomodulation

Disadvantages to blood substitutes include:

- Vasoactivity: increases in systemic and pulmonary arterial pressure and increases in systemic and pulmonary vascular resistance occur with the use of HBOCs
- Nephrotoxicity
- Interference in macrophage function
- Activation of complement, kinin, and coagulation
- Gastrointestinal distress
- Neurotoxicity

The development of a satisfactory blood substitute will enhance the appropriate use of blood components. The issues associated with blood substitutes have not changed since the inception of the idea. The disadvantages need resolution in order for these products to be acceptable in the medical community.

Storage of Components

Storage temperatures of components are summarized in Table 11-2. The FDA and AABB create and modify guidelines for storage of blood components, monitoring parameters, storage temperatures, and maintenance of equipment for storage and transportation of the blood components. As discussed in Chapter 3, all equipment must be monitored, parameters documented, and the records maintained. Written procedures must exist for all of these procedures. All procedures must be readily available for all staff members involved with this maintenance. Maintenance for component storage must include the following:

- Temperatures of refrigerators, freezers, platelet incubators, water baths, and room temperature must be monitored.

- All calibrated thermometers must be checked against reference thermometers.

- Recorders must monitor temperature every four hours.

- Audible alarms must be set to ensure an alert every 24 hours. The alarms must be set to trigger before the temperature is out of range.

- All alarms must be checked on a routine basis.

Transportation of Components

Blood components must be transported between institutions for optimum use of available resources. Guidelines for transportation are outlined by the AABB. The CFR sets guidelines for transportation. These guidelines state: "whole blood must be placed in storage at a temperature between 1 and 6°C immediately after collection unless the blood is to be further processed into another component or the blood must be transported from the donor center to the processing laboratory. If transported, the blood must be placed in temporary storage having sufficient refrigeration capacity to cool the blood continuously toward a temperature between 1 and 10°C until arrival at the processing laboratory. At the processing laboratory, the blood must be stored at a temperature between 1 and 6°C. Blood from which a component is to be prepared must be held in an environment maintained at a temperature range specified for that component in the directions for use for the blood collecting, processing, and storage system."

Each institution must maintain records of the transportation process. When a shipment of blood or blood components is received, the temperature and outward appearance of the units are recorded as part of the quality assurance program. Any irregularities encountered in the shipment process should be recorded and the shipping facility notified. Questionable units should be quarantined until determined acceptable for transfusion.

Whole blood and red cells are transported with the following guidelines:

- Temperature 1 to 10°C

- Plastic bags with wet ice approximately equal to the volume of the component being shipped

- Enough wet ice to maintain the temperature for 24 hours

- Containers must be periodically validated for maintenance of temperature at a variety of temperature ranges

Frozen components are shipped on dry ice. Frozen components should be packed carefully, as the frozen plastic bags are fragile. All frozen components should always be handled with care. The frozen plastic bags are fragile and will crack easily. In addition, frozen components should be handled with insulated gloves to prevent cold burns.

Platelets are maintained as close to 20 to 24°C as possible. The platelets may be maintained without agitation during transportation for as long as 24 hours.

LABELING COMPONENTS

International Society of Blood Transfusion (ISBT) Recommendations (ISBT 128)

The move to an international standard labeling system has evolved over many years. The ISBT structured a set of recommendations for uniform labeling of blood products. This set of recommendations was entitled **ISBT 128**. The objectives of ISBT 128 include:

- Improving unit traceability and look-back tracking.

- Aiding in detection and prevention of errors in data entry by using data identifiers and check characters.

- Special testing results may be encoded, e.g. CMV results and RBC phenotyping.

- Computerized method to follow donor/unit information.

ISBT 128 Components

The purpose of ISBT 128 was to provide a unique identification to be applied to any donation worldwide. The label provides a series of bar coded areas. Each bar

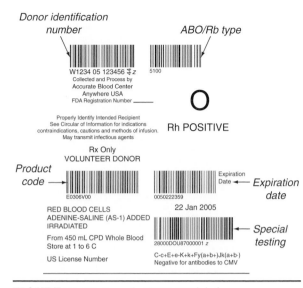

Donor identification number

ABO/Rb type

W1234 05 123456 ⅌ z   5100
Collected and Process by
Accurate Blood Center
Anywhere USA
FDA Registration Number

O

Properly Identify Intended Recipient
See Circular of Information for indications
contraindications, cautions and methods of infusion.
May transmit infectious agents

Rh POSITIVE

Rx Only
VOLUNTEER DONOR

Product code

E0306V00

Expiration Date

Expiration date

0050222359

RED BLOOD CELLS
ADENINE-SALINE (AS-1) ADDED
IRRADIATED

22 Jan 2005

From 450 mL CPD Whole Blood
Store at 1 to 6 C

US License Number

28000DOU87000001 z

Special testing

C-c+E+e-K+k+Fy(a+b+)Jk(a+b-)
Negative for antibodies to CMV

FIGURE 11-12 Sample ISBT 128 label
Source: **Delmar, Cengage Learning**

coded area provides a single piece of information (see Figure 11-12). A summary of the bar coded areas is:

1. Donor Identification Number
2. ABO/Rh Blood Groups
3. Product Code
4. Expiration Date and Time
5. Special Testing

Donor Identification Number (DIN). The

labeling system uses a 13-character identifier. The donor identification number (DIN) cannot be repeated anywhere in the world for 100 years. The DIN is composed of three elements:

■ The first part represents the country. It consists of a letter (A, B, C, etc.) followed by four numeric digits.

■ The second part is the year. For example: 06 = 2006.

■ The third part is a sequence number for the donation. This number is assigned by the collection facility. This is a six-digit character.

■ A sample is A123408812000.

ABO and Rh Barcode. The ABO/Rh barcode

allows for inventory control. It is in line with the DIN so that these two bar codes can be read together. This

process of reading two bar codes as a single message is **concatenation**.

Expiration Date and Product Code. Ex-

piration date is in line with the product code. If the product code changes, as with irradiation of the unit, the expiration date may also change. This placement allows for concatenation of these two components. This placement also allows these two components to be replaced without overlaying the ABO/Rh label. See Figures 11-12 and 11-13 for examples of ISBT labeling.

Special Testing. The lower right quadrant of the

label allows space for two bar codes. These bar codes may include information on RBC antigen typing, other special testing information, or both.

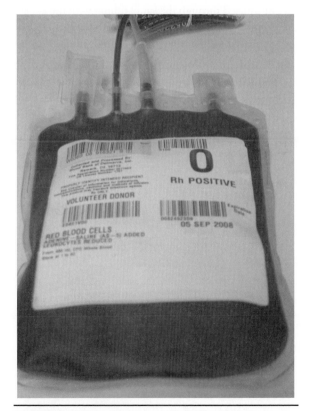

FIGURE 11-13 Example of blood bag labeling.
Reprinted with permission of the Blood Bank of Delmarva.

GUIDELINES FOR TRANSFUSION OF BLOOD COMPONENTS

A summary of guidelines for transfusion of whole blood and blood components is found in the *Circular of Information for the use of Human Blood and Blood Components.* The basic guidelines include:

1. The intended recipient and the blood container must be properly identified before the transfusion is started.

2. Sterility must be maintained.

3. All blood components must be transfused through a filter designed to remove clots and aggregates (generally a standard 170-260 micro filter). See Figure 11-14 for a sample.

4. Blood and components should be mixed thoroughly before use.

5. No medications or solutions may be routinely added or infused through the same tubing with the exception of 0.9% sodium chloride unless the FDA has approved the solution for this application.

6. Blood and components must be inspected immediately prior to administration. If the appearance is abnormal, the units should not be used for transfusion.

7. Transfusion should be completed within four hours and prior to component expiration.

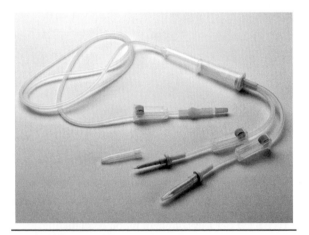

FIGURE 11-14 Example of filter used for infusion of blood products. *Reprinted with permission of Terumo Medical, Somerset, NJ.*

CRITICAL THINKING ACTIVITY

For each of the following scenarios, determine the possible components for transfusion. Explain the reason for each of the components chosen.

1. A trauma patient received eight units of leukocyte-reduced red cells. The trauma surgeon noticed some bleeding at the incision site. What component or components should be transfused to correct this post-surgical bleeding? Explain your choice.

2. A six-year-old leukemic patient has a platelet count of 6.0×10^{12}/L.

DONOR BLOOD TESTING

All donor blood and components are tested prior to issue for transfusion. The testing includes serological testing and infectious disease screening. All testing is completed and test results documented by the collection facility. Serological testing includes ABO grouping, Rh typing, weak D typing through the antiglobulin phase, if required, and antibody screening with reflex to antibody identification, if required. All donor units are labeled with the ABO and Rh type. The serological testing results should be negative, with some rare exceptions.

Infectious Disease Testing

Infectious disease screening is an important component of testing performed on a unit of blood, plasma, or platelets before release for transfusion to a recipient. Testing ensures that the components have the smallest possible risk of transmitting TTDs to the recipient. These TTDs include bacterial, **viral**, **parasitic**, and **prion** pathogens. The FDA dictates stringent testing to significantly decrease the risk of TTDs.

After collection of a donor unit, serological testing performed include tests to detect Hepatitis B and C viruses, HIV I and II, HTLV I and II, and Syphilis. In addition to these pathogens, some blood centers also screen for West Nile Virus (WNV), and Chagas Disease. Cytomegalovirus (CMV) testing is performed on select units. Additional potential TTDs may be included in donor blood screening, for example, Human Parvovirus B19.

Testing is performed using a variety of methods including nucleic acid amplification testing (NAT), polymerase chain reaction (PCR), Western blot, and recombinant immunoblot assay (RIBA). Testing methods are extremely sensitive, and most include a confirmation method that is both sensitive and specific. This combination of methods allows detection of small quantities of potential TTDs, while trying to minimize false positives, which would exclude the donor from future donations.

Hepatitis

Background

Hepatitis is a general term used to describe inflammation of the liver. Causative agents for hepatic inflammation include bacterial infections, alcohol abuse, and autoimmune processes. Transfusion-associated hepatitis is viral in origin. Hepatitis B and C viruses are detected in donor screening tests. These two viruses are transmitted parenterally. Hepatitis B and C may cause significant disease in transfusion recipients. Immunocompromised patients are particularly susceptible to the physiological effects of the hepatitis virus.

The Hepatitis B virus (HBV) is a double-stranded DNA virus, belonging to the *Hepadnaviridae* family. HBV was first discovered in 1965 in patients with hemophilia who had received multiple blood transfusions. Retrospective studies performed following the discovery provided evidence for association of the Hepatitis B surface antigen (HBsAg) discovered in 1965 and patients with post-transfusion hepatitis (PTH). Routine screening for HBsAg was initiated in 1971.

The Hepatitis C virus (HCV) is small single-stranded RNA virus, belonging to the *Flaviviridae* family. HCV was discovered after it became apparent that PTH cases were occurring that were caused by known viral agents such as HBV, Hepatitis A virus (HAV), or other known viral agents. These hepatitis infections were labeled non-A, non-B hepatitis (NANBH). In 1988, the presence of the HCV was discovered using molecular techniques. Within one year, a specific antigen detection assay was developed.

Testing

In order to prevent the transmission of HBV and HCV, five possible screening tests include: HbsAg, the antibody to Hepatitis B core (anti-HBc), alanine aminotransferase (ALT), the antibody to Hepatitis C virus (anti-HCV), and NAT testing for the presence of HCV.

The first screening test for hepatitis, to test for HBV, was the HbsAg assay introduced in 1975. HbsAg is a protein antigen produced by HBV. It is frequently the first indicator of infection and may be detected before the development of overt symptoms. HbsAg testing is performed using enzyme linked immunosorbent assay (ELISA). See Figure 11-15 for a summary of the ELISA test for Hepatitis B Surface Antigen. Confirmation of a positive HbsAg test is typically accomplished with a neutralization assay. This neutralization assay utilizes the principle that antibodies to HbsAg are incubated with the donor serum that may contain the HbsAg, an antigen-antibody complex will be formed. When this mixture is added to the test wells that are coated with antibody, the antigen will not be free to attach to this bound antibody since it has been "neutralized." Hence, less indicator substance will be detected in the final measurement. Therefore, a significant reduction in the test value, typically >50%, compared to the non-neutralized test indicates a positive result.

In an effort to eliminate transfusion-associated infections due to the transfusion of units with low, undetectable levels of HbsAg, anti-HBc and ALT testing was added. anti-HBc detects antibodies formed to the protein found in the inner portion or core of the virus. These antibodies typically begin formation prior to the development of symptoms but after the presence of detectable levels of HbsAg anti-HBc levels may persist for many years following acute infection (see Figure 11-16). These levels are, therefore, useful in eliminating potentially infectious donors who are not presenting with acute HBV infection at the time of infection. Anti-HBc is detected using enzyme immunoassay technique. This test method reacts the antibody with antigen coated on a microplate. Following incubation an indicator solution is added that is detected at wavelength 615-630 nm. The quantity of anti-HBc is directly proportional to the amount of color development detected. See Figure 11-17 for a summary of the test method. ALT testing was previously used as a screening test for liver inflammation: hence, inflammation and increased ALT levels are present in hepatitis, but limited to hepatitis. Elevated levels of ALT are also present in other diseases of the liver such as cirrhosis. As HBV testing has become more sensitive and specific, the use of ALT as a donor-screening test has been eliminated.

Hepatitis B surface antigen ELISA detection.

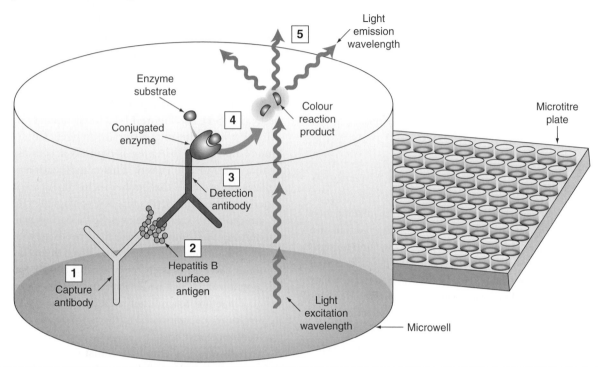

FIGURE 11-15 A Summary of the ELISA Test for Hepatitis B Surface Antigen. The wells are coated with antibodies that recognize the Hepatitis B Surface Antigen. The patient's plasma is added. If the plasma contains antigen, it binds to the attached antibody. A second detection antibody is added. The detection antibody is attached to enzyme. A substrate for the detection antibody is added. This substrate-enzyme reaction results in color development. The color development is measured with emitted light.

Source: Delmar, Cengage Learning

WEB ACTIVITIES

1. Proceed to http://depts.washington.edu/hepstudy/hepB
2. Choose: Serologic and Virologic Markers of Hepatitis B Virus Infection.
3. Choose: Discussion.
4. Choose: Figure 3 in the right-hand column.
5. Choose each of the items in the upper right of the screen. Watch the development of each marker. Read the accompanying text.

WEB ACTIVITIES

1. Go to www.cdc.gov
2. On the A-Z Index, choose "V."
3. Choose "Viral Hepatitis."
4. Choose "Hepatitis B."
5. Choose "For Health Care Professionals."
6. Under "Frequently Asked Questions," choose "Hepatitis B Serology."
7. Review the Hepatitis B Markers and note the significance of each.

Hepatitis B Serology

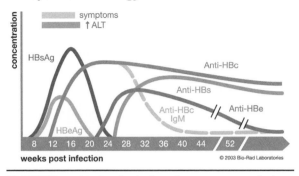

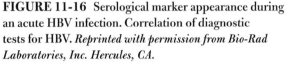

FIGURE 11-16 Serological marker appearance during an acute HBV infection. Correlation of diagnostic tests for HBV. *Reprinted with permission from Bio-Rad Laboratories, Inc. Hercules, CA.*

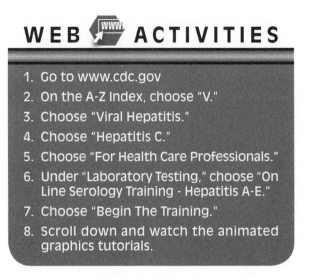

WEB ACTIVITIES

1. Go to www.cdc.gov
2. On the A-Z Index, choose "V."
3. Choose "Viral Hepatitis."
4. Choose "Hepatitis C."
5. Choose "For Health Care Professionals."
6. Under "Laboratory Testing," choose "On Line Serology Training - Hepatitis A-E."
7. Choose "Begin The Training."
8. Scroll down and watch the animated graphics tutorials.

HCV testing was introduced in 1989 with the anti-HCV assay. The anti-HCV assay is typically an ELISA assay that detects the presence of antibodies to HCV. A positive anti-HCV test is confirmed using a RIBA (see Figure 11-18). In this test recombinant HCV antigens are immobilized on a nitrocellulose strip. The strip is incubated with the patient's serum. If the serum contains HCV antibodies, they will bind to the antigens on the strip. A positive RIBA is a strong indicator of an active HCV infection.

The major technical issue with anti-HCV testing is the long window period from the time of infection until antibodies are present and levels detectable, approximately 70 to 80 days. During this window, an infected donor will continue to exhibit a negative test for HCV and may donate blood products. The development of NAT testing for HCV provided a method with increased sensitivity. Testing for HCV using NAT was adopted beginning in 1999 with over 99% of centers participating by 2000. The introduction of NAT testing has been demonstrated to prevent more than 50 cases of HCV infection annually. Combined with anti-HCV testing, the residual risk of HCV infection has decreased to 1 in 2 million units of blood.

HIV

Background

Human Immunodeficiency Virus-1 (HIV-1) and Human Immunodeficiency Virus-2 (HIV-2) are the etiology of acquired immunodeficiency syndrome (**AIDS**). HIV is a retrovirus. A retrovirus contains the reverse transcriptase

enzyme, which permits the virus to copy its own RNA to produce DNA. The DNA produced becomes integrated into the host DNA.

The presence of AIDS was first reported in the early 1980s. AIDS was identified in persons with hemophilia who had received multiple transfusions of human blood products. The causative agent was identified in late 1984. It was determined that the HIV virus was transmitted by sexual contact and exposure to contaminated blood products. The causative agent of the majority of HIV infections in the United States is HIV-1, while HIV-2 is found primarily in western Africa. Donor screening for HIV-1 began in 1985 with HIV-2 testing added to the test menu in 1992.

Testing

Historically, testing for antibodies to HIV-1 and 2 may be performed concurrently with a combined EIA test. A positive test for HIV antibodies is confirmed using a Western blot, which confirms the specificity of the antibodies. The 22-day window period from time of infection to antibody detection allows for numerous potential infections.

Antigen testing began in 1996 with a test to detect the p24 antigen, a core protein of HIV. This antigen test was added to the protocol for HIV screening (see Figure 11-19). This p24 assay decreased the window period to 17 days. The introduction of NAT for HIV RNA in 2002 has led to further reduction in the window period, to 12 days, and made the p24 antigen test obsolete. The current NAT assays have a sensitivity of

Bio-Rad Laboratories MONOLISA™ Anti-HBc EIA Testing Procedure

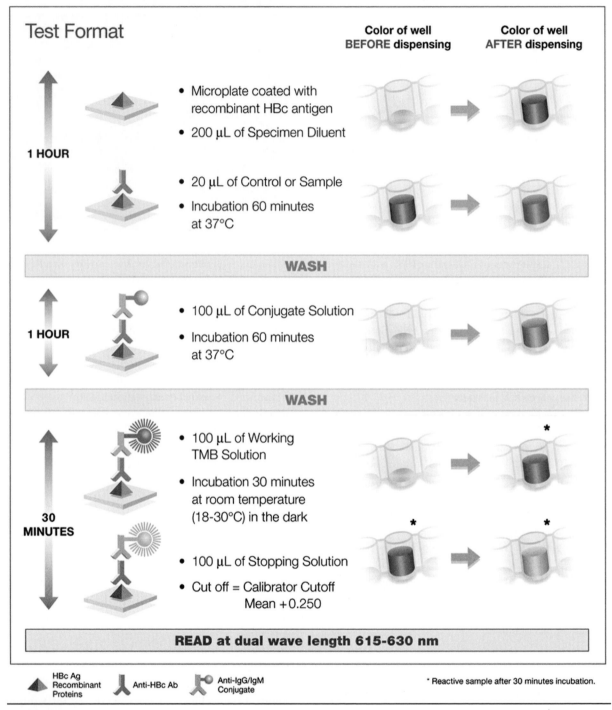

FIGURE 11-17 Test method for quantitation of anti-HBc. *Reprinted with permission from Bio-Rad Laboratories, Inc. Hercules, CA.*

Hepatitis C

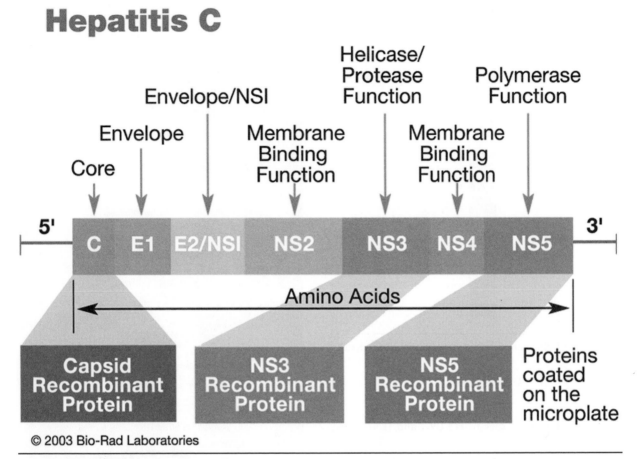

FIGURE 11-18 RIBA for Hepatitis C. *Reprinted with permission from Bio-Rad Laboratories, Inc. Hercules, CA.*

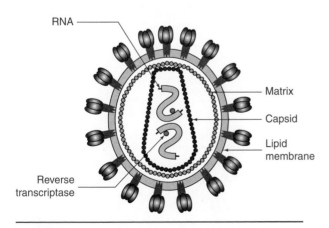

FIGURE 11-19 Schematic structure of HIV 1
Source: Delmar, Cengage Learning

approximately 30 to 60 copies/mL. A sample NAT assay is illustrated in Box 11-5. This increased sensitivity has decreased the risk of acquiring HIV to approximately 1 in every 2 million donations. Confirmation of HIV is accomplished with Western Blot (see Figure 11-20).

NAT testing is often performed using mini-pool testing. A mini-pool is the combination of 16 donor samples that are tested as a batch. Although this slightly decreases the sensitivity of the assay, it allows for a cost-effective alternative.

Human T-Lymphotropic Virus (HTLV)

HTLV I and II are RNA retroviruses demonstrated to be a causative agent for leukemia, including adult T-cell leukemia and a variant of hairy cell leukemia. Once integrated in the host DNA, the virus has the potential to complete its replication cycle or remain latent in the host for years. HTLV is spread both sexually and parenterally.

HIV WESTERN BLOT STRIP*

ENV
- p160
- p120
- p41

POL
- p68
- p53
- p32

GAG
- p55
- p40
- p24
- p18

FIGURE 11-20 Sample Western blot strip. Individual bands
Source: Delmar, Cengage Learning

Tests for antibodies to HTLV-I and II are performed concurrently in a combined assay. This assay is an EIA that is confirmed using a Western blot. The Western Blot determines the specificity of the HTLV antibodies.

West Nile Virus (WNV)

The WNV is a single-stranded RNA virus commonly found in Africa and the Middle East. Typically spread by a mosquito bite, the WNV may also be spread parenterally. The first cases of WNV in the western hemisphere occurred in New York 1999. Since 1999, the CDC have reported cases of WNV in all 48 contiguous states. Although most cases of WNV are subclinical, the virus demonstrates a continuum of symptoms that span from mild flu-like symptoms to encephalitis.

Beginning in July 2003 following the demonstration of transfusion-associated infections, NAT for WNV was implemented. This test methodology has been successful in identifying potentially infectious units of blood. WNV testing is performed on all units of blood donated in the United States.

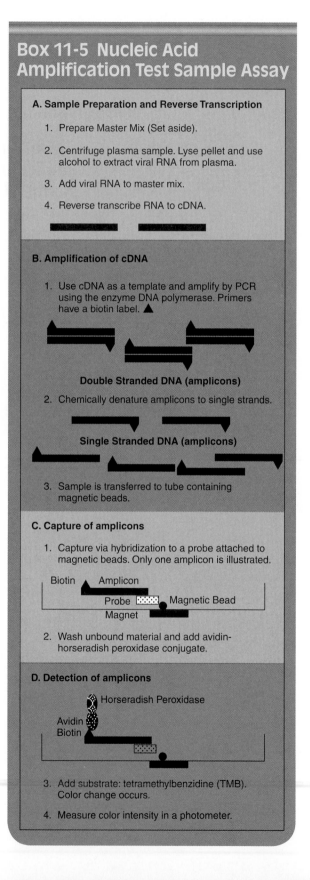

Box 11-5 Nucleic Acid Amplification Test Sample Assay

A. Sample Preparation and Reverse Transcription

1. Prepare Master Mix (Set aside).
2. Centrifuge plasma sample. Lyse pellet and use alcohol to extract viral RNA from plasma.
3. Add viral RNA to master mix.
4. Reverse transcribe RNA to cDNA.

B. Amplification of cDNA

1. Use cDNA as a template and amplify by PCR using the enzyme DNA polymerase. Primers have a biotin label. ▲

Double Stranded DNA (amplicons)

2. Chemically denature amplicons to single strands.

Single Stranded DNA (amplicons)

3. Sample is transferred to tube containing magnetic beads.

C. Capture of amplicons

1. Capture via hybridization to a probe attached to magnetic beads. Only one amplicon is illustrated.

Biotin Amplicon
Probe   Magnetic Bead
Magnet

2. Wash unbound material and add avidin-horseradish peroxidase conjugate.

D. Detection of amplicons

Horseradish Peroxidase
Avidin
Biotin

3. Add substrate: tetramethylbenzidine (TMB). Color change occurs.
4. Measure color intensity in a photometer.

Syphilis

Syphilis is a sexually transmitted disease caused by the bacterial spirochete *Treponema pallidum*. Refrigerated conditions are toxic to *T. pallidum*. *T. pallidum* can, however, survive in blood products, such as platelets, that are stored at room temperature. Syphilis testing is performed as a part of mandatory donor testing, in spite of recommendations that this testing be discontinued.

T. pallidum testing is usually performed using the Rapid Plasma Reagin (RPR) test. The RPR test is not specific for *T. pallidum*. The test detects reagin, an antibody-like substance, present in numerous infections including untreated syphilis. Confirmation testing may be performed by specific methods including hemagglutination and fluorescent treponemal antibody absorption.

Cytomegalovirus (CMV)

CMV is a double-stranded DNA virus found ubiquitously in the United States. By age 40, an estimated 85% of the adult population has been exposed, with most of the cases being subclinical. The virus is known to lay dormant in the host. CMV positive units may contain latent virus, they are not transfused to patients at risk for contracting an infection. Patients without a competent immune system, such as bone marrow transplant recipients, individuals infected with HIV, and infants are at increased risk for contracting a CMV infection through a transfusion.

Screening for CMV is not performed on all donor units, since the virus does not present a risk for most transfusion recipients. Many blood banks screen a small percentage of O negative units for CMV, and reserve the negative units for transfusion to immunocompromised patients. Detection of antibodies to CMV is performed utilizing an ELISA test.

Chagas Disease

Chagas disease, American trypanosomiasis, is an infection transmitted by the bite of the reduviid bug. The causative agent is the protozoan parasite *Trypanosoma cruzi*. Transfusion-transmission is a potential risk. Seroprevalence in the United States is extremely low, with the exception of areas such as Los Angeles and Miami, where there are high numbers of immigrants from endemic Latin American countries.

Beginning in 2007, blood centers began testing for *T. cruzi* following the FDA approval of a screening test for Chagas disease. Through the use of an ELISA test, blood units are being screened for the presence of antibodies to *T. cruzi*. Although not currently required, there exists a potential for future mandatory donor screening for Chagas disease.

Future Testing

The future screening of donor blood includes tests directed at reducing the core window associated with known pathogens. The tests under investigation include the expansion of NAT testing for HBV and the use of multiplex PCR for the concurrent detection of HBV, HCV, and HIV. Multiplex PCR would allow for the detection of all three viruses using one assay, in a highly sensitive and specific manner, while reducing operating costs. The development of sensitive NAT methodologies will reduce the window periods for transfusion-transmitted viral infections, therefore increasing the safety of the blood supply.

Emerging diseases are a major concern for the American blood supply. Adaptations of pathogens allowing for transmission from animals to humans as well as an increase in human-to-human transmission have altered the degree of concern with regard to transfusion transmission. Population dynamics and migration patterns are changing, hence permitting pathogens to move into new geographic areas. Environmental changes foster the growth of the pathogen vectors. Emerging pathogens that present a risk to the blood supply are malaria, *Babesia*, Dengue Virus, Human Parvovirus B19, Human Herpes Virus-8, Avian Flu, and variant CJD. As these diseases and accompanying serious sequelæ become apparent as they relate to the U.S. blood supply, it becomes necessary to weigh the risks of disease transmission versus the expense of testing. By developing donor testing and deferral criteria, the goal is to maintain a safe blood supply. Ongoing research continues in an attempt to maintain the safety of the blood supply. Monitoring of the blood supply continues as pathogens are recognized and test methods developed.

SUMMARY

- Components available for transfusion originate from whole blood. When a unit of whole blood is divided into individual components, the products are able to serve multiple patients and provide optimal benefits for each patient. The first step for fractionation of a unit of whole blood is to centrifuge the unit of whole blood. Following this separation, the individual components are removed and stored according to the optimal storage temperature range. The component is labeled with an expiration date. The shelf life of components is dependent on the method of preparation, anticoagulant-preservative solution, and additional treatments such as additive solutions and irradiation.

- Good manufacturing practices and quality control practices are followed throughout all steps of collection, preparation, storage, and distribution of all components. The FDA and AABB monitor all of these practices.

- Transfusion of all components is accomplished in a controlled environment. The identification of the recipient and all of the components must be confirmed and documented. Administration of components is performed with filtration. Any untoward reactions are documented and follow up performed.

  Infectious disease testing is performed on all donor units. This testing includes methods that detect:

- Hepatitis B and C
- HIV 1 and HIV 2
- HLTV I and II
- Syphilis
- CMV
- WNV
- Chagas Disease

BLOOD COMPONENTS AND INDICATIONS FOR TRANSFUSION

COMPONENT	INDICATIONS FOR TRANSFUSION
Whole Blood	Rarely implicated; Replacement of volume and increase in oxygen carrying capacity
Red Blood Cells	Increase oxygen carrying capacity; Anemia; Replacement for blood loss
Leukocyte Reduced Red Blood Cells	Increase oxygen carrying capacity; Anemia; Replacement for blood loss; Avoid febrile non-hemolytic reactions and prevent alloimmunization to leukocyte
Washed Red Cells	Reduce concentration of plasma proteins; Avoid allergic and anaphylactic reactions
Frozen Red Cells	Rare blood storage; Reduce concentration of plasma proteins, white blood cells and platelets; Avoid allergic and anaphylactic reactions
Fresh Frozen Plasma	Replacement of all coagulation factors; Consumption coagulopathy
Cryoprecipitated Antihemophilic Factor	Treatment of deficiency of Factors VII, XIII, and von Willebrand's Factor
Platelets Granulocytes	Thrombocytopenia or consumption coagulopathy

REVIEW QUESTIONS

1. Which of the following is *not* a method for preparation of leukocyte reduced red cells:
   a. differential centrifugation
   b. filtration
   c. freezing and deglycerolization
   d. washing of red cells

2. Pheresis may be used to collect all of the following *except*:
   a. leukocytes
   b. platelets
   c. plasma
   d. cryoprecipitate

3. Additive solutions are added to a unit of blood:
   a. immediately after collection of whole blood
   b. immediately before transfusion
   c. after plasma is removed from the cells
   d. as a part of the freezing process

4. Post-transfusion red blood cell survival requirements are:
   a. 90% survival 24 hours post-transfusion
   b. 80% survival 12 hours post-transfusion
   c. 75% survival 24 hours post-transfusion
   d. 50% survival 12 hours post-transfusion

5. Whole blood is to be collected from a donor weighing 95 lb. How much anticoagulant should be removed from a bag containing 63 ml of anticoagulant?
   a. 9 ml
   b. 12 ml
   c. 39 ml
   d. 43 ml

6. A donor unit is collected on May 1 in CPDA anticoagulant. AS1 is added to the red cells. The last day that this unit may be transfused is:
   a. May 29
   b. June 5
   c. June 12
   d. June 26

7. Which of the following contain one or more labile coagulation factors:
   1. stored plasma
   2. FFP
   3. Cryoprecipitate
   4. platelet concentrate
   a. 1 and 3 are correct
   b. 1 and 4 are correct
   c. 2 and 3 are correct
   d. 2 and 4 are correct
   e. 1, 2, and 3 are correct
   f. 1, 2, 3, and 4 are correct

8. Whole blood is shipped:
   1. 1 to 6°C
   2. 1 to 10°C
   3. unrefrigerated
   4. with wet ice
   5. with dry ice
   a. only 3 is correct
   b. 1 and 4 are correct
   c. 1 and 5 are correct
   d. 2 and 4 are correct
   e. 2 and 5 are correct

9. Cryoprecipitate may be used to correct a deficiency of all the following *except*:
   a. Factor I
   b. Factor VII
   c. Factor VIII
   d. VonWillebrand's factor

10. Examine the following ISBT 128 number. The country of origin is designated by

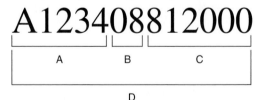

Source: Delmar, Cengage Learning

   a. part A
   b. part B
   c. part C
   d. part D

11. The marker that is determined using a neutralization assay is:
   a. HBsAg
   b. HBc
   c. Anti-HCV
   d. HCV

12. The clinical condition that is *not* transmitted sexually and parenterally is:
    a. Chagas Disease
    b. Hepatitis B
    c. Hepatitis C
    d. syphilis

13. A mini-pool methodology is used to screen for:
    a. CMV
    b. HAV

    c. HIV
    d. HTLV

14. Reduction of the window period in testing will:
    a. make testing less expensive
    b. apply more advanced technology to the testing methodologies
    c. detect the pathogen earlier in the disease process
    d. consolidate tests for multiple pathogens into one panel

15–20 Choose the component most likely to be transfused for each of the conditions listed.

_____ 15. Chronic anemia

_____ 16. Hemophilia A

_____ 17. Thrombocytopenia

_____ 18. Anemic neonate

_____ 19. Anemic renal transplant recipient

_____ 20. Hereditary deficiency of coagulation factor I

a. cryoprecipitate
b. platelet concentrate
c. washed red cells
d. irradiated red cells
e. packed red cells
f. fresh frozen plasma
g. whole blood

CASE STUDY

1. You are working in the component lab of the local Blood Bank. A large snowstorm has paralyzed the entire east coast. A local hospital calls and asks for a large shipment of both cryoprecipitate and fresh frozen plasma for two critically ill patients. These patients are both group AB. A technologist asks you if the AB units of whole blood that were collected yesterday at a local blood drive can each be used to produced BOTH cryoprecipitate and fresh frozen plasma.
   a. Provide a detailed answer to the technologists query.
   b. Is there an alternative suggestion for a successful outcome for both patients? If so, what is it?
   c. Is there an alternate ABO group that may provide plasma products to this patient?

2. A local Blood Bank collects and prepares all components for transfusion that are used by a local hospital. The local hospital has had to return several units of platelet concentrates due to visible agglutinates in the units.
   a. What causes these agglutinates?
   b. What step(s) should be taken to correct this problem?

REFERENCES

Alter, Harvy J, Stramer, Susan L, and Dodd, Roger Y. "Emerging Infectious Diseases That Threaten the Blood Supply." *Seminars in Hematology*. Vol. 44, Issue 1, 2007, pp. 32–41.

"An Introduction to ISBT 128." Available at www.iccbba.org.

Blaney, Kathy and Howard, Paula. *Basic and Applied Concepts of Immunohematology*. Mosby, Philadelphia, 2000.

Blumberg, Neil and Heal, Joanna M. "Universal Leukocyte Reduction of Blood Transfusions." *Clinical Infectious Diseases*. Vol. 45, 2007, pp. 1014–1015.

Brecher, Mark, editor. *American Association of Blood Banks Technical Manual 15th edition*. AABB, 2005.

Burnouf, Thierry. "Modern Plasma Fractionation." *Transfusion Medicine Reviews*. Vol. 21, Issue 2, 2007, pp. 101–117.

Busch, Michael P. "Transfusion-transmitted viral infections: building bridges to transfusion medicine to reduce risks and understand epidemiology and pathogenesis." *Transfusion*. Vol. 46, Issue 9, 2006, pp. 1624–1640.

Butch, S. H., Distler, P. B. "ISBT 128 Blood Labeling: Introduction and Reference Laboratory Applications." *Immunohematology*. Vol. 22, No. 1, 2006, pp. 30–36.

Candotti, D, Allain, JP. "The Utility of Multiplex NAT in Blood Screening." *Developments in Biologicals*. Vol. 127, 2007, pp. 71–86.

Centers for Disease Control and Prevention: West Nile Virus Case Counts: 1999–2008. Available at *www.cdc.gov/ncidod/dvbid/westnile*. Accessed September 17, 2008.

CFR: Title 21, Section 640. "Additional Standards for Human Blood and Blood Products." Available at www.accessdata.fda.gov

CFR: Title 21, Section 606, 607, 610, and 640. "Revisions to the Requirements Applicable to Blood, Blood Components and Source Plasma." August 2007.

Circular of Information: For the use of Human Blood and Blood Components. Available at www.aabb.org

Dimino, Michael L. "Hemoglobin-Based O2 Carrier O2Affinity and Capillary Inlet pO2 are Important Factors that Influence O2 Transport in a Capillary."

Biotechnology Progress. Vol. 23, No. 4, 2007, pp. 921–931.

Fasano, Ross, MD, Luban, Naomi L. C. MD. "Blood Component Therapy." *Pediatric Clinics of North America*. Vol. 55, 2008, pp. 421–445.

Fiebig, Eberhard, et al. "Dynamics of HIV Viremia and Antibody Seroconversion in Plasma Donors: Implications for Diagnosis and Staging of Primary HIV Infection." *AIDS*. Vol. 17, Issue 13, 2003, pp. 1871–1879.

Hess, J. R. "An Update on Solutions for Red Cell Storage." *Vox Sanguinis*. Vol. 91, 2006, pp. 13–19.

Jahr, Jonathan S. "Blood Substitutes as Pharmacotherapies in Clinical Practice." *Current Opinion in Anesthesiology*. Vol. 20, No. 4, pp. 325–330.

McCullough, Jeffrey. *Transfusion Medicine 2nd edition*. Elsevier. 2005.

Osby, Melanie, A., et al. "Safe Handling and Administration of Blood Components." *Archives of Pathology of Laboratory Medicine*. Vol. 131, 2007, pp. 690–695.

Price, Thomas H. Editorial: "Granulocyte Transfusion Therapy: It's Time for an Answer." *Transfusion*. Vol. 46, 2006, pp. 1–3.

"Revisions to the Requirements Applicable to Blood, Blood Components and Source Plasma; Confirmation of Effective Date and Technical Amendment. Direct Final Rule; Confirmation of Effective Date and Technical Amendment. *Federal Register*. 2008. pp. 7463–7464.

Standards for Blood Banks and Transfusion Services, 25th Edition. AABB, Bethesda, MD. 2008.

Stramer, S. L. "NAT Update: Where Are We Today." *Developments in Biologicals*. Vol. 108, 2002, pp. 41–56.

Tabor, Edward, Epstein, Jay S. "NAT screening of Blood and Plasma Donations: Evolution of Technology and Regulatory Policy." *Transfusion*. Vol. 42, Issue 9, September 2002, pp. 1230–1237.

Van der Meer, Pieter F., Eijzen, Marjan, Rietersz, Ruby N. I., "Comparison of two Sterile Connection Devices and the Effect of Sterile Connections on Blood Component Quality." *Transfusion*. Vol. 46, 2006, pp. 418–423.

Adverse Reaction to Transfusion

LEARNING OUTCOMES

At the completion of this chapter, the reader should be able to:

- Outline and describe the major categories of transfusion reactions.
- Differentiate transfusion-related acute lung injury (TRALI) from circulatory overload.
- Compare and contrast acute and delayed hemolytic transfusion reactions (HTR).
- Outline characteristics of allergic transfusion reactions to include urticarial and anaphylactic reactions.
- List viral and non-viral infectious diseases that may be transmitted via transfusion.
- Discuss the physiological effects of red blood cell hemolysis.
- Discuss the components of a transfusion reaction investigation.
- Relate the severity of a transfusion reaction to the level of response necessary.
- Discuss the need for monitoring recipients of blood transfusions.
- Discuss prevention of HTR.

GLOSSARY

anaphylactic   intense allergic reaction including bronchial constriction and collapse

febrile   having a fever

hemoglobinemia   presence of free hemoglobin in the serum or plasma

hemoglobinuria   presence of hemoglobin in the urine

hemolytic transfusion reactions (HTR)   adverse reaction to transfusion most often resulting from an interaction between antigens of the donor and antibodies of the recipient

hemolysis   destruction of red blood cells with release of hemoglobin

hemosiderosis   accumulation of excess iron in macrophages in various tissues

icterus   yellow color in serum; indicates increased bilirubin in the serum

post-transfusion   after transfusion

post-transfusion purpura (PTP)   appearance of red or purple discolorations on the skin at any time after transfusion has been completed; purpura are usually caused by bleeding under the skin

pre-transfusion   before transfusion

sepsis presence of bacterial infection in the circulatory system

transfusion reaction any unfavorable response in a blood or blood product recipient

urticaria hives

INTRODUCTION

The main purpose of blood banks and transfusion services is to provide blood products for transfusion and follow the transfusion process to assure that the products are administered in the safest possible manner. In addition, transfusion of any blood product should provide maximum benefit to its recipient with minimum complications or side effects. The entire process, beginning with donor recruitment and screening through post-transfusion monitoring of the recipient, is focused on a positive, uneventful outcome. A transfusion reaction is defined as any unfavorable response in a blood or blood product recipient. Transfusion reactions display a range of symptoms from mild exacerbation up to and including death. Major categories of transfusion reactions are summarized in Table 12-1.

TABLE 12-1 Categories of Transfusion Reactions

Acute Immune Mediated Reactions

Hemolytic

Febrile

Anaphylactic

Urticaria

TRALI (Transfusion-Related Acute Lung Injury)

Acute Non-Immune-Mediated

Circulatory Overload

Bacterial Contamination

Physical Red Blood Cell Damage

Delayed Immune Medicated Reactions

Hemolytic

Graft vs. Host Disease (GVHD)

Post-transfusion Purpura (PTP)

Delayed Non-Immune Mediated

Disease Transmission

Hemosiderosis (Iron Overload)

OVERVIEW OF TRANSFUSION REACTIONS

As defined, a transfusion reaction is any unfavorable response in a blood or blood product recipient. Historically, acute hemolytic transfusion reactions (HTR) resulting from ABO incompatibility are the reactions that have claimed the most attention both within and outside of the medical community. In spite of the notoriety, transfusion of ABO incompatible blood occurs infrequently with actual rates difficult to determine. Discrepancies in published rates are attributed to voluntary reporting that is often inaccurate. With Human Immunodeficiency Virus (HIV) coming to the forefront in the 1980s, the blood supply came under attack for transmission of infectious disease. Since that time, in addition to HIV, Hepatitis C, Human T-Cell Lymphotropic Virus (HTLV) Types I and II, Chagas disease, and West Nile Virus (WNV) have been added to the donor-test menu—in addition to syphilis serology that has been historically performed.

In addition to the notorious issues of ABO incompatibility and infectious disease transmission, many other effects of transfusion are included under the broad category of adverse transfusion reactions. As outlined in Table 12-1, transfusion reactions can be divided into categories. The most common divisions are acute vs. delayed and immune vs. non-immune. These categories are not firm and cross-over exists with some types of reactions. A synopsis of the categories includes:

1. Acute and delayed: Acute reactions occur in a short time frame from the initiation of the transfusion. Delayed reactions occur hours, days, or (rarely) weeks after the completion of the transfusion.

2. Hemolytic vs. non-hemolytic: Hemolytic reactions are those that result in the destruction of red blood cells. The hemolysis may result from an immune process or physical or chemical damage to the red cells. Non-hemolytic reactions do not involve the destruction of red cells. Theoretically, any reaction

WEB ACTIVITIES

1. Type www.virtualmedicalcentre.com into your browser.
2. Search for "transfusion reactions."
3. Review information for transfusion reactions on this web site.
4. Continue to refer to this web site while reading this chapter and working the included activities.

that does not result in red cell destruction is non-hemolytic. Some examples include transfusion-related acute lung injury, allergic reactions, and post-transfusion purpura (PTP).

3. Immune-mediated vs. non-immune mediated: Immune reactions involve antigen-antibody reactions. Complement may be involved, but it is not necessarily a part of the reaction. The antigen-antibody reaction may involve red cells, white cells, or platelets.

4. Infectious vs. non-infectious: Infectious reactions result in the transmission of disease. The etiology may be bacterial, viral, or parasitic.

Immune Reaction to *in vivo* Red Blood Cell Destruction

The most severe and dreaded transfusion reactions result from the destruction of donor's red cells as they enter the recipient circulation. Historically, this type of reaction was first described when the medical community began to experiment with blood transfusion. This *in vivo* destruction can occur in varying time frames. Those that occur within minutes are classified as an immediate or acute HTR. ABO incompatibility is the *clinical* scenario for the majority of HTR's while clerical error is the most frequent *technical* cause of this type of incompatibility. The reaction may also be "delayed" from hours to days after completion of the transfusion. An anamnestic antibody response may cause a delayed reaction. Antibodies to the Kidd blood group system, known as the *treacherous Kidds*, are notorious for these delayed reactions. Hemolytic reactions are immune in nature and non-infectious. The laboratory investigation of transfusion

reactions is focused on the signs and symptoms of the hemolytic reaction.

Mechanisms of Red Cell Destruction

The most common cause of transfusion-related red cell destruction is an antigen-antibody interaction. The immune reaction proceeds as follows:

1. Antibody attaches to a specific antigen on the surface of the red cell
2. Complement is activated
3. Additional components are activated, including cytokines
4. Coagulation cascade is activated
5. Organ failure (e.g. renal) and shock occur

Mechanical hemolysis may be of two types: complement-mediated intravascular destruction of red blood cells and IgG antibody-mediated extravascular destruction of red blood cells. These two mechanisms are summarized in Figure 12-1.

Impact of Antigen-Antibody Reactions and Immunological Components. Properties of antigens and antibodies were discussed in Chapter 1. The sequential steps of a HTR begin with the combination of antibodies from the recipient's serum with antigens on the transfused red cells.

- Antibody: The antibody may be IgG or IgM. IgM antibodies provide the most significant reaction resulting from the ability of IgM antibodies to activate the complement pathway.

- ABO antibodies are most often IgM with small amounts of IgG.

- Both IgM and IgG ABO antibodies are capable of binding complement.

- IgG antibodies can also interact with Fc receptors for phagocytes. This will affect the activation of phagocytosis and other cellular processes.

- Antibody concentration, or titer, plays a role in the amount of antigen-antibody interaction. A high titer antibody, such as anti-A, will create many more antigen-antibody complexes than a low titer antibody with fewer antibody molecules.

- Antigen: The antigens are found on the surface of the red blood cells. The greater the number of

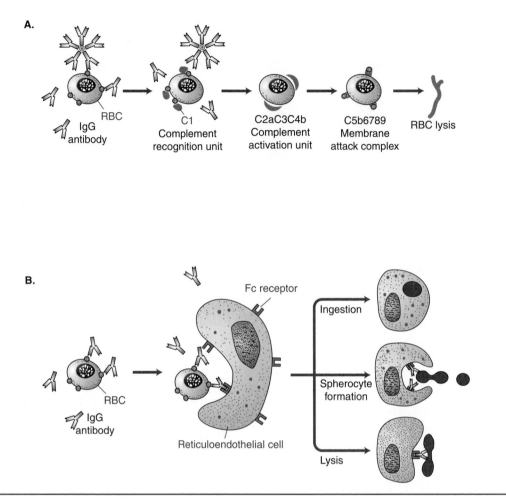

FIGURE 12-1 **A. Complement-mediated intravascular destruction of red blood cells.**
B. IgG antibody-mediated extravascular destruction of red blood cells.
Source: Delmar, Cengage Learning

antigens on the surface of each cell, the stronger the reaction with the antibody. In addition, when antigens are found in clusters on the red cell surface, there is increased likelihood that complement will be activated.

- Complement: Once the complement cascade is activated, the red cell hemolysis occurs with complete activation to the C9 component. Other effects of complement activation are:

    - The destruction of the red cell membrane with release of free hemoglobin and red cell stroma (membrane debris) into the plasma.

    - Free hemoglobin binds with haptoglobin. This decreases serum haptoglobin levels. When the

binding capacity of haptoglobin is exceeded, hemoglobinemia and hemoglobinuria may be present.

- C3 and C5 trigger the release of vasoactive amines, such as serotonin and histamine, from mast cells and basophils. Increased vascular permeability is cumulative effect of the release of these amines. As a result, the recipient will exhibit hypotension.

- Cytokines: In addition to the release of serotonin and histamine triggered by complement, additional cytokines include:

    - Bradykinin released as a result of immune complex formation. Bradykinin is a potent vasodilator that contributes to hypotension.

- Norepinephrine release is stimulated by the formation of the immune complex. This substance will contribute to vasoconstriction in the kidneys and lungs. This factor also contributes to the impending renal failure that is exhibited in a hemolytic episode.

- Coagulation Activation: The complex of antigen-antibody-complement will stimulate the coagulation cascade as well as the fibrinolytic system. Activation of these two systems may result in disseminated intravascular coagulation (DIC). This is a consumption coagulopathy that consumes coagulation factors and platelets. Finally, diffuse microvascular bleeding may cause tissue ischemia. This tissue ischemia will release additional tissue factors and promote the continuation of the DIC process.

Symptoms of Acute and Delayed HTR

Hemolytic reactions to the transfusion of red cell products may present as either acute or delayed. The acute presentation will occur rapidly and symptoms may span from mild to severe. Suspected acute reactions warrant immediate discontinuation of the transfused unit and medical evaluation of the patient. Delayed reactions occur up to two weeks following the infusion of the red cell products.

The clinical symptoms of a HTR are secondary to "cytokine generation after complement activation as well as cellular interaction between antibody-or complement-coated RBCs and phagocytic cells." A summary of symptoms and laboratory test results for all hemolytic reactions is included in Table 12-2.

The symptoms listed in Table 12-2 are objective signs of a transfusion reaction. There are also subjective signs of a reaction, which are summarized in Table 12-3. Subjective signs are in the "gray area" of diagnostic criteria. However, subjective signs are frequently the initial indication of an impending reaction and provide valuable diagnostic information. Patients receiving a transfusion should be monitored closely at the onset of

TABLE 12-2 Comparison of Acute and Delayed HTR

	ACUTE	DELAYED
Time Frame	Rapid; within minutes of starting transfusion	5 to 14 days post-transfusion; administration of antigen-negative blood for future transfusions
Symptoms	■ Burning or pain at site of infusion ■ Flushing ■ Lower back pain ■ Fever and chills ■ Tachycardia ■ Tachypnea ■ Hypotension	■ Fever; possibly with chills ■ Unexplained decrease in hemoglobin or hematocrit ■ Possible jaundice
Laboratory Test Results	■ DAT; may be + or negative ■ Hemoglobinuria ■ Increased free hemoglobin in plasma (hemoglobinemia) ■ Increase serum bilirubin ■ Decreased haptoglobin	■ DAT: + ■ Decreased hemoglobin or hematocrit ■ Antibody screen: +
Major Complications	■ Renal failure ■ DIC ■ Shock ■ Possibly death	■ No major complications
Treatment	■ Treat symptoms; hypotension, DIC ■ Dialysis, if indicated	■ No additional treatment necessary

the transfusion. Subjective signs will not be observed in anesthetized or comatose patients, which may contribute to a more severe reaction in these individuals.

Immune Causes of Non-hemolytic Transfusion Reactions

Immunological causes of transfusion reactions may not result in red cell hemolysis. These reactions typically involve antibodies that react with non-red cell components in the recipient. The specificity of the antibodies may be directed to antigens on the surface of platelets, granulocytes, the human leukocyte antigen (HLA) system, or human neutrophil antigens (HNA). The reaction severity is a continuum from mild (urticaria or hives) to severe or very life-threatening reactions, such as graft vs. host disease (GVHD). A summary of the major points of these reactions is found in Table 12-4.

TABLE 12-3 Subjective Signs of a HTR

- Restlessness
- Anxiety
- Feeling of impending doom
- Headache
- Nausea vomiting
- Chest or abdominal pain

WEB ACTIVITIES

1. Type www.merck.com into your browser.
2. Search for "Complications of Transfusion."
3. Choose this topic when the results of the search appear.
4. Review contained material taking special notice of the treatment for HTR.
5. Continue to refer to this material as you continue to read and complete activities in this chapter.

Allergic Reactions

Allergic reactions vary from very mild cases of urticaria or hives to life-threatening anaphylactic reactions. Urticarial reactions may be caused by multiple factors and the causes are usually indeterminate. Appropriate treatment is antihistamine and continuing the transfusion.

Anaphylactoid reactions that mimic anaphylaxis may be noted. IgE does not mediate these reactions. Anaphylactic reactions occur very rapidly as the transfusion is commencing. It requires immediate intervention. These two categories (anaphylactoid and anaphylactic) are indistinguishable and hence are described as anaphylactic. Anaphylactic reactions are most often a rapid antibody response directed against a plasma protein lacking in the recipient. However, the true etiology of most reactions is not known. Future transfusions require the transfusion of red cells with no plasma. Frozen-thawed or deglycerolized red cells are the best choice.

Febrile Reactions

A febrile reaction is one of the most common transfusion reactions. A febrile reaction is an increase of at least 1°C in temperature during the course of the transfusion, and is caused by antibodies to antigens on white cells or platelets. The recipient exhibits fever and chills. The symptoms are attributed to pyrogenic cytokines and intracellular contents released from donor leukocytes or infused with the blood component. These substances react with leukocyte reactive antibodies produced by the recipient. The vital step in evaluation of a febrile reaction is to rule out the presence of a more severe reaction. While uncomfortable for the patient, a febrile transfusion reaction is not life-threatening. Treatment should include termination of the transfusion and treatment of the symptoms.

Reducing the level of leukocyte contamination in transfused units will decrease the number of febrile reactions. This is best accomplished by reducing the leukocyte population as part of the processing procedure of all red cell units. See Chapter 11 for a summary of leukoreduction techniques.

TRALI

TRALI is a rare complication of blood transfusion. The physiological cause of TRALI is not known. Projected causes include "endothelial damage when leukocyte-reactive antibodies, usually with HLA class I or II are

TABLE 12-4 Major Points of Non-hemolytic Transfusion Reactions

Category	*Specifics*
Febrile Transfusion Reactions	
Clinical Signs/Symptoms	■ Major symptoms: fever, chills
	■ Additional symptoms: nausea, vomiting, headache, back pain
Causes	■ HLA antibodies in recipient to antigens on donor white cells
	■ Cytokines released by white blood cells during blood product storage
Laboratory Tests	■ DAT = negative
	■ Hemolysis = no visible hemolysis
Prevention	Leukocyte reduced red cell products
Treatment	Symptom control; antipyretics, acetaminophen
Urticarial Transfusion Reactions	
Clinical Signs/Symptoms	Hives, itching, erythema
Causes	Antibodies in recipient to foreign plasma proteins or other substances in donor blood
Laboratory Tests	■ DAT = negative
	■ Hemolysis = no visible hemolysis
Prevention	■ If history exists, premedicate with antihistamines
	■ Transfusion washed cellular products
Treatment	■ Interrupt (not discontinue) transfusion
	■ Administer antihistamine
Anaphylactic Transfusion Reactions	
Clinical Signs/Symptoms	■ Rapid onset and progression
	■ Wheezing, coughing, dyspnea, bronchospasm, respiratory distress, vascular instability
	■ Afebrile
Causes	■ IgA deficiency in recipient
	■ An IgG anti-IgA in recipient; complement binding antibody
Laboratory Tests	■ DAT = negative
	■ Hemolysis = no visible hemolysis
Prevention	■ Washed or deglycerolized red cell products
	■ Plasma products from IgA deficient donors
Treatment	■ Stop transfusion
	■ Administer epinephrine
	■ Maintain airway
TRALI	
Clinical Signs/Symptoms	■ Rapid onset
	■ Marked respiratory distress
	■ Fever, chills
	■ Hypotension
	■ Cyanosis

(Continued)

TABLE 12-4 Major Points of Non-hemolytic Transfusion Reactions (Continued)

TRALI (Continued)

Causes	■ Interaction of granulocytes and specific *donor* antibodies
	■ Clinical comorbidities
	■ Host factors of C3 regulation, antigen expression on white cells and cytokine responsiveness
Laboratory Tests	■ DAT = negative
	■ Hemolysis = no visible hemolysis
Prevention	■ Donor screening
	■ Decrease in use of units of multiparous women
Treatment	■ Steroid administration
	■ Respiratory support

Transfusion-Associated GVHD

Clinical Signs/Symptoms	■ Post-transfusion—3 to 30 days
	■ Fever
	■ Maculopapular rash
	■ Nausea, vomiting, diarrhea, abdominal pain
	■ Jaundice, abnormal liver function
Causes	■ Immunologic response in recipient
	■ Cause: Immunocompetent T-lymphocytes
Laboratory Tests	■ DAT = negative
	■ Hemolysis = no visible hemolysis
	■ Confirmation by HLA typing to show disparity between donor lymphocytes and recipient tissues
Prevention	■ Transfused HLA matched platelets
	■ Irradiation of blood products before transfusion in patients who are at risk
	■ Irradiation of donor lymphocytes to prevent blast transformation
	■ Identifying candidates for irradiated blood products: bone marrow or stem cell transplant patients, infants, fetuses receiving intrauterine transfusions, any immunocompromised patients
Treatment	■ None, usually unresponsive to interventions

transfused and activate antigen-positive neutrophils in the pulmonary capillaries" or "patients, as a result of their disease or treatment, are in an inflammatory 'alert' state in which neutrophils are assembled and primed in the pulmonary capillary beds" or a combination of both factors. These patients exhibit acute respiratory distress within two to four hours of transfusion. All blood components and intravenous immunoglobulins (IVIG) have been implicated in TRALI. The causative leukocyte-reactive antibodies are often found in multiparous women. Plasma containing components, such as fresh frozen plasma (FFP) and platelet concentrate, from donors with leukocyte-reactive antibodies are more frequently implicated than red cell containing components. The severity of symptoms is on a continuum of asymptomatic to fatal.

GVHD

Transfusion associated GVHD is a rare, but serious complication of blood transfusion. It is fatal in about 90% of cases. It occurs when donor lymphocytes are transfused to a severely immunocompromised individual. The donor lymphocytes engraft and react against recipient tissues. Symptoms include fever, skin rash, diarrhea, and bone marrow failure within seven to ten days post-transfusion. When properly identified pretransfusion, at-risk recipients should receive cellular blood components irradiated with 15 Gy gamma radiation.

At risk recipients include individuals with congenital or acquired immunodeficiencies, fetuses and infants less than four months old, and recipients of directed donations from first- or second-degree relatives. Recipients of directed donations are at risk because they are unable to eliminate transfused lymphocytes with shared HLA haplotypes.

PTP

PTP is a rare occurrence found in a multiparous female population. PTP should be suspected when a platelet-containing blood component is transfused and a significant decrease in the recipient's platelet count is noted within one week post-transfusion. Additional symptoms include purpura and an increase in bleeding episodes. PTP is an anamnestic response resulting from previous sensitization to a high incidence platelet antigen (Pl^{a1} or HPA-1a). Antigen-negative females are sensitized by multiple pregnancies. On subsequent exposure, the individual responds by destroying not only the transfused-antigen positive platelets, but also the recipient's own antigen negative cells. Treatment may include plasmapheresis, exchange transfusion and administration of intravenous IgG (IVIG).

Non-immune Causes of Transfusion Complications

Transfusion complications that are non-immune in nature consist of a compilation of miscellaneous etiologies. Some of these complications include effects on red cell survival. Others are random adverse effects that may be long term or short lived. Additionally, these effects may be minor or serious in nature.

Additional Red Cell Destruction Mechanisms

Red cell destruction may occur by mechanisms that are not immune in nature. When alloantibodies are

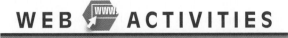

WEB ACTIVITIES

Using an appropriate search engine, research intravenous IgG (IVIg). Briefly summarize the manufacturing process for this product. List five conditions that are treated with this product.

TABLE 12-5 Summary of Non-Immune Red Blood Cell Destruction Mechanisms

- Hemolysis in the transfused unit
- Exposure of the red cells by exposure to extreme temperatures
- Less than 0°C
- Greater than 50°C
- Improper deglycerolization of frozen red blood cells
- Incompatible solution—addition of solution to unit of red cells that may affect the osmotic pressure and result in hemolysis. Examples include:
  - Medications
  - Ringers lactate
  - Half-strength saline
- Transfusion of bacterially contaminated blood products
- Mechanical destruction of red blood cells
- Mechanical heart valves
- Administration through small bore needles
- Excessive pressure to units being administered with force
- Clinical condition with red cell defect
- Sickle cell anemia
- Hereditary spherocytosis
- Paroxysmal nocturnal hemoglobinuria (PNH)
- Burn patients

not implicated, an alternate mechanism for destruction of the cells should be investigated. A summary of possible non-immune causes for hemolysis is provided in Table 12-5.

Bacterial Contamination of Blood Products

Transfusion of bacterial contaminants is a serious complication of transfusion. Sources of bacterial contamination include improper cleansing of the donor's skin during blood collection or a transient bacteremia in the donor. Bacterial endotoxins accumulate while the unit is in storage. Upon transfusion, the recipient rapidly becomes symptomatic and progresses to shock. Clinical symptoms may mimic a HTR. The bacterial load parallels the severity of symptoms. Grading of severity of septic reactions on a scale of zero to five is summarized

TABLE 12-6 Grading System for Septic Transfusion Reaction

GRADE	REACTION TYPE	DETAILS
0	None	■ No clinical or laboratory evidence of a septic reaction after receiving a contaminated unit
1	Mild	■ Mild febrile reaction (1 to 2°C) *or* ■ Asymptomatic with positive blood culture *or* ■ Development of leukocytosis
2	Moderate	■ Transient change in vital signs (fever, etc.) *or* ■ Clinical status that resolved within 24 hours with minimal intervention or no intervention
3	Severe	■ Change in vital symptoms; requires intervention; resolves without lasting effects
4	Life-Threatening	■ Severe reaction with septic shock *or* ■ Impairment of organ function
5	Fatal	■ Severe reaction with death partly or entirely attributable to the contaminated transfusion

in Table 12-6. Treatment with broad-spectrum antibiotics may be initiated before confirmation of diagnosis. Bacteria detected in components stored at refrigerator temperatures must remain viable at 4°C. Some examples include *Pseudomonas species, Yersinia enterocolitica, Enterobacter cloacae, Staphylococcus epidermidis* and *Bacillus cereus.*

Diagnosis methods include recipient blood cultures and cultures of the blood bag from the unit transfused. Careful inspection of blood products by transfusion personnel at the time of issue may prevent some of these reactions. As previously described in Chapter 9, inspection of a unit of blood should include examination for discoloration, clots, or hemolysis. Prior to the time of issue or administration, careful cleansing of the phlebotomy site by collection personnel aids in prevention of bacterial contamination of donor units.

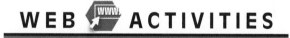

WEB ACTIVITIES

1. Proceed to www.aabb.org
2. Search for "Bacterial Contamination of Platelet Concentrates."
3. Review the historical listing of articles related to this topic.
4. Discuss results with classmates.

Contamination in platelet concentrates that are stored at room temperature (20 to 24°C) has been determined to cause a higher incidence of bacterial sepsis than red cell products. *AABB Standards for Blood Banks and Transfusion Services, 25th Edition* requires that "the blood bank or transfusion service shall have methods to limit and detect bacterial contamination in all platelet components." In addition, the standards require preparation of the venipuncture site to minimize the risk of bacterial contamination.

Circulatory Overload

Circulatory overload occurs when the volume of the cardiopulmonary system is exceeded. Symptoms include dypsnea, headache, peripheral edema, and congestive heart failure in close proximity to transfusion. Compromised cardiac and pulmonary status impair the recipient's ability to tolerate elevations in blood volume. These recipients are more susceptible to circulatory overload. Differentiation from TRALI is necessary in order to initiate appropriate treatment. A comparison of the symptoms of TRALI and circulatory overload is found in Table 12-7. Aggressive treatment with oxygen and diuretics may prevent further complications. This type of reaction may lead to fatality, but most often is resolved with diuresis.

Prevention of circulatory overload begins with identification of susceptible patients. These patients

TABLE 12-7 Differentiation of Circulatory Overload and TRALI

CRITERIA	TRANSFUSION-RELATED ACUTE LUNG INJURY (TRALI)	TRANSFUSION-ASSOCIATED CIRCULATORY OVERLOAD (TACO)
Pulmonary Edema	Yes	Yes
Dypsnea	Yes	Yes
Respiratory Distress	Yes	Yes
Hypoxia	Yes	Yes
Hypotension	Yes	No
Hypertension	No	Yes
Jugular Distension	No	Yes
Increased Central Venous Pressure	No	Yes
Improve with Diuresis	No	Yes
BNP* Level	Normal range	>500 pg/ml or post-transfusion to pre-transfusion ratio of >2.0
WBC Count	Decreases	Increases

* BNP = B-natriuretic peptide

should receive packed red cell units transfused slowly over four to six hours. Infusion of large volumes of plasma or other fluids should be avoided in these patients.

Transmission of Infectious Disease

Disease transmission through transfusion of blood components has historically been an issue as it relates both to donor screening and testing and with regard to the recipient. The transmission of infectious diseases came to the forefront in the 1980s when HIV was discovered and it became apparent that transmission could occur via blood products. Since that time, the testing of blood components for infectious agents has escalated. Chapter 11 summarizes infectious agent testing that is performed in the blood bank. Infectious agents transmitted via blood or blood components are found in Table 12-8.

TABLE 12-8 Transfusion Transmitted Disease

Viral
- HIV
- Hepatitis B and C (Hepatitis A rarely)
- HTLV I and II
- Cytomegalovirus
- Epstein-Barr Virus
- Human Parvovirus B19
- WNV

Non-viral
- Syphilis
- Malaria
- Babesiosis
- Leishmaniasis
- Creutzfeldt-Jakob Disease (CJD)
- Bacteria
- Chagas disease

CRITICAL THINKING ACTIVITY

Research each non-viral infectious agent that may be transmitted via transfusion. Determine the organism that is the causative agent for each of these agents. Record the genus and species for each. Compare with a partner.

Iron Overload

Iron overload or hemosiderosis is the result of accumulation of excess iron in reticuloendothelial cells and parenchymal cells. In transfusion, the iron intake is approximately 250 mg/unit. This intake exceeds the daily excretion of iron (1 mg/day). The human body has no physiologic means for elimination of excess iron. This accumulation may create end-organ damage. The most significant damage occurs in the hepatic, cardiac, and endocrine systems. Complications related to organ damage may not be evident until end-organ damage has occurred. This damage is found most often in patients with chronic conditions requiring frequent transfusion therapy. Diagnoses include thalassemia and sickle cell anemia.

Citrate Toxicity

Transfusion of large quantities of citrated blood may cause citrate toxicity in the recipient. Citrate, by action, binds ionized calcium. This toxicity may be due to large amounts of citrate transfused in massive transfusion situations or transfusions administered to individuals with impaired liver function. This toxicity can be corrected with injections of calcium in an acceptable formulation.

INVESTIGATION OF TRANSFUSION REACTIONS

Investigation of transfusion reactions requires immediate action both by the administering personnel and the laboratory. The technician will not be involved with detection of symptoms of a transfusion reaction nor will he or she initiate the immediate steps to stop the transfusion and begin an investigation or institute treatment. The focus of this investigation focuses on the detection of a hemolytic reaction. The investigative process varies by institution. A general system for investigation is discussed in the following sections and summarized in a flow chart in Figure 12-2.

Response to Transfusion Reaction

As soon as a transfusion reaction is suspected, the transfusion is discontinued and the administering personnel

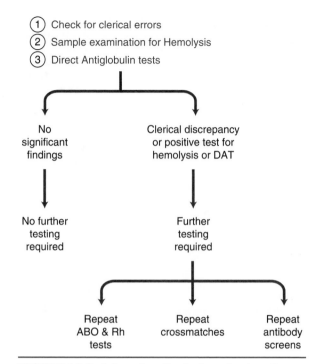

FIGURE 12-2 A flow chart for the investigation of a transfusion reaction
Source: Delmar, Cengage Learning

begin an investigation. The investigation is initiated and should include the following steps:

- Reidentification of the recipient and the unit being incriminated. If a discrepancy is detected, it is documented and reported to the physician.

- Recipient's physician and the transfusion service are notified.

- The physician assesses the recipient's symptoms and initiates intervention if necessary.

- The intravenous line is kept open and saline or other FDA approved solution is infused.

- If the signs and symptoms indicate that the possibility of a serious complication—such as acute HTR, TRALI, sepsis, anaphylaxis or other serious complication—the following items should be forwarded to the transfusion service for evaluation:

  - A post-reaction blood sample; sample should be properly collected and labeled

  - Transfusion container and administration set

  - Attached intravenous solutions

  - All related forms and labels

- First voided post-reaction urine (in some circumstances)

If the signs and symptoms indicate uritcara or circulatory overload, post reaction samples are not indicated.

Laboratory Role

The laboratory designate any transfusion reaction as a high priority. A clerical check for errors is immediately initiated in recipient samples, blood components, and records when required items arrive in the laboratory. If any discrepancies are observed, the recipient's physician is notified immediately.

All samples are centrifuged and examined for hemolysis. Red or pink plasma or serum indicates hemoglobinemia. If hemoglobinemia is present in the post-transfusion sample, but not in the pre-transfusion sample, an intense investigation ensues. Icterus or an increase in bilirubin in the serum or plasma may appear if the transfusion took place over a three to four hour period.

Direct antiglobulin testing (DAT) is an integral part of the immediate investigation of a transfusion reaction. A DAT is performed on the post-transfusion sample. This test may be positive with a mixed field reaction, if an immune reaction is occurring in the recipient. If the reacting cells are being rapidly cleared from the system, the DAT may be negative in spite of an active immune reaction. The physician should be notified immediately if a positive DAT is detected.

Further Testing

Additional testing may be initiated, dependent on the results of the initial investigation. Some examples of key findings include a clerical error such as misidentification, hemolysis in the post-transfusion sample, or a positive post-transfusion DAT. The testing performed in the investigation is summarized in Table 12-9. If all of the above items are negative and no discrepancies encountered, an immune cause may be eliminated. Further investigation is not necessary. If all initial tests are negative but the physician still detects symptoms of a HTR, the remaining steps of the testing process may be necessary.

Post-transfusion monitoring includes observation to detect a change in hematologic status, such as a decrease in hemoglobin or hematocrit. This may indicate that hemolysis is occurring. The presence of free hemoglobin in the urine with absence of other incriminating clinical findings may indicate that intravascular

TABLE 12-9 Tests for Investigation of Transfusion Reaction
ABO and Rh Tests
Patient's Pre-Transfusion Sample
Patient's Post-Transfusion Sample
Donor Segment
Compatibility Testing
Pre-Transfusion Sample and Donor Segment
Post-Transfusion Sample and Donor Segment
Antibody Screen
Pre-Transfusion Sample
Post-Transfusion Sample
Donor Segment
Additional Tests
Serum Haptoglobin and Bilirubin
Urine Hemoglobin
Hemoglobin and Hematocrit
Inspection of Donor Unit
Gram Stain and Blood Culture
Culture of the Transfused Unit

hemolysis is occurring. A decrease in haptoglobin levels may also indicate hemolysis.

Pre-transfusion and post-transfusion samples are tested in parallel to confirm the initial test results and prove that mixed populations of cells or previously undetected antibodies are not preset in the post-transfusion sample. Discrepancies should be reported to the physician. Continuation of the extended work up would be imperative to identify the root of the discrepancy. When repeating the antibody screen on the post-transfusion sample, additional enhancement techniques may be required for detection of an antibody resulting from an anamnestic response. The antibody titer might initially be undetectable since the antibody may be absorbed out by the transfused cells. Checking the donor cells for the presence of antigens corresponding to the incriminating antibody could also provide useful information. As discussed in Chapter 8, antigen typing of the recipient red cells may only be performed if the recipient has not been transfused within the last 90 days.

Microbiologic techniques employed in the extended workup include culture of the patient and the transfused unit. Should any of these tests yield positive results, gram stain of the positive cultures should be performed. This helps to rapidly identify the causative organism.

Transfusion Reaction Records

All alleged transfusion reactions should be documented in the patient's record. Transfusion reaction records are maintained indefinitely in the blood bank. If bacterial contamination or a transfusion-transmitted disease is detected, the blood collection facility must be notified. Fatalities that are attributed to a transfusion must be reported to the FDA according to their published guidelines.

SUMMARY

Adverse reactions to transfusions are typically categorized. Two ways of categorizing are hemolytic vs. nonhemolytic and immune versus non-immune. The reactions are then placed into each of the categories as appropriate by etiology. Within each of the categories, a specific cause for each class of reaction can be defined. Major adverse reactions and the most common causes are:

- Immune Mediated Reactions
- Acute hemolytic—most often ABO incompatiblities
- Delayed hemolytic—alloantibodies
- Febrile—white blood cell antibodies
- Urticarial—allergen
- Anaphylactic—Anti-IgA in IgA-deficient individual
- TRALI—white blood cells
- GVHD—donor lymphocytes
- Non-Immune Mediated

- Circulatory overload—too much fluid volume transfused
- Bacterial contamination—bacteria in transfused unit
- Iron overload—transfusing more iron than the recipient can excrete
- Disease
- Citrate toxicity

Investigation of alleged transfusion reactions should be conducted in an organized and timely fashion. Any discrepancies discovered in the investigation process should be documented and reported to the individuals treating the patient. This investigation protocol should include cross-check of patient and donor identification, documentation, units transfused, and testing. All testing should be documented and the documentation retained indefinitely.

REVIEW QUESTIONS

1. A common cause of an anaphylactic transfusion reaction is a (an):
   a. previously undetected alloantibody
   b. immunocompetent lymphocytes
   c. anti-IgA reacting with transfused IgA
   d. transfusion of excessive fluid volume

2. HTRs may present with which of the following sets of symptoms?
   a. shortness of breath and pulmonary infiltrates
   b. hives, itching, and erythema
   c. burning at site of infusion, hypotension
   d. decrease in white cell count and increase in BNP

3. Hemolytic transfusion reactions will present with all of the following clinical results *except*:
   a. lipemia
   b. hemoglobinemia
   c. hemoglobinuria
   d. decreased haptoglobin

4. Mechanical destruction of red cells may result from:
   a. saline addition to blood unit
   b. heart valve shearing
   c. alloantibody attachment
   d. change in osmotic pressure

5. Circulatory overload can be differentiated from TRALI by which of the following assessments:
   a. blood pressure
   b. oxygen saturation
   c. temperature
   d. chest x-ray

6. Accumulation of excess iron in the tissues of the body may be seen in:
   a. malaria
   b. sepsis
   c. PNH
   d. thalassemia

7. A technician receives a transfusion work up in the blood bank for assessment. The technician should do which of the following tests?
   1. examine blood bag
   2. check patient identification on samples
   3. compare blood tag with patient identification
   4. compare pre-transfusion plasma for color
   5. DAT on post-transfusion sample
   a. only 1, 3, 4, and 5 are correct
   b. only 1, 2, 3, and 5 are correct
   c. only 2, 3, 4, and 5 are correct
   d. only 2 and 3 are correct
   e. all are correct

8. A delayed HTR may result from which of the following antibodies:
   a. anti-Le^a
   b. anti-M
   c. anti-Jk^a
   d. anti-I

9. Transfusion associated GVHD will most like present in a (an):
   a. newborn
   b. multiparous female
   c. sickle cell anemia patient
   d. platelet transfusion recipient

10. A 35-year-old mother of four had a bowel resection during which she received blood component therapy. One week later she presented to the emergency department of the local hospital with purpura and oozing at the incision site. This complication is most likely related to the transfusion of:
    a. whole blood
    b. packed red cells

c. cryoprecipitate
d. platelet concentrate

11. The product that is most often incriminated for bacterial contamination is:
    a. packed red blood cells
    b. deglycerolized cells
    c. platelet concentrate
    d. leukocyte concentrate

12. A patient presents with hives and itching ½ hour into his transfusion of packed red blood cells. The following step should be taken:
    a. discontinue the transfusion and proceed with a transfusion reaction work up
    b. discontinue the transfusion until all symptoms resolve
    c. continue transfusion after medicating with antihistamine
    d. continue monitoring patient after medicating with broad spectrum antibiotics

13. Factors that affect the severity of a HTR include:
    1. antibody concentration
    2. antigen density on red cell
    3. complement concentration in serum
    4. initial concentration of bradykinin
    5. amount of donor plasma in unit
    a. 1, 2, and 4 are correct
    b. 1, 3, and 5 are correct
    c. 2, 3, and 4 are correct
    d. 1 and 2 are correct
    e. 3 and 5 are correct

14. The renal failure that occurs as a result of an acute HTR directly results as an effect of:
    a. IgM antibody binding to renal cells
    b. bradykinin release
    c. norepinephrine release
    d. histamine release from basophils and mast cells

15. Post-transfusion DAT will be negative in all of the following *except*:
    a. acute HTR
    b. febrile reaction
    c. anaphylactic reaction
    d. urticarial reaction

CASE STUDY

1. A patient originally seen in the trauma unit following a multi-car collision was sent to the OR. The patient collectively received 12 units of packed red cells and 4 units of fresh frozen plasma. All units were type specific and compatible at all phases of testing. The patient was preparing for discharge 5 days later when a 4 gram drop in hemoglobin was noted with some mild jaundice. No hemorrhaging was present and the patient appeared well.

   a. Provide a transfusion-related explanation for these findings.

   b. Suggest testing to prove your theory. Outline the results that you expect to find.

2. A 10-day-old infant was admitted for a transfusion following a hospital stay with significant blood drawing. The hematologist ordered 100 cc of irradiated packed red cells. The hospital must request irradiated cells from a local trauma center. This request is made on a Saturday morning and you are reluctant to make this request as it requires paid couriers and your administration is concerned about expenses.

   a. Is it necessary to provide irradiated blood? If so, why?

   b. Is packed red cells an acceptable alternative?

REFERENCES

Blaney, Kathy and Howard, Paula. *Basic and Applied Concepts of Immunohematology*. Mosby, Philadelphia, 2000.

Brecher, Mark, editor. *American Association of Blood Banks Technical Manual 15th Edition*. AABB, 2005.

Bryan, Sandra, RN, CPAN, "Hemolytic Transfusion Reaction: Safeguards for Practice." *Journal of Perianesthesia Nursing*. Vol. 17, No. 6, 2002, pp. 399–403.

Bux, Jurgen. "The Pathogenesis of Transfusion-Related Acute Lung Injury (TRALI)." *British Journal of Haematology*. Vol. 136, No. 6, 2007, pp. 788–799.

Cherry, Tad. "Transfusion-Related Acute Lung Injury: Past, Present and Future." *American Journal of Clinical Pathology*. Vol. 129, No. 2, 2008, pp. 287–297.

Circular of Information: For the Use of Human Blood and Blood Components. Available at www.aabb.org

Davis, Amanda. "A touch of TRALI." *Transfusion*. Vol. 48, No. 3, 2008, pp. 541–545.

Eder, Anne F. PhD and Chambers, Linda A. MD. "Noninfectious Complications of Blood Transfusion." *Archives of Pathology Laboratory Medicine*. Vol. 131, 2007, pp. 708–718.

Eder, Anne F., et al. "Bacterial Screening of Apheresis Platelets and the Residual Risk of Septic Transfusion Reactions: The American Red Cross Experience (2004-2006)." *Transfusion*. Vol. 47, 2007, pp. 1134–1142.

Jacobs, Michael R., et al. "Relationship between Bacterial Load, Species Virulence, and Transfusion Reaction with Transfusion of Bacterially Contaminated Platelets." *Clinical Infectious Diseases*. Vol. 46, 2008, pp. 1214–1220.

McCullough, Jeffrey. *Transfusion Medicine 2nd Edition*. Elsevier. 2005.

Niu, Manette, et al. "Transfusion-Transmitted *Klebsiella pneumoniae* Fatalities, 1995-2004." *Transfusion Medicine Reviews*. Vol. 20, No. 2, 2006, pp. 149–157.

Prowse, C. "Zero Tolerance." Editorial. *Transfusion*. Vol. 47, 2007, pp. 1106–1109.

Standards for Blood Banks and Transfusion Services, 25th Edition. AABB, Bethesda, MD. 2008.

Uhl, L, and Johnson, S. T. "Evaluation and Management of Acute Hemolytic Transfusion Reactions." *Immunohematology*. Vol. 23, No. 3, 2007, pp. 93–99.

UNIT 5

Hemolytic Disease of the Newborn

Hemolytic Disease of the Fetus and Newborn

LEARNING OUTCOMES

At the completion of this chapter, the reader should be able to:

- Outline criteria for diagnosis and treatment of hemolytic disease of the fetus and newborn (HDFN).
- Describe tests to diagnose presence of HDFN.
- Define and discuss fetomaternal hemorrhage including diagnosis and maternal treatment.
- Compare diagnosis, treatment, and prevention of HDFN caused by ABO, Rh, and other significant antibodies.
- Discuss causes and treatment of fetal and neonatal anemia.
- Compare and contrast HDFN caused by Kell and Rh antibodies
- Describe and discuss Rh immune globulin.
- Discuss antenatal and postpartum administration of Rh immune globulin.
- Outline prenatal and postpartum maternal testing.
- Outline postpartum neonate testing.
- Differentiate invasive and noninvasive methods for diagnosis of HDFN.
- Diagram and interpret Liley graphs.
- Discuss the diagnostic and predictive values of Doppler ultrasonography, flow cytometry, and cell-free fetal DNA techniques
- Outline a plan for prevention of HDFN.
- Differentiate qualitative and quantitative fetal screening methods.
- Describe *in utero* and exchange transfusion indications and techniques.

GLOSSARY

amniocentesis   procedure for removing amniotic fluid for analysis

anemia   decreased oxygen carrying capacity due to low hemoglobin level

antenatal   before birth

Cell-Free Fetal DNA (cff-DNA)   acellular fetal DNA; may be detected in the maternal circulation and used for fetal genotyping

chorionic villus sampling (CVS)   removal of a small piece of placenta tissue (chorionic villi) from the uterus during early pregnancy

cordocentesis   synonym for Percutaneous Umbilical Blood Sampling (PUBS)

erythroblastosis fetalis   a condition in a fetus or neonate where immature red cells, known as erythrobasts, are found in the peripheral circulation

exchange transfusion   transfusion of cells performed after birth that uses a system where some of the infant's cells are removed for each portion of transfused cells that are administered

fetomaternal hemorrhage   fetal bleeding into the maternal circulation

hemolytic disease of the fetus and newborn (HDFN)   clinical condition involving the fetus and the neonate that results in hemolysis of red cells due to maternal antibody coating the red cells of the baby

hydops fetalis   a condition where fluid accumulates in the pleural and peritoneal cavities

in utero   while the fetus is in the uterus

intrauterine transfusion   transfusion administered to a fetus still in the uterus

kernicterus   permanent brain damage resulting from the accumulation of bilirubin in the brain tissue

Kleihauer-Betke acid elution stain   stain with a low pH that will stain fetal cells a dark pink while causing the adult cells to lyse and appear as pale-staining ghost cells

Liley graph   a graph used to evaluate data on spectophotometric analysis of amniotic fluid at 450 nm; the optical density (OD) is plotted against the gestational age

parallel testing   series of tests performed under identical conditions to the patient or control tests; used to rule out contamination or other interferences

Percutaneous Umbilical Blood Sampling (PUBS)   aspiration of a fetal blood sample from the umbilical vein

phototherapy   treatment using lights

postpartum   after giving birth

qualitative   establishes presence of a substance but does not determine the quantity

quantitative   determines the amount of a substance present

Rh immune globulin   concentrated anti-D commercially processed for administration prevent Rh hemolytic disease of the newborn

rosette   clump of cells consisting of a central cell surrounded by other cells

serial amniocentesis   the process of multiple comparative amniocentesis procedures to monitor changes in the status of the *in utero* fetus

titer   measurement of strength of an antibody by testing its reactivity with decreasing amounts of the appropriate antigen; reciprocal of the highest dilution that shows agglutination is the titer

Wharton's jelly   sticky connective tissue substance found on the umbilical cord

INTRODUCTION

Hemolytic disease of the fetus and newborn (HDFN), also known as erythroblastosis fetalis, is an anemic condition in neonates and fetuses. This is a condition where maternal antibody crosses the placental barrier and sensitizes the fetal red blood cells. The fetus or neonate destroys these antibody-coated cells. The red cell destruction produces a clinical condition with severity on a continuum from mild anemia to death of the infant. The transfusion service provides the obstetrical service with assistance in the prediction, prevention, diagnosis, and treatment of this condition.

MECHANISM FOR HDFN

During pregnancy, the mother's body, as well as the body of the developing fetus, is not static or without interaction. The placenta is a multi-purpose organ that creates a barrier between mother and infant. The organ also functions to exchange oxygen, nutrients, and waste.

While not impervious to fetal cells, the barrier serves to limit the passage of cells from the fetus to mother. A feto-maternal hemorrhage occurs when some fetal cells pass into the maternal circulation. Passage of fetal cells most often occurs at the time of separation of the placenta from the uterine wall. This passage of fetal cells may occur at other times such as amniocentesis, chorionic villi sampling (CVS), or as a result of maternal abdominal trauma.

Whether fetal cells cross the placenta during the pregnancy or at the time of delivery, they may stimulate antibody production by the mother. If the antibody is IgG, in nature, it has the ability to cross the placenta. If the antibody is produced during an existing pregnancy, it may not have a significant effect on the *in utero* fetus, but will impact a subsequent pregnancy with an antigen positive fetus. The antibody may also be a naturally occurring antibody, such as anti-A. The causative antibodies of HDFN may be placed into three categories. These are summarized in Table 13-1.

Regardless of the origin of the antibody, while the fetus is *in utero*, the antibody may cross the placenta and attach to the corresponding antigens on the red blood cells of the fetus. Red blood cell destruction occurs in the liver and spleen of the fetus. Hemoglobin released from the red blood cells is metabolized to indirect bilirubin. This bilirubin is actively transported across the placenta. The mother's liver conjugates the bilirubin and the mother excretes the water soluble, direct bilirubin. Maternal secretion of the waste products of hemolysis diminishes or alleviates the detrimental effects on the fetus. See Figure 13-1 for a summary of this process.

As hemolysis continues, the infant becomes increasingly anemic. The anemia leads to additional detrimental effects. The fetus may be at risk for cardiac failure. Progression of anemia results in resumption of extramedullary erythropoiesis in the infant's spleen and liver. This physiologic adjustment occurs to help compensate for the ongoing hemolysis. As the anemia progresses, organs enlarge and fluid accumulates in the pleural and peritoneal cavities creating a condition known as hydops fetalis. Immature cells (erythrobasts) are released into the fetal circulation.

Transfusion therapy to treat the advancing anemia may begin *in utero*. Treatment, whether *in utero* or post-partum, focuses on correction of anemia and bilirubinemia. After delivery, red blood cell destruction continues with the release and accumulation of indirect bilirubin. Bilirubin is no longer conjugated and excreted by the mother. As a result, the neonate must independently conjugate the accumulating bilirubin. The neonate may not have the enzyme, known as glucuronyl transferase, that is required for conjugation of bilirubin. The unconjugated, indirect, bilirubin accumulates in the tissues. Since this form of bilirubin is lipid soluble, it can bind to the tissues of the central nervous system. When indirect bilirubin levels rise to critical levels, it can cause brain damage or kernicterus.

ABO HDFN

ABO HDFN is the most common, while Rh hemolytic disease is usually the most severe. ABO HDFN may affect a first pregnancy whereas Rh HDFN is rarely exhibited in the initial pregnancy. Clinical findings and test results for ABO and Rh HDFN are summarized in Table 13-2. HDFN caused by other antibodies is uncommon, but may be severe. Causative antibodies, other than ABO antibodies and anti-RhD, are summarized in Table 13-4.

The most common scenario for ABO hemolytic disease is a group O mother and a group A infant, although other combinations of maternal and infant blood groups may also result in HDFN. The causative antibodies are in the maternal circulation. The antibodies cross the placenta and attach to the red cells of the infant if the corresponding antigen is present. In spite of high antibody titers, the decreased severity of ABO HDFN may be related to the following factors:

- ABO antigens are not well developed on the red cells of a fetus or newborn

- The number of antigen sites is reduced in newborns

- A and B substances may be found in secretions. These soluble substances will neutralize the antibodies. This reduces the severity of the reaction.

These infants may show mild elevations in bilirubin and jaundice. Phototherapy or exchange transfusion

TABLE 13-1 Categories of Hemolytic Disease of the Fetus and Newborn

Rh HDFN (Anti-RhD)
ABO HDFN
HDFN Caused by Other Antibodies

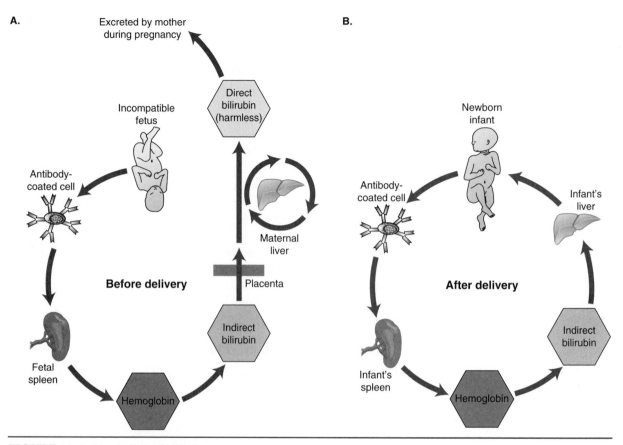

FIGURE 13-1 Metabolism of bilirubin.
A. Prior to delivery, bilirubin is metabolized by the maternal liver and excreted safely.
B. Following delivery, the infant's immature liver cannot conjugate the bilirubin since the enzyme, glucuronyl transferase, is not produced. This unconjugated bilirubin accumulates in the tissues with potentially dangerous sequelae, brain damage or kernicterus.
Reprinted from Blood Group Antigens and Antibodies as Applied to Hemolytic Disease of the Newborn. *Ortho Diagnostics, 1968, Raritan, NJ.*

may be necessary. Testing and investigation incorporates the same tests as Rh hemolytic disease and will be discussed in a later section.

Rh HDFN

A typical scenario for Rh HDFN is summarized in Table 13-3. Potential for Rh HDFN is determined by testing all expectant mothers. ABO, Rh, and antibody screen testing are performed. Typically, the antibody develops as a result of the first (or a previous) pregnancy. The newly developed antibody will rarely have effects during the initial pregnancy. If anti-D is identified in the serum, a titer is performed to determine the origin as natural or passively acquired from administration of RhIg.

In subsequent pregnancies with Rh positive infants, the antibody crosses the placenta and binds to the Rh positive red cells. The infant may be affected to varying degrees. If anti-D is in the serum during the pregnancy, an extended test panel including antibody screen and antibody titers will be performed on the mother throughout the pregnancy. The fetus may require transfusion *in utero* or treatment may not be required until the postpartum period. Postpartum, the infant will be monitored for rising bilirubin levels and increasing anemia. Exchange transfusion may be instituted if the bilirubin levels rise to critical levels.

TABLE 13-2 Clinical Observations and Test Results for ABO and Rh Hemolytic Disease of the Newborn

	NORMAL INFANT	ABO HDFN	RH HDFN
Clinical Findings			
Jaundice	Physiologic	None to Mild	Mild to Severe
Hepatosplenomegaly	No	No	Mild to Severe
Edema	No	No	Mild to Severe
Serologic Results			
ABO Group	Any ABO Group	Mother Group O Newborn A or B	Any ABO Group
Rh type	Any Rh Type	Any Rh type	Mother D-negative Newborn D-positive
DAT	Negative	Negative or Weakly Positive	Positive
Antibody	None	Anti-A, Anti-B, Anti-A,B	Anti-D
Hematology Results			
Hemoglobin	16 to 28 g/dl	Mild: >13 g/dl	Mild: >13 g/dl Moderate: 8–13 g/dl Severe: <8 g/dl
Reticulocyte Count	2 to 6%	Mild Increase	Greatly increased
Blood Smear Morphology	Normal	Spherocytes	Macrocytes, Hypochromia
NRBC/100 WBC's	10 to −20%	Mild Increase	Greatly Increased
Chemistry Results			
Bilirubin	1 to 3 mg/dl	Mild Increase	Often >20 mg/dl
Value of Prenatal Testing		None	Useful
Occurrence in First Pregnancy		Often	Rare

This article was published in Basic and Applied Concepts of Immunohematology, *Blaney, Kathy D. and Howard, Paula R., Mosby, p. 287, Copyright Elsevier (2000).*

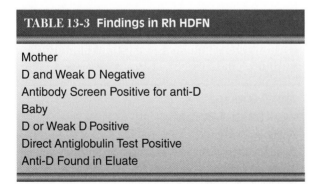

TABLE 13-3 Findings in Rh HDFN

Mother
D and Weak D Negative
Antibody Screen Positive for anti-D
Baby
D or Weak D Positive
Direct Antiglobulin Test Positive
Anti-D Found in Eluate

Additional Alloantibodies Causing HDFN

Any antibody that crosses the placenta has the potential to cause HDFN in an infant with antigen positive cells.

As with RhD, the potential for hemolytic disease can be determined by screening the mother early in the pregnancy. "*KEL1* (K) antigen of the Kell Blood group system is second to RhD as a cause of hemolytic disease of the fetus and newborn (HDFN)." Anti-K is followed in frequency of HDFN by anti-c.

Antibodies to the Kell system warrant additional discussion. Anti-K, as a causative antibody for HDFN, is encountered second in frequency to anti-D. The severity of the Kell system antibodies parallels that of anti-D. The determination of severity of HDFN caused by the Kell system antibodies requires different parameters. The parameters used to predict HDFN caused by Rh antibodies do not have the same predictive value for Kell antibodies. The Kell antigens are developed early in the gestational period. The mechanism of fetal anemia in Kell sensitization is projected to be both hemolysis and

TABLE 13-4 Antibodies That Cause Hemolytic Disease of the Newborn

Rh Antibodies
Anti-C
Anti-E
Anti-c*
Anti-e
Kell System Antibodies
Anti-K*
Anti-k
Duffy System Antibodies
Anti-Fy^a
Anti-Fy^b
Kidd System Antibodies
Anti-Jk^a
Anti-Jk^b
MNSs System Antibodies
Anti-S
Anti-s

Most frequently encountered after anti-D

erythropoietic suppression. Anti-Kell antibodies have a lower level of reticulocytosis and erythroblastosis. The inverse relationship between fetal hematocrit and reticulocyte count encountered in anti-D sensitized pregnancies is not encountered in Kell sensitized pregnancies. Due to the severity of HDFN with Kell antibodies, it has been proposed that women of child-bearing age be transfused with phenotypically identical blood for the Kell system antigens.

As molecular diagnostic techniques have developed, it is possible to determine the genetic makeup of the fetus while *in utero*. The blood bank can predict and provide antenatal intervention for affected infants. The specific diagnostic tools will be discussed later in this chapter.

PREDICTION OF HDFN

Historically, prenatal testing for prediction of HDFN has focused on the mother. ABO and RhD testing, as well as antibody screen and identification, comprise the panel of prenatal tests. As molecular diagnostic techniques have developed, available test methods and accuracy of diagnosis have expanded. The purpose of testing, however, has not changed. The laboratory is still focused on:

1. Identifying RhD negative women to determine women who are candidates for Rh immune globulin.

2. Determining the presence of an antibody that may place the fetus at risk for HDFN.

3. In the presence of a potentially harmful antibody, testing the father for the presence of antigens that could place the fetus at risk for HDFN.

Prenatal testing should be performed early in the pregnancy. Women with clinically significant antibodies should be followed through the course of the pregnancy. A summary of prenatal testing for predicting HDFN is presented in Table 13-5.

Obstetrical History

An accurate obstetrical history is imperative to determine risk to the fetus. History of delivery of an affected infant will increase the risk of subsequent infants being affected by the same antigen-antibody combination. While obstetrical history is not the responsibility of the blood bank laboratory, advance information provides notice that an affected infant may be presenting either prior to delivery or postpartum. If an atypical antibody is detected in the maternal plasma, the father should be tested for the corresponding antigen. If the paternal cells are antigen negative, monitoring throughout the pregnancy is not necessary.

TABLE 13-5 Summary of Maternal Laboratory Testing for Prediction of HDFN

ABO and Rh test
Weak D Test, if indicated
Antibody Screen
Antibody Identification, if indicated by antibody screen
Antibody Titration, if indicated by identification of a clinically significant antibody
Paternal Antigen Testing, if indicated by presence of HDFN causative antibody
Follow-Up Testing
Repeat Titration, if indicated

Antibody Titration

Historically, identification of an antibody in the maternal serum indicates need for periodic monitoring of antibody titer throughout the pregnancy. Serial dilutions of the mother's serum tested with antigen positive cells are performed to determine the antibody titer or amount of antibody present. Each serum sample should be aliquoted (divided) and frozen when the initial testing is complete. These frozen aliquots are then used for parallel testing. For purposes of comparison, an aliquot of the previous test serum is tested concurrently with the current test sample. The results of the two sera are compared to determine a change in the amount or titer of antibody present in the maternal serum. This principle of parallel titers is performed each time a new sample is tested. For an example of a titer with results (see Figure 13-2). Testing should begin early in the pregnancy and be repeated every 4 weeks up to the 28th week. After that point, titers should be performed weekly until delivery of the fetus.

As the pregnancy progresses and titers are performed, the physician will evaluate the results for an increase in the level of the titer. A significant change in titer

	Dilution Strength							
	1:1	1:2	1:4	1:8	1:16	1:32	1:64	1:128
Sample #1	4+	4+	3+	2+	1+	0	0	0
Sample #2 (4 weeks later)	4+	4+	4+	3+	2+	1+	1+	0

FIGURE 13-2 Sample titer results from a plasma containing anti-RhD
Source: Delmar, Cengage Learning

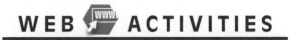

WEB ACTIVITIES

1. Type www.traqprogram.ca into your browser.
2. Choose "Continuing Education." Then from the drop-down choose "Case Studies."
3. Scroll down and choose "View Level A Case Studies."
4. Choose Case A3 "Multiple antibodies in a mother delivering twins."
5. Choose each of the available sets of test results.
6. Return to "Case Studies."
7. Scroll down and choose "View Level B Case Studies."
8. Choose Case B2 "Positive DAT in a neonate."
9. Choose each of the available sets of test results.
10. Search the remaining areas of the web site and review appropriate material.

CRITICAL THINKING ACTIVITY

interpret the following titer results:

1. Antibody Identified: Anti-E

	1:2	1:4	1:8	1:16	1:32	1:64	1:128	1:256
Titer #4	4+	4+	4+	2+	1+	0	0	0
Titer #3	4+	3+	1+	0	0	0	0	0

2. Antibody Identified: Anti-K

	1:2	1:4	1:8	1:16	1:32	1:64	1:128	1:256
Titer #3	4+	4+	4+	2+	0	0	0	0
Titer #2	4+	1+	1+	0	0	0	0	0

3. Antibody Identified: Anti-D

	1:2	1:4	1:8	1:16	1:32	1:64	1:128	1:256
Titer #4	4+	4+	1+	1+	0	0	0	0
Titer #3	4+	3+	1+	0	0	0	0	0

For each example:
Decide if the results are significant and suggest treatment for each newborn.

is indicated by an increase of two or more tubes. If the titer remains stable, it is likely that the fetus does not possess the antigen that corresponds to the antibody in the maternal serum. For Rh and other significant antibodies, a value of 32 or greater is significant and an amniocentesis should be considered. For anti-K and anti-k a titer of eight is considered a significant finding.

If the titer demonstrates a significant increase, additional testing and treatment of the fetus may be necessary. Interventions may occur before delivery and/or postpartum. Intrauterine transfusion takes place before birth while exchange transfusion is a postpartum treatment option. For both procedures, crossmatch is performed using the mother's plasma which contains the original antibody.

Invasive Procedures

Invasive procedures for diagnosis and monitoring of HDFN include amniocentesis and chorionic villus sampling (CVS). These procedures are performed to obtain additional clinical information related to the infant and the status of hemolysis as the pregnancy progresses.

Amniocentesis

Amniocentesis is the removal of a small amount of amniotic fluid for analysis. A sample of amniotic fluid is extracted by insertion of a needle through the abdominal wall and uterus. The fluid is scanned spectophotmetrically from 350 to 700 nm. The change in optical density (OD) at 450 nm will indicate bilirubin pigments in the fluid. A comparison is made between the baseline at 450 nm and the actual reading of the amniotic fluid. This diagnostic tool does not have good predictive value of the severity of HDFN in the Kell alloimmunized pregnancy where lower levels of bilirubin are exhibited in the amniotic fluid (see Figure 13-3).

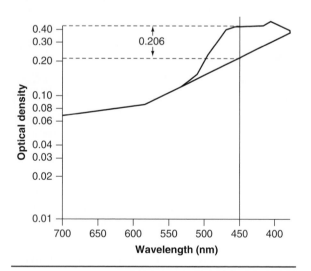

FIGURE 13-3 The difference in OD between a baseline and the amniotic fluid is plotted and compared. The result is plotted on a Liley graph to determine the correct course of treatment. *Adapted from: Blaney and Howard, Basic and Applied Concepts of Immunohematology.*

The ΔOD is plotted on a Liley graph. The Liley graph is a plot of Δ 450 and weeks of gestation. Interpretation of the Liley graph will estimate the severity of the HDFN. A reading of 0.206 at 35 weeks correlates with severe HDFN (see Figure 13-4). The upper zone correlates to severe HDFN while the midzone correlates with moderate disease. Information obtained from this analysis are used to monitor the pregnancy and determine the clinical course. Amniocentesis is repeated periodically over the course of an affected pregnancy. This process is serial amniocentesis.

Amniocentesis is an invasive procedure that carries risk of fetal death, fetal or maternal hemorrhage, spontaneous abortion, and increased risk of fetomaternal hemorrhage. Fetomaternal hemorrhage may expose the mother to antigen incompatible cells and the risk of additional red cell stimulated antibodies. Noninvasive procedures carry less risk, but may not be available in all clinical settings.

CVS

CVS is the removal of a small piece of placental tissue (chorionic villi) early in the pregnancy. This procedure may be performed either through the cervix or through the abdominal wall. The antigen status of the fetus may be determined with CVS. As with amniocentesis, CVS is invasive and carries risks for both the fetus and mother.

Percutaneous Umbilical Blood Sampling (PUBS)

Percutaneous Umbilical Blood Sampling (PUBS) or cordocentesis is a collection method for *in utero* fetal blood sampling. An ultrasound is used to guide a needle into the umbilical vein near the point of placental insertion, and a blood sample is aspirated. The sample may be used for hemoglobin and hematocrit determinations as a direct measurement of anemia, bilirubin levels, or other chemical variables. The sample may also be used to determine the genetic composition of the fetus. Phenotyping the blood and comparing to the maternal phenotype is done to verify that the sample is fetal in origin. This procedure may be used for infusion of red cells, if necessary.

Noninvasive Procedures

Doppler Ultrasonography

A noninvasive procedure for determination of fetal anemia was introduced by Mari and coworkers. Measurement of

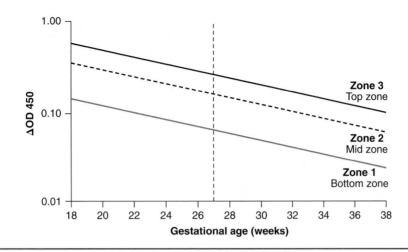

FIGURE 13-4 The Liley graph is used to interpret results of spectophotometric analysis of amniotic fluid. The difference in OD at 450 nm is plotted and compared to the three zones. The endpoint zone will determine the course of treatment.
Source: Delmar, Cengage Learning

peak velocity of blood flow in the fetal middle cerebral artery is determined with Dopler ultrasonography. An anemic fetus, presents with increased cardiac output, increased blood velocity and low blood viscosity. The blood velocity is evaluated on the middle cerebral artery (MCA). The blood velocity is measured in multiples of the median (MoMs). A threshold value of 1.5 MoMs for the peak MA velocity is used to predict moderate to severe anemia. These fetal adaptations will oxygenate peripheral tissues. The degree of anemia can be predicted with 100% sensitivity and a false positive rate of 10%.

Cell-Free Fetal DNA Testing (cff DNA)

Cell-Free Fetal DNA (cff-DNA) can be detected in maternal plasma as early as the seventh week of gestation. The amount of cff-DNA increases with gestational age. Utilizing polymerase chain reaction (PCR) on maternal plasma, cff-DNA can be detected and the genotype of the fetus determined. If the fetus carries the antigen corresponding to the maternal antibody, additional monitoring and treatment may be necessary throughout the pregnancy.

POSTPARTUM TESTING OF NEONATES

A diagnosis of HDFN has been made while the fetus is *in utero*. Postpartum, the cord blood or capillary sample, is used to perform initial testing on the neonate. If a cord blood sample is used, the sample should be washed several times to remove the connective tissue substance, Wharton's jelly. Wharton's jelly may cause false positive agglutination if present in the sample. ABO forward grouping, Rh typing, and direct antiglobulin testing are included in the initial neonatal test battery. Neonates born of Rh negative mothers are tested to determine the need for administration of Rh immune globulin to the mother.

ABO Testing

The forward ABO grouping is performed on neonates. ABO antigens may not be fully developed on the red cells of newborns. Hence, weaker reactions may be seen when testing neonates as compared to those seen in adult patients. Antisera should be used according to manufacturers instructions.

Since antibody production has not yet begun in a neonate, reverse grouping is not performed.

Rh Testing

Rh testing of neonates should be interpreted with caution if a positive DAT exists. The Rh antigen sites could be blocked with maternal antibody. This would prevent the antibodies in the antisera from attaching to the antigens on the red cells and result in a false negative reaction. False positive results may also result from a positive DAT. Elution and identification of the antibody would resolve typing discrepancies. Use of appropriate reagent controls supports the validity of an Rh positive result. Manufacturers' instructions will provide information on control procedures.

DAT

A DAT should be performed on every newborn suspected of having an incompatibility that may result in HDFN. Careful observation of the DAT is necessary for detection of weak reactions. Weak reactions in the DAT test is especially problematic with ABO HDFN. If the DAT is positive, an eluate may be performed on the sample. Elution may be optional if antibody identification studies are performed on the mother at the time of admission.

If a newborn's DAT is positive and the maternal antibody screen is negative, ABO HDFN may be suspected. This can be confirmed with either a freeze-thaw or heat elution test. The eluate is tested against A_1, B, and O cells using an antiglobulin technique. A positive reaction in either A_1 or B cells confirms ABO HDFN. It the eluate is negative, further exploration of antibody specificity should be performed.

PREVENTION OF RH HEMOLYTIC DISEASE OF THE FETUS AND NEWBORN

The development of any IgG antibody directed against a red cell antigen may create serious consequences for an infant that carries the specific antigen for the maternal antibody. The development of an antibody via exposure in pregnancy or transfusion represents a permanent condition that cannot be reversed. Avoiding immunization to red cell antigens, especially anti-RhD, is important in women of child-bearing age. The development and administration of Rh immune globulin has significantly reduced the number of cases of Rh HDFN by preventing development of anti-D in the mother. Criteria for administration of Rh immune globulin are summarized in Table 13-6.

Rh Immune Globulin (RhIg)

Rh immune globulin (RhIg) is concentrated anti-D prepared from pools of human plasma. The antibody is a human product commercially purified, titered, and packaged for sale under trade names. The product is

TABLE 13-6 Criteria for Administration of Rh Immune Globulin

Mother
Rh negative, Weak D Negative
Antibody Screen for anti-D (Prior to 28-Week Administration)
Infant
Rh Positive (Or Potentially Rh Positive)

administered via intramuscular injection or intravenously to Rh negative women at 28 weeks of gestation (antenatal) and again within 72 hours of delivery of an Rh positive infant (postpartum). There should be postpartum confirmation of the presence of the D antigen on the surface of the red cells of any infant born to an Rh negative mother. Postpartum mothers having received a 28-week administration of RhIg should receive another full dose within 72 hours of delivery of an Rh positive infant. The presence of IgG antibodies other than anti-D does not require the administration of this product.

Rh immune globulin is packaged in 300 μg doses for use with any pregnancy progressing beyond the first trimester. A 300 μg dose will counteract up to 15 ml of Rh positive red cells (30 ml of Rh positive whole blood). Rh immune globulin is also administered to an Rh negative mother following the termination of any pregnancy, amniocentesis, chorionic villus sampling, PUBS, intrauterine transfusion, or abdominal trauma.

Smaller doses of 50 μg are commercially available and may to be administered up to the end of the first trimester. The criterion for administration is potential for red blood cell exposure (feto-maternal hemorrhage) before 12 weeks of gestation when the fetal blood volume is less than 2.5 ml.

Determining Dosage of Rh Immune Globulin

Events before or during delivery may result in a fetomaternal hemorrhage (FMH) of more than 30 ml of fetal blood. When this occurs, greater than one vial of Rh immune globulin must be administered to prevent the mother from developing the anti-D antibody. All Rh negative postpartum mothers should be tested for evidence of significant FMH. Tests methods available include: the rosette test and Kleihauer-Betke acid elution stain (both available in kit form). The rosette test is a qualitative test. Positive results must be quantitated. The Kleihauer-Betke test is a quantitative test to determine the quantity of the fetal bleed. Flow cytometry for quantitation of cells with fetal hemoglobin is a more accurate method for determining the volume of fetal cells present in the maternal circulation.

Fetal Screen Methods

Fetal screen kits use a method that exhibits production of rosettes in a positive test. A maternal sample of anticoagulated blood is used. The cells are incubated with anti-D. This allows attachment of the antibody to any fetal cells in the sample. Following incubation, the cells are washed to remove excess antibody. Indicator cells are added to the washed patient sample. The indicator cells are Rh positive cells. If the fetal cells are antibody coated during incubation, the Rh-positive indicator cells will attach to the free arm of the anti-D molecules that have bound to the fetal cells. The indicator cells will surround the fetal cells and appear as a rosette. See Figure 13-5 for a pictorial explanation of rosette formation.

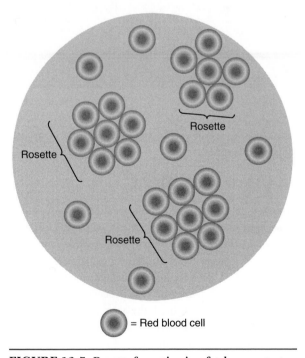

FIGURE 13-5 Rosette formation in a fetal screen test
Source: Delmar, Cengage Learning

After the addition of indicator cells, the mixture is centrifuged and examined microscopically. The appearance of rosettes is considered a positive result. Positive and negative controls are used. When interpreting the patient's test results, a comparison to the controls is made. A quantitative test method is performed on all positive fetal screens.

Quantifying the Fetomaternal Hemorhage

The Kleihauer-Betke acid elution stain is a method that quantifies the volume of fetomaternal hemorrhage. The method consists of a buffer with an acid pH. When applied to thin smears of a maternal sample, this buffer will cause the adult cells to lose their hemoglobin. The hemoglobin F present in fetal cells will be resistant to this loss of hemoglobin. The smear is stained and examined under oil immersion. Adult cells appear as pale ghost cells while the fetal cells will stain dark pink. See Figure 13-6 for a visual comparison of fetal and adult cells in an acid elution procedure. The calculations used to determine volume of fetal bleed and dose of RhIg required are summarized in Table 13-7.

For a final determination of the number of doses, the calculated number must be converted to a whole number. Since this method has a large margin of error, the final dose should be "padded" to be certain that a sufficient dose of RhIg has been administered. If the decimal is less than five, the number should be rounded down and one dose added. If the decimal is equal to or greater than five, the number should be rounded up and one dose added. In the above example, 3.3 is rounded down to three and one dose added. This provides a final dose of four vials of RhIg.

Flow Cytometry

Rosetting techniques and acid elution stains are methods historically used for screening and quantifying FMH. Both methods are imprecise. Flow cytometric methods for quantitation of fetal RBC have been cleared through the FDA. There are two flow methods that may be used:

1. Anti-HbF method: Intracellular staining of red blood cells for the level of hemoglobin F.

2. Anti-D method: Presence or absence of the D antigen on the red blood cell surface using anti-D.

SAMPLE PROCEDURE 13-1

1. Label three tubes for the rosette test: patient, positive control, and negative control.
2. Add one drop of patient cells to the patient tube.
3. Add one drop of the appropriate control cell to the appropriate tube.
4. Add one drop of fetal screen antibody reagent to each of the three tubes.
5. Incubate the tubes at 37°C for 20 minutes.
6. Wash all tubes with saline three times. Following the third wash, blot the tubes with gauze before reinverting the tubes.
7. Add one drop of indicator cells to the three tubes.
8. Read tubes macroscopically and microscopically.
9. Observe for rosettes
10. Record results on the appropriate worksheet or appropriate field in the laboratory information system.

Interpretation

Patient	Positive Control	Negative Control	
Negative (less than 7 clumps in 5 fields)	+	O	Bleed has not occurred
Positive (greater than 7 clumps in 5 fields	+	O	Bleed has occurred; perform Kleihauer
O	+	+	Invalid; repeat test
+	+	+	Invalid; repeat test
O	O	O	**Invalid**; repeat test

The anti-Hb-F method uses monoclonal antibodies and flow cytometry to detect high levels of hemoglobin F in the fetal cells. This method correlates very well with the acid elution stain and provides accurate at quantitation of FMH. The anti-D method is applicable for detection of Rh incompatibility and support of Rh immune globulin therapy and may offer more wide reaching applications.

TREATMENT OF HEMOLYTIC DISEASE OF THE FETUS AND NEWBORN

Treatment of HDFN will parallel the severity of the disease as it progresses through pregnancy and the symptoms displayed postpartum. The percentage of successful outcomes for the affected fetus parallels the prompt initiation of treatment.

In Utero Treatment

Assessing the results of the diagnostic tools previously described, the medical team will develop and initiate a plan of action for treatment of the fetus while in utero. If warranted by severity, intrauterine transfusion (IUT) may be initiated. IUTs were historically administered by intraperiotoneal transfusion. This process was performed by passing a needle through the abdomen of the mother and into the peritoneal cavity of the fetus. The blood was infused into the peritoneum of the fetus. It was absorbed from the peritoneum into the circulation. Disadvantages included inability to transfuse prior to 25 weeks of gestation and the uncertainty of volume absorbed from the peritoneum. Development of PUBS has introduced the

TABLE 13-7 Calculations for Quantifying FMH

1. Percentage of Fetal Cells = Number of Fetal Cells/Total Cells Counted
2. Volume of Fetal Cells = Percentage of Fetal Cells × 50
3. Dose of RhIg = Volume of the FMH/30 = Number of Doses of RhIg
4. Final Calculation:
   - Decimal = less than 5 → round down and add one dose
   - Decimal = equal to or greater than 5 → round up and add one dose

Example

Results of Kleihauer-Betke Test: 20 fetal cells/1000 cells counted = 2.0%

Volume of FMH: 2.0 × 50 = 100 ml of Rh Positive fetal blood

Required doses of RhIg: 100/30 = 3.3 doses

Final Calculation = 3 doses (rounded down) + 1 = 4 doses for administration

CRITICAL THINKING ACTIVITY

Calculate the required dose of Rh immune globulin for each of the following scenarios:

1. Kleihauer-Betke Test: 4 fetal cells/1000 cells counted
2. Kleihauer-Betke Test: 329 fetal cells/1000 cells counted
3. Kleihauer-Betke Test: 150 fetal cells/1000 cells counted

application of this process for transfusion of red cells directly into the fetus via the umbilical vein. This method is advantageous since it allows transfusion as early as 17 weeks. It also allows for determination of hematocrit in the fetus. This permits more accurate monitoring and determination of the volume of red cells to transfuse.

Component selection for transfusion consists of group O, D negative red blood cells that are less than seven days old. The unit should be screened and found to be negative for CMV and hemoglobin S. The red blood cells are packed to a hematocrit of 75 to 80%. This packing prevents overload and allows for a sufficient blood viscosity to allow the cells to be transfused without hemolysis. The unit should be irradiated to prevent graft vs. host disease (GVHD). These donor cells are crossmatched using the maternal plasma. Multiple transfusions of O negative cells *in utero* may result in a neonate that presents as O negative at birth due to the presence of donor cells and the absence of the neonates own cells.

Postpartum Treatment

Treatment of the affected neonate will be dependent on *in utero* treatment and the severity of anemia and jaundice at birth. The treatment regimen may change as the neonates own physiologic systems begin to function. The neonate's ability to metabolize and compensate for the anemic process may not be sufficient to clear the waste products and keep up with the rate of hemolysis. The need for additional intervention will be determined by monitoring progressing anemia and increasing jaundice.

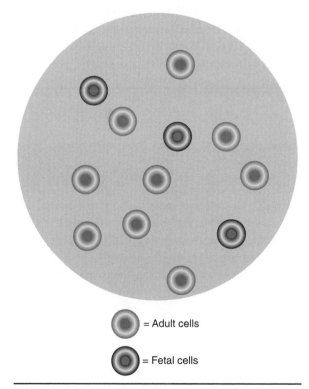

= Adult cells

= Fetal cells

FIGURE 13-6 Kleihauer-Betke staining of fetal and adult cells. Fetal cells stain dark while the adult cells are pale ghost cells
Source: Delmar, Cengage Learning

Phototherapy

Neonates experiencing HDFN may continue to accumulate bilirubin after birth, bilirubinemia. When the bilirubin level approaches a level where the infant is in danger of developing kernicterus, treatment for the bilirubinemia will be initiated. Phototherapy, or the use of ultraviolet lights, is used to conjugate bilirubin deposited near the skin. The neonate is exposed to fluorescent blue light in the 420 to 475 nm range. The unconjugated bilirubin undergoes photoisomerization to photobilirubin. The formed isomers are carried to the liver and excreted in the bile. ABO hemolytic disease is often responsive to phototherapy with no need for additional treatment. If the jaundice does not resolve with phototherapy, exchange transfusion may be necessary.

Exchange Transfusion

Anemia and hyperbilirubinemia are the major complications of HDFN. While hyperbilirubinemia is treatable with phototherapy, anemia requires correction with transfusion. Hyperbilirubinemia may be severe enough to require additional treatment. Exchange transfusion will correct both of these complications of HDFN. Exchange involves transfusing small amounts of red cells and removing equal portions. The criteria for initiating exchange transfusion is summarized in Table 13-8.

Additional considerations for initiating exchange transfusion include prematurity, low birth weight, sepsis, or deterioration of the CNS system. Premature infants have lower threshold for bilirubin toxicity. One or more existing criteria may lead the medical staff to initiate exchange the infant with lower bilirubin levels.

Selection of Blood and Pretransfusion Testing for Exchange Transfusion. The neonate's ABO and Rh type are determined at birth. As previously discussed, a neonate transfused *in utero* will often type as O negative. The blood bank personnel should be aware of previous transfusion with O negative cells. Plasma from the mother or infant may be used for the antibody screen. Often, the mother's sample is used since it is readily available and is the source of maternal antibody with the highest titer. The red cells to be transfused should be antigen negative for the antigen corresponding to the causative antibody. Cells that are ABO compatible with both mother and infant may be chosen for transfusion. If a non-group O infant receives A or B cells, the serum of the infant must be tested against A_1 and B cells using the indirect antiglobulin technique. If anti-A or anti-B is detected, Group O cells should be transfused. Institutional policy may exclusively use O negative red cells.

The red cells may be reconstituted with fresh frozen plasma (FFP). A hematocrit of 40 to 50% is achieved with the FFP. Group specific (or group AB) FFP is employed for this purpose. Additional criteria for selection of blood for exchange transfusion are summarized in Table 13-9.

TABLE 13-8 Criteria for Exchange Transfusion

- Cord blood bilirubin is 5 mg/dl at birth
- Plasma bilirubin rising to 11.5 mg/dl within 12 hours after birth *or* above 16 mg/dl within 24 hours after birth
- Rate of increase of plasma bilirubin is greater than 0.5 mg/dl
- Hemoglobin <14.0 g/dl

TABLE 13-9 Criteria for Blood Selection for Exchange Transfusion

- ABO compatible or group O D-negative blood
- Fresh red cells (less than seven days old)
- Irradiated blood (prevent GVHD)
- CMV and hemoglobin S negative
- Compatible with maternal serum; including antigen negative

SUMMARY

HDFN is a condition that results from a maternal antibody that corresponds to antigens on the fetal cells. Antibodies must be IgG in nature have the ability to cross the placenta. Specific antibodies include:

- ABO
- Rh
- Other Blood Group Antibodies: Kell, Duffy, Kidd, for example

Prenatal testing for maternal samples include: ABO, Rh, antibody screen, and identification, if indicated. Antibody titers may be performed at regular intervals throughout the pregnancy. Paternal testing may be performed if indicated by the maternal results.

After the antibodies cross the placenta and coat the red blood cells, the physiologic issues include red cell hemolysis, increased bilirubin, and anemia. Maternal excretion of waste products helps to minimize detrimental effects of the fetus. As the anemia increases,

intrauterine transfusion may be utilized as a treatment method. Diagnostic techniques for the fetus include:

- Amniocentesis
- CVS
- Doppler Ultrasonography
- Flow Cytometry
- Cell Free DNA Analysis

Postpartum testing of maternal and neonatal samples will confirm the presence and indicate the severity of HDFN. Treatment of an affected newborn includes phototherapy and exchange transfusion.

Rh hemolytic disease may be prevented with Rh immune globulin. This is administered antenatally and postpartum. Postpartum maternal screening includes resetting techniques and Kleihauer-Betke staining. Dosage of Rh immune globulin may be calculated based on the results of the screening tests.

REVIEW QUESTIONS

1. Phototherapy is most useful for which of the following antibodies:
   a. Anti-A
   b. Anti-D
   c. Anti-K
   d. Anti-S

2. Hyperbilirubinemia *in utero* may be corrected by:
   a. amniocentesis
   b. exchange transfusion
   c. maternal conjugation
   d. ultrasonography

3. All of the following tests are used for prediction of HDFN *except:*
   a. Rh typing
   b. weak D testing
   c. antibody screen
   d. Kleihauer-Betke

4. An antibody is identified in a prenatal maternal sample. From the following list choose the antibody (ies) that could cause HDFN:
   1. Anti-C
   2. Anti-M

3. Anti-Fy^a
4. Anti-P
5. Anti-Le^a
   a. 1, 2, and 3 are correct
   b. 2, 4, and 5 are correct
   c. 1 and 3 are correct
   d. 2 and 4 are correct
   e. 1 and 5 are correct
   f. Only 1 is correct

5. From the following prenatal testing scenarios, choose the mother that is eligible for administration of Rh immune globulin:
   a. Rh negative, with anti-K identified; Rh positive father
   b. Rh negative, with anti-D identified; Rh negative father
   c. Rh negative, with anti-D identified; Father unavailable for testing
   d. Rh positive, with anti-K identified; Rh negative father

6. Parallel testing is performed for:
   a. weak D
   b. antibody screen
   c. antibody identification
   d. antibody titer

7. Amniocentesis is performed and the fluid scanned from 350 to 700 nm. The results are interpreted by:
   a. plotting OD vs. antibody titer changes over time
   b. comparing 450 nm reading of fluid to baseline
   c. drawing a graph of readings at 20 nm intervals and noting the point of maximum absorbance
   d. performing multiple scans and averaging the readings at 450 nm

8. Doppler ultrasonography is used for diagnosis of fetal anemia. The criteria that will appear when this anemia is present are:
   1. increased cardiac input
   2. decreased cardiac input
   3. increased blood velocity
   4. decreased blood velocity
   5. low blood viscosity
   6. high blood viscosity
   a. 1, 3, and 5 are correct
   b. 1, 4, and 5 are correct
   c. 1, 3, and 6 are correct
   d. 2, 4, and 6 are correct
   e. 2, 3, and 5 are correct
   f. 2, 4 and 5 are correct

9. During the gestation period, the phenotype of the fetus can be determined by:
   a. cell-free fetal DNA testing
   b. cordocentesis
   c. Doppler ultrasonography
   d. exchange transfusion

10. Maternal evaluation for fetal bleed include:
    a. qualitative rosette testing and qualitative Kleihauer-Betke test
    b. qualitative rosette testing and quantitative Kleihauer-Betke test
    c. quantitative rosette testing and qualitative Kleihauer-Betke test
    d. quantitative rosette testing and quantitative Kleihauer-Betke test

11. In an Rh negative mother who has delivered an Rh positive infant, it was determined that the volume of fetal bleed is 35 ml. The number of vials to be administered is:
    a. 1 vial
    b. 2 vials
    c. 3 vials
    d. 4 vials

12. Intrauterine transfusion may be performed by:
    1. cordocentesis
    2. removing a small amount and replacing it with an equal volume
    3. intraperitoneal infusion into the fetus
    4. direct placental infusion
    a. 1 and 2 are correct
    b. 1 and 3 are correct
    c. 1 and 4 are correct
    d. 2 and 3 are correct
    e. 2 and 4 are correct
    f. 3 and 4 are correct

13. Which of the following is *not* necessary screening on blood used for intrauterine transfusion:
    a. screened for CMV
    b. screened for Hemoglobin S
    c. irradiated prior to transfusion
    d. packed to 50%

14. Criteria for exchange transfusion includes:
    a. cord blood bilirubin >1 mg/dl
    b. plasma bilirubin 12 g/dl in a 2-day-old infant
    c. hemoglobin 12 g/dl 6 hours postpartum
    d. maternal antibody level demonstrated a 2 tube rise 2 days before delivery

15. Most desirable sample used for crossmatch for an exchange transfusion is:
    a. maternal plasma
    b. cord serum
    c. neonate plasma
    d. no crossmatch necessary

CASE STUDY

1. An obstetric patient who received all of the appropriate pre-natal care delivered a healthy full term 7-pound baby boy. Initial maternal testing: O negative with a negative antibody screen. She received a 300 μg dose of Rh immune globulin. The baby's cord blood was:

Anti-A	Anti-B	Anti-D	A₁ Cells	B Cells	Interpretation	DAT
4+	0	3+	0	4+	A positive	+w

The baby's hemoglobin was 18.0 g/dl and bilirubin is 0.4 mg/dl.
A Freeze-Thaw elution was performed and the results were

A cells	B cells	O cells
1+	0	0

a. What should be done with the infant?
b. Does the infant have HDN? What additional steps, if any, should be taken to treat the infant?
c. Should RH immune globulin be administered?

REFERENCES

Boturao-Neto, Edmir, et al. "Anti-KEL7 (anti-Jsᵇ) Alloimmunization Diagnostic Supported by Molecular Kel*6,7 typing in a Pregnant Woman with Previous Intrauterine Deaths." *Transfusion and Apheresis Science.* Vol. 35, 2006, pp. 217–221.

Brennand, Janet and Cameron, Alan. "Fetal Anemia: Diagnosis and Management." *Best Practice and Research Clinical Obstetrics and Gynecology.* Vol. 22, No. 1, 2008, pp. 15–29.

Bullock, R, et al. "Prediction of Fetal Anemia in Pregnancies with Red-Cell Alloimmunization: Comparison of Middle Cerebral Artery Peak Systolic Velocity and Amniotic Fluid OD 450." *Ultrasound Obstetrics and Gynecology.* Vol. 25, 2005, pp. 331–334.

Davis, Bruce, MD and Davis, Kathleen T. "Laboratory Assessment of Fetomaternal Hemorrhage is Improved Using Flow Cytometry." *Laboratory Medicine.* Vol. 38, No. 6, 2007, pp. 365–371.

Denomme, Gregory A. and Fernandes, Bernard J. "Fetal Blood Group Genotyping." *Transfusion.* Vol. 47 Supplement, 2007, pp. 64S–67S. "Noninvasive

Prenatal Diagnosis: Current Practice and Future Perspectives." *Current Opinion in Obstetrics and Gynecology.* Vol. 20, 2008, pp. 146–151.

Finning, Kirstin, et al. "Fetal Genotyping for the K (Kell) and Rh C, c, and E Blood Groups on Cell-Free Fetal DNA in Maternal Plasma." *Transfusion.* Vol. 47, 2007, pp. 2126–2133.

Hahn, Sinuhe and Chitty, Lyn. "Noninvasive Prenatal Diagnosis: Current Practice and Future Perspectives." *Current Opinions in Obstetrics and Gynecology.* Lippincott, Williams and Wilkins, Vol. 20, 2008, pp. 1146–1151.

Mari, G., et al, "Non-Invasive Diagnosis by Doppler Ultrasonography of Fetal Anemia due to Maternal Red-Cell Immunization." *New England Journal of Medicine.* Vol. 342, 2000, pp. 9–14.

Moise, Kenneth J. "Fetal Anemia Due to non-Rhesus-D Red Cell Alloimmunization." *Seminars in Fetal and Neonatal Medicine.* Vol. 13, Issue 4, 2008, pp. 207–214.

Moise, Kenneth J. "Diagnosing Hemolytic Disease of the Fetus—Time to Put the Needles Away?" *The New*

England Journal of Medicine. Vol. 355, No. 2, 2006, pp. 192–194.

Moise, Kenneth J. "Non-anti-D Antibodies in Red-Cell Alloimmunization." *European Journal of Obstetrics and Gynecology and Reproductive Biology.* Vol. 92, 2000, pp. 75–81.

Moise, Kenneth J. "Red Blood Cell Alloimmunization in Pregnancy." *Seminars in Hematology.* Vol. 10, 2005, pp. 169–178.

Moise, Kenneth J. "The Usefulness of Middle Cerebral Artery Doppler Assessment in the Treatment of the Fetus at Risk for Anemia." *American Journal of Obstetrics and Gynecology.* 2008, pp. 161.e1–161.e4.

Nielsen, Leif K., et al. "In vitro Assessment of Recombinant, Mutant Immunoglobulin G anti-D Devoid of Hemolytic Activity for Treatment of Ongoing Hemolytic Disease of the Fetus and Newborn." *Immunohematology.* Vol. 48, 2008, pp. 12–19.

Orinska, K., et al. "Preliminary results of fetal Rhc Examination in Plasma of Pregnant Women with anti-c." *Prenatal Diagnosis.* Vol. 28, 2008, pp. 335–337.

Package Insert. *Immucor: Fetal Bleed Screening Test.* 12/05, Immucor, Atlanta, Ga.

Sloan, S. R. "Technical Issues in Neonatal Transfusions." *Immunohematology.* Vol. 24, No. 1, 2008, pp. 4–8.

Smits-Wintjens, V. E. H. J., Walther, F. J., and Lopriore, E. "Rhesus Haemolytic Disease of the Newborn: Postnatal Management, Associated Morbidity and Long-Term Outcome." *Seminars in Fetal and Neonatal Medicine.* Vol. 13, 2008, pp. 265–271.

Swindell, Christine, et al. "Washing of Irradiated Red Blood Cells Prevents Hyperkalaemia During Cardiopulmonary Bypass in Neonates and Infants Undergoing Surgery for Complex Congenital Heart Disease." *European Journal of Cardio-Thoracic Surgery.* Vol. 31, 2007, pp. 659–664.

Van der Schoot, C. Ellen, et al. "Prenatal Typing of Rh and Kell Blood Group System Antigens." *Transfusion Medicine Reviews.* Vol. 17, No. 1, 2003, pp. 31–44.

Wu, YanYan and Stack, Gary. "Blood Product Replacement in the Perinatal Period." *Seminars in Perinatology.* 2007, pp. 262–271.

Glossary

A

acquired immunity response by lymphocytes in response to antigen exposure; response is specific for the stimulating antigen

active immunization stimulation of antibody production by direct antigen contact

agammaglobulinemia the absence of gamma globulins in the plasma

agglutination clumping of red blood cells or particulate matter resulting from the interaction of antibody and the corresponding antigen

agglutinogen group of antigens or factors in the Weiner inheritance theory

AIDS complex of symptoms and diseases that result from damage to the immune system of the host; caused by the Human Immunodeficiency Virus (HIV)

allele one or more different form of a gene that occupies a specific locus on a chromosome

alloantibody antibody directed at antigens not present on an individual's red cells

allogeneic adsorption adsorption of antibody from serum with selective cells that are not autologous cells

allogeneic donation blood or tissue from the same species that is not genetically identical

amniocentesis procedure for removing amniotic fluid for analysis

amorph a gene does not code for the production of any detectable product

analytical relating to analysis or testing; during the testing process of the laboratory test

anamnestic response antibody response stimulated by secondary exposure to an antigen; the response is accentuated and a rapid rise in antibody is exhibited

anaphylactic intense allergic reaction including bronchial constriction and collapse

anemia decreased oxygen carrying capacity due to low hemoglobin level

antecubital the area of the arm in front of the elbow

antenatal before birth

antibody proteins produced in response to stimulation by an antigen and interacts with the stimulating antigen

antibodies proteins produced in response to stimulation by an antigen which then reacts with that antigen

antibody identification test performed using a panel of cells with known antigen content; when reacted with serum, eluate, or other body fluid the panel of cells creates a pattern of reactivity that can be used to identify the specific antibody or combination of antibodies in the fluid being tested

antibody screen test performed by mixing patient or donor serum with cells of known antigen content to detect the presence of atypical antibodies

anticoagulant chemical substance that will prevent the clotting (coagulation) of blood

anticoagulant-preservative solution chemical solution that serves to prevent clotting of whole blood and provide metabolic support during storage

antigen biochemical substance recognized as foreign; stimulates an immune response

antigram chart describing the antigen content of the cells used for antibody screen and antibody identification tests

anti-human globulin (AHG) sera reagent sera produced in a species other than human (usually a rabbit) that contains antibodies directed against human globulins; used to aid in the detection of antibody coated cells in test procedures

anti-human globulin test test method that uses antibodies directed against human globulins to aid in detection of antibody coated cells; used in specific tests in the blood bank

antithetical opposite allele

apheresis removal of a specific component of the blood; the remaining components are returned to the donor

atypical antibodies antibodies found either in the serum or on the cells that are unanticipated or not found under normal circumstances

275

atypical antibodies   antibodies found either in the serum or on the cells that are unanticipated or not found under normal circumstances

audit trail   system of paper records that recreates all steps in a process

audits   investigation of compliance with policies and procedures

autoagglutinins   antibodies that agglutinate an individual's own cells

autoantibodies   antibodies directed against antigens on an individual's red cells

autocontrol   mixture of serum and cells from the same individual; used to determine the presence of antibody coating the patient's red cells

autologous donation   donation by a donor that is reserved for the same donor's use at a later time

autosomes   chromosomes that are not sex chromosomes; humans have 22 pairs

B

biohazardous   having the ability to cause infections in humans

blood bank   major division in the hospital laboratory that performs blood type determinations, preparation and testing of components for transfusion, and screens serum for atypical antibodies

Bombay phenotype   phenotype in an individual who does not possess the gene to produce the H antigen; designated O_h

C

cell-free fetal DNA (cff-DNA)   acellular fetal DNA; may be detected in the maternal circulation and used for fetal genotyping

cell-mediated immunity   immunity involving cellular components such as macrophages, natural killer cells, T lymphocytes and cytokines

chemical mediators   substances secreted by cells that are then involved in an inflammatory response

chorionic villus sampling (CVS)   removal of a small piece of placenta tissue (chorionic villi) from the uterus during early pregnancy

chromosome   nuclear structures made of DNA that carry genetic information

Chronic Granulomatous Disease (CGD)   an inherited disorder of phagocytic cells in which the cells do not properly capture and destroy foreign invaders, leading to recurrent life-threatening bacterial and fungal infections

cis   two or more genes on the same chromosome of a homologous pair

closed system   blood collection system that allows for fractionation of the unit without breaking the seal and exposing the blood products to the environment

codominant   two inherited alleles that are expressed concurrently

cold hemagglutinin disease   autoimmune disease with high concentrations of antibodies to red blood cells; the antibodies react at temperatures below body temperature

compatible   no evidence of agglutination or hemolysis in a crossmatch when recipient's serum and donor's cells are combined

compatibility test (crossmatch)   the mixing of donor red cells and recipient serum to determine if *in vitro* reactions that may indicate potential for an *in vivo* reaction between the donor's cells and the recipient's serum

complement   a series of proteins in the serum that are activated sequentially; following activation, bacterial and red cell lysis may occur

components   fractions of a unit of whole blood that are used for transfusion

compound or cis-product antigens   antigens found as a result of two genes being found on the same chromosome

concatenation   reading of two bar codes as a single message

continuous quality improvement (CQI)   a process for review, evaluation, and effecting change within the laboratory on an ongoing basis

Coombs control cells (check cells)   cells coated with an antibody used to confirm negative results obtained in indirect or direct antiglobulin tests

Coomb's sera   synonym for AHG sera

cordocentesis   synonym for percutaneous umbilical blood sampling (PUBS)

corrected count increment   anticipated increase in platelet count adjusted for the number of platelets infused and the size on the patient

crossing over   physical exchange of genetic material between two chromosomes

crossmatch   the mixing of donor red cells and recipient serum to determine if *in vitro* reactions that may indicate potential for an *in vivo* reaction between the donor's cells and the recipient's serum

cryoprecipitate   concentrated coagulation factor VIII and fibrinogen extracted from fresh frozen plasma

cytokines   chemical mediators that stimulate tissue response to invading pathogens

D

decline phase   phase of antibody production where the level of detectable antibody is decreasing due to catabolism

deferral   non-acceptance of a potential donor

deglycerolized red cells   cells that have been frozen in glycerol, thawed, and washed

diastolic pressure   the second sound heard while taking a blood pressure; it represents the filling of the heart chamber

differential centrifugation   centrifuging at varying speeds to separate a whole unit of blood into individual parts or components; the principle of this separation is by the different specific gravities of the components

direct antiglobulin test (DAT)   test that detects the presence of antibody on the surface of red cells

DNA deoxyribonucleic acid; chromosomes are made of this substance

dominant an allele that is expressed while its inherited counterpart is silent

Donath-Landsteiner antibody an IgG autoantibody that binds to red cells in the cold and fixes complement; lysis occurs when cells are warmed to 37°C

dosage a situation where an antibody reacts more strongly with red cells that a double dose of an antigen (homozygous) than with those that have a single dose of an antigen (heterozygous)

E

eluate liquid harvested after an elution is performed

elution method used to remove antibodies from the surface of red cells for testing purposes

epitope single antigenic determinate; physically the part of the antigen that combines with the antibody

erythroblastosis fetalis a condition in a fetus or neonate where immature red cells, erythroblasts, are found in the peripheral circulation

erythrocyte mature red blood cell; cell that transports oxygen and carbon dioxide

exchange transfusion transfusion of cells performed after birth that uses a system where some of the infant's cells are removed for each portion of transfused cells that are administered

external proficiency testing specimens for evaluation of test methods that are distributed to laboratories by an outside agency

F

febrile having a fever

fetomaternal hemorrhage fetal bleeding into the maternal circulation

flocculation soluble antigen and soluble antibody combine to fall out of solution in flakes

foreign recognized by the immune system as non-self

fractionation dividing a whole into parts or fractions

fresh frozen plasma fluid portion of one unit of blood that has been centrifuged, separated, and frozen solid at –18°C (or colder) within six hours of collection

frozen thawed red cells cells that have been frozen in glycerol and thawed when ready for transfusion

G

gene basic unit of inheritance on a chromosome; an area of DNA that controls a trait or characteristic

gene chip glass or a silicon chip to which the probes are attached

genetic loci the location of a specific gene on the chromosome

genetics a discipline of biology is the science of heredity

genotype the genetic constitution of a cell, an organism, or an individual

glycophorin a glycoprotein that projects through a red cell membrane; may carry blood group antigens

Good Manufacturing Practices a series of procedures published in the Code of Federal Regulations used by blood banks and transfusion services as a guideline for work practices

Graft vs. Host Disease (GVFD) functional immune cells received from a donor become engrafted in the recipient; these cells then recognize the recipient as "foreign" and mount an immunologic attack

H

haplotype set of genes inherited together because of their proximity to one another on a chromosome

hapten a small molecule that can elicit an immune response only when attached to a large carrier such as a protein

hemagglutination the clumping of red blood cells; used to visualize antigen-antibody reactions

hemapheresis whole blood removed from a donor and separated into components; one or more of the components are retained; the remainder is returned to the donor

hepatitis inflammation of the liver, frequently due to bacterial or viral infections

hemoglobinemia presence of free hemoglobin in the serum or plasma

hemoglobinuria presence of hemoglobin in the urine

hemolysis disruption of the membrane of a red blood cell; results in release of the contents into the plasma

hemolytic disease of the fetus and newborn (HDFN) clinical condition involving the fetus and the neonate that results in hemolysis of red cells due to maternal antibody coating the red cells of the baby

hemolytic transfusion reactions (HTR) adverse reaction to transfusion most often resulting from an interaction between antigens of the donor and antibodies of the recipient

hemosiderosis accumulation of excess iron in macrophages in various tissues

heterozygous two different alleles for a single trait inherited on homologous chromosomes

homozygous two identical alleles for a single trait on homologous chromosomes

Human Leukocyte Antigens (HLA) antigens present on leukocytes and tissues; genes that code for these antigens are part of the major histocompatibility complex (MHC) gene systems

humoral immunity immune response resulting in the production of antibodies

hydatid cyst fluid fluid from a cyst of the liver (hydatid cyst) caused by a tapeworm; the fluid is used to inhibit anti-P_1

hydops fetalis a condition where fluid accumulates in the pleural and peritoneal cavities

hypogammaglobulinemia decreased production of gamma globulins; results in decreased quantities in the plasma

I

icterus   yellow color in serum; indicating increased bilirubin in the serum

idiopathic   without a detectable cause

immediate spin crossmatch   mixing donor and recipient blood and reading for agglutination after the first spin without incubation or enhancement media

immune antibody   antibody produced by direct stimulation with an antigen

immunogen   synonym for antigen; substance that prompts the generation of antibodies and can cause an immune response

immunoglobulin   gamma globulin protein found in blood or bodily fluids and used by the immune system to identify and neutralize foreign objects, such as bacteria and viruses

Immunohematology   study of blood related antigens and antibodies as they may be applied to situations encountered in blood bank and transfusion service

Immunology   study of components and processes of the immune system

in utero   while the fetus is in the uterus

in vitro   outside of the body; in glass

in vivo   in the body

incompatible   no evidence of agglutination or hemolysis in a compatibility test where recipient's serum and donor's red cells are tested in combination; these units should not be transfused

independent assortment   traits are inherited separately and expressed discreetly from one another

independent segregation   transmission of a trait from on generation to the next in a predictable fashion

indirect antiglobulin test   test method that promotes antibody attachment to cells *in vitro* and uses an anti-human globulin to bridge the antibody molecules on the cells; varied specific test applications

innate immunity   first line of defense for invading pathogens; cells and mechanisms that defend the host from infection by other organisms; a non-specific defense

internal proficiency testing   specimens for evaluation of test methods that originate within the laboratory

intrauterine transfusion   transfusion administered to a fetus still in the uterus

ISBT 128   a system of labeling blood components that will provide an international standard

isoagglutinin   an antibody present in the plasma of an individual that may cause agglutination of the red blood cells of another individual of the same species

K

kernicterus   permanent brain damage resulting from the accumulation of bilirubin in the brain tissue

Kleihauer-Betke acid elution stain   stain with a low pH that will stain fetal cells a dark pink while causing the adult cells to lyse and appear as pale-staining ghost cells

L

labile   not stable; will disintegrate upon storage or standing

lag phase   first phase of immune response where the levels of antibody are not detectable by testing

lectin   protein originating from a seed extract; the protein has antibody specificity

leukapheresis   the removal of whole blood from a donor; the blood is separated into components; the leukocytes are retained and the remaining components returned to the donor

leukocyte concentrate   white blood cells collected by pheresis from a single donor

leukocyte reduced red cells   red cell products prepared by one of several methods to create a product that has a decreased amount of white blood cells

leukocytes   white blood cells

Liley graph   a graph used to evaluate data on spectophotometric analysis of amniotic fluid at 450nm; the OD is plotted against the gestational age

linkage disequilibrium   genes inherited as a set occur more frequently than would be expected by chance

locus   location of a gene on a chromosome

log phase   second phase of a immune response where antibody production occurs in a logarithmic fashion

lymphocyte   mononuclear leukocyte that mediates cellular and humoral immunity

M

major crossmatch   compatibility test combining recipient's serum with donor's cells

Major Histocompatibility Complex (MHC)   a group of linked genes on Chromosome 6 that determine the expression of complement proteins and leukocyte antigens

massive transfusion   a total blood volume exchange by transfusion within a 24-hour period

microarray   a DNA detection method in which a probe is attached to solid surface and binds to the target sequence of DNA, allowing for detection, usually through fluorescence

minor crossmatch   compatibility test combining recipient's cells with donor's serum

molecular diagnostics   tests for nucleic acid targets found in various settings in medicine; three areas of testing are genetics, hematopathology, and infectious disease

monoclonal   originating from a single clone of cells; antibody that will have increased specificity for an antigen as a result of the use of a single clone

monoclonal antisera   antisera where the antibodies are derived from a single clone of cells

mononuclear phagocytes   leukocytes that are involved in phagocytosis and antigen presenting; these include monocytes (circulating cells) and macrophages (fixed cells)

monospecific AHG   anti-human globulin sera containing only a single component

murine   related to a mouse

N

natural antibody antibody produced without known exposure to the antigen

neutralization combination of two substances where one has the capability to combine with and render the other inactive in future reactions

nonsecretor individual who genetically does not produce soluble antigens to be released into the body fluids

O

oligosaccharide a polymer composed of simple saccharides (sugars)

P

packed red cells donor unit of red cells from which the plasma has been removed

panel series of cells from different donors used in the antibody identification test

parallel testing series of tests performed under identical conditions to the patient or control tests; used to rule out contamination or other interferences

parasite eukaryotic organism that infects a host to its benefit, while harming the host

parenterally route of entry of a substance into the body other than by the digestive tract; e.g. by injection

paroxysmal cold hemoglobinuria (PCH) PCH is a cryopathic hemolytic syndrome, it is an autoimmune hemolytic anemia due to cold-reacting autoantibodies

partial D phenotype of the D antigen that is missing a part of the antigenic determinant or epitope of the D antigen

passive antibody antibody administered to an individual

pedigree chart schematic illustration of an inheritance pattern of a specific trait within a family

peer review evaluation of a laboratory, specific department in the laboratory, or a specific procedure by a group consisting of ones equals

Percutaneous Umbilical Blood Sampling (PUBS) aspiration of a fetal blood sample from the umbilical vein

phenotype outward expression of inherited characteristics

phototherapy treatment using lights

plasma liquid portion of whole blood containing water, electrolytes, glucose, proteins, fats, and gases; refers also to the liquid portion of a blood sample collected with an anticoagulant

plasmapheresis the removal of whole blood from a donor; the blood is separated into components; the plasma is retained and the remaining components returned to the donor

plateau phase response phase where antibody production is constant and detectable at stable levels

platelet concentrate platelets removed from whole blood and stored for transfusion

platelet-rich plasma (PRP) plasma prepared from whole blood with a "light spin"; the platelets are remaining in the plasma after the centrifugation step; the plasma is removed to a satellite bag

plateletpheresis the removal of whole blood from a donor; the blood is separated into components; the platelets are retained and the remaining components returned to the donor

polymerase chain reaction (PCR) a molecular technique for the amplification of a specific target sequence of DNA

polymorphic system possessing multiple allelic forms at a single locus

polymorphism the expression of more than one phenotype

polymorphonuclear neutrophil a granulocytic white blood cell that phagocytizes invading microorganisms to provide protection to the host

polyspecific AHG anti-human globulin sera with multiple components; usually anti-IgG and anti-complement while anti-IgM and IgA may be included

post-analytical time after the testing procedure; post-analytical factors include reporting, result delivery, and interpretation of results

postpartum after giving birth

post-transfusion after transfusion

post-transfusion purpura (PTP) appearance red or purple discolorations of the skin at any time after transfusion has been completed; purpura are usually caused by bleeding under the skin red or purple discolorations on the skin

pre-analytical time prior to the performance of the testing procedure; pre-analytical factors include specimen collection, specimen handling, interfering substances and patient factors

pre-transfusion before transfusion

precipitation the condensation of a solid from a liquid

preservative chemical substance that provides substances to prevent deterioration of the cells

primary response antibody response following initial antigen exposure

primer pieces of single-stranded DNA, that are complementary to the end sequences of the target, and mark the sequence of DNA to be amplified

prion presumptive infectious agent composed entirely of protein

probe single-stranded piece of labeled DNA, that is complementary to the target sequence, and binds to a targeted DNA site to allow for the detection of a specific DNA

proenzyme an inactive enzyme precursor that requires a chemical change to become active

prozone phenomenon incomplete lattice formation with a lack of agglutination; results from antibody excess in comparison to antigen

Punnett Square a diagram used to determine the probability of an offspring having a particular genotype when two parents are crossed

Q

qualitative   establishes presence of a substance but does not determine the quantity

quality assurance   efforts of all personnel to monitor and evaluate all aspects of laboratory testing to improve patient care

quality control   series of procedures to monitor test system

quantitative   determines the amount of a substance present

R

recessive   an allele that is not expressed when inherited in combination with another allele that is expressed

recipient   individual who receive a transfusion of blood or its components

recovered plasma   plasma that does not qualify as fresh frozen plasma

red cell pheresis   the removal of red cells from a donor via pheresis

refractory   resistant to ordinary treatment

Rh immune globulin   concentrated anti-D commercially processed for administration to prevent Rh hemolytic disease of the newborn

Rh null   phenotype with a lack of Rh antigens on the surface of the red cells

rosette   clump of cells consisting of a central cell surrounded by other cells

rouleaux   coin-like stacking of red cells in the presence of abnormal plasma proteins

S

secondary response (anamnestic response)   antibody response that follows any antigen exposure other than the first

secretors   individuals who have a gene causing soluble forms of antigens to be released into the body fluids

sepsis   presence of bacterial infection in the circulatory system

serial amniocentesis   the process of multiple comparative amniocentesis procedures to monitor changes in the status of the *in utero* fetus

serum   liquid portion of the blood after coagulation

sialoglycoproteins   glycoproteins that carry sialic acid; the sialic acid lends a negative charge to the red blood cell membrane

single donor plasma   plasma extracted from red cells after the time frame allowable for fresh frozen plasma or plasma with the cryoprecipitate removed; used for volume replacement

single nucleotide polymorphism (SNP)   a genetic variation in which only one base pair differs between two strands of DNA

solid phase adherence   testing method where one component of testing is adhered (attached) to a solid phase such as a microtiter plate; the patient's sample is added and when the

test is completed a final assessment is made by examining the wells of the plate

specificity   state of having a certain nature or action

steric   related to the spatial arrangement of the molecules

subclinical   an infection that produces no overt symptoms or only mild nonspecific symptoms

sublocus   location within the gene locus

red cell pheresis   the removal of red cells from a donor via pheresis

syncope   fainting

systolic pressure   the first sound heard when taking a blood pressure; the contraction of the heart

T

T cytotoxic (T_C) cells   a sub-group of lymphocytes that kill other cells

T helper (T_H) cells   a sub-group of lymphocytes that plays an important role in activating and directing other immune cells

thrombocytes   anucleate cell fragments called platelets; these cells play a key role in blood clotting

titer   measurement of strength of an antibody by testing its reactivity with decreasing amounts of the appropriate antigen; reciprocal of the highest dilution that shows agglutination is the titer

total quality management (TQM)   a strategy to create an awareness of quality in all processes in the establishment

transferase   enzyme that catalyzes the transfer of atoms from one chemical compound to another chemical compound

transfusion reaction   untoward effect of transfusion

trans   alleles found on different chromosomes of a homologous pair

U

universal antigen   an antigen found on the red cells of a large percentage of the population approaching 100%

universal donor   group O individual who provides red blood cells that may be transfused to a recipient of any ABO blood group

universal precautions   set of guidelines developed to protect health care workers from exposure to infectious agents

universal recipient   group AB individual who may receive red blood cells of any ABO blood group

urticaria   hives

V

validation   assessment that a procedure or product consistently produces the defined product or result

virus   an infectious agent, consisting of nucleic acid, either DNA or RNA, and a protein based protective covering called a capsid

W

warm autoimmune hemolytic anemia (WAIHA)   anemia caused by hemolysis of red cells caused by an antibody directed against autologous cells; the etiology of the antibody is a warm-reacting antibody

Wharton's jelly   connective tissue substance coating the umbilical cord

whole blood   blood that contains all components

Z

zeta potential   difference in charge density between the inner and outer ion cloud surrounding the surface of the red blood cells in an electrolyte solution

zone of equivalence   when both reactants are present in amounts to create optimal reaction conditions

zygosity   the similarity or dissimilarity of genes at an allelic position on two homologous chromosomes

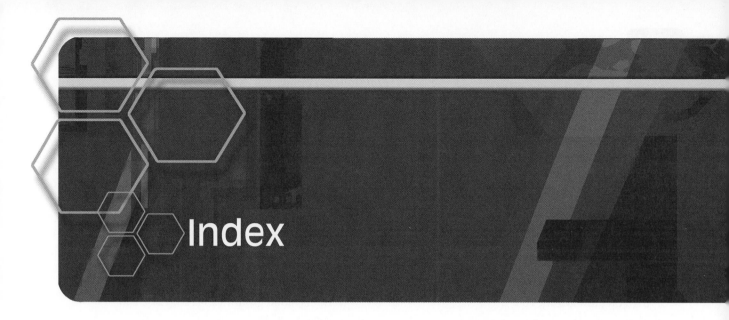

Index

Note: page numbers followed by *b*, *f*, or *t* refer to Boxes, Figures, or Tables respectively

K

L

M